ELECTROBIOLOGY OF NERVE, SYNAPSE, AND MUSCLE

Electrobiology
of
Nerve, Synapse, and Muscle

In Honor of Harry Grundfest

Editors

John P. Reuben, Ph.D.
Laboratory of Neurophysiology
Department of Neurology
College of Physicians and
* Surgeons*
Columbia University
New York, New York

Dominick P. Purpura, M.D.
Department of Neuroscience and
Rose F. Kennedy Center for
* Research in Mental Retardation*
* and Human Development*
Albert Einstein College of Medicine
New York, New York

Michael V. L. Bennett, D. Phil.
Department of Anatomy and
Rose F. Kennedy Center for
* Research in Mental Retardation*
* and Human Development*
Albert Einstein College of Medicine
New York, New York

Eric R. Kandel, M.D., Ph.D.
Division of Neurobiology and
* Behavior*
College of Physicians and
* Surgeons*
Columbia University
New York, New York

Raven Press ▪ New York

Raven Press, 1140 Avenue of the Americas, New York, New York 10036

Made in the United States of America

International Standard Book Number 0-89004-030-3
Library of Congress Catalog Card Number 75-14587

Contents

CONTENTS   vii

Contributors

Joseph Bastian
Department of Biological Sciences
Purdue University
West Lafayette, Indiana 47907

Arturo Jorge Bekerman
Instituto de Biologia Celular
Facultad de Medicina
Universidad de Buenos Aires
Paraguay 2155
Buenos Aires, Argentina

Michael V. L. Bennett
Department of Anatomy and
Rose F. Kennedy Center for
  Research in Mental
  Retardation and Human
  Development
Albert Einstein College of Medicine
Bronx, New York 10411

Philip W. Brandt
Laboratory of Neurophysiology
Department of Anatomy
College of Physicians and Surgeons
Columbia University
New York, New York 10032

Theodore Holmes Bullock
Department of Neurosciences
School of Medicine
and
Neurobiology Unit
Scripps Institution of Oceanography
University of California–San Diego
La Jolla, California 92037

T. J. Carew
Division of Neurobiology and Behavior
College of Physicians and Surgeons
Columbia University
New York, New York 10032

D. J. Chiarandini
Department of Ophthalmology
New York University Medical Center
New York, New York 10016

Stanley M. Crain
Departments of Neuroscience and
  Physiology and
Rose F. Kennedy Center for Research
  in Mental Retardation and Human
  Development
Albert Einstein College of Medicine
Bronx, New York 10461

Abraham B. Eastwood
Laboratory of Neurophysiology
Department of Neurology
College of Physicians and Surgeons
Columbia University
New York, New York 10032

René Epstein
Instituto de Biologia Celular
Facultad de Medicina
Universidad de Buenos Aires
Paraguay 2155
Buenos Aires, Argentina

Alan R. Freeman
Department of Physiology
Temple University School of Medicine
3420 North Broad Street
Philadelphia, Pennsylvania 19140

Harold Gainer
Behavioral Biology Branch
National Institute of Child Health and
  Human Development
National Institutes of Health
Bethesda, Maryland 20014

Vivian S. Gainer
Marine Biological Laboratory
Woods Hole, Massachusetts 02543

Lucien Girardier
Département de Physiologie
Ecole de Médecine
Université de Genéve
Geneva, Switzerland

Stephen M. Highstein
Department of Neuroscience
Albert Einstein College of Medicine
Bronx, New York 10461

L. Janiszewski
Department of Animal Physiology
Institute of Biology
N. Copernicus University
Toruń, Poland

Eric R. Kandel
Division of Neurobiology and Behavior
College of Physicians and Surgeons
Columbia University
New York, New York 10032

George M. Katz
Laboratory of Neurophysiology
Department of Neurology
College of Physicians and Surgeons
Columbia University
New York, New York 10032

Nobufumi Kawai
Department of Neurobiology
Tokyo Metropolitan Institute for
   Neurosciences
2–6 Fuchu City,
Tokyo, Japan

R. D. Keynes
Physiological Laboratory
University of Cambridge
Cambridge, England

J. Koester
Division of Neurobiology and Behavior
College of Physicians and Surgeons
Columbia University
New York, New York 10032

K. Kusano
Department of Biology
Illinois Institute of Technology
Chicago, Illinois 60616

Alexander Mauro
The Rockefeller University
New York, New York 10021

Pat G. Model
Department of Neuroscience
Albert Einstein College of Medicine
Bronx, New York 10461

Fumiaki Motokizawa
Department of Physiology
Nara Medical College
Kashihara, Nara 634
Japan

Shigehiro Nakajima
Department of Biological Sciences
Purdue University
West Lafayette, Indiana 47907

S. Obara
Department of Physiology
Teikyo University
School of Medicine
Itabashi-ku, Tokyo 173, Japan

Morton Orentlicher
Laboratory of Neurophysiology
Department of Neurology
College of Physicians and Surgeons
Columbia University
New York, New York 10032

Masahiro Ozeki
Department of Biology
Faculty of Education
Yamanashi University
Kofu 400, Japan

Dominick P. Purpura
Department of Neuroscience and
Rose F. Kennedy Center for Research
   in Mental Retardation and Human
   Development
Albert Einstein College of Medicine
New York, New York 10411

John P. Reuben
Laboratory of Neurophysiology
Department of Neurology
College of Physicians and Surgeons
Columbia University
New York, New York 10032

Michelangelo Rossetto
The Rockefeller University
New York, New York 10021

Vladimir I. Skok
Bogomoletz Institute of Physiology
Kiev, U.S.S.R.

A. L. Sorenson
Departamento de Farmacologia
Instituto de Ciencias Biomedicas

Universidade Federal do Rio de
  Janeiro
Rio de Janeiro, Brazil

E. Stefani
Departamento de Fisiologia
Centro de Investigación y Estudios
  Avanzados del IPN
Mexico City, Mexico

Sidney Steinberg
Laboratory of Neurophysiology
Department of Neurology
College of Physicians and Surgeons
Columbia University
New York, New York 10032

G. Suarez-Kurtz
Departamento de Farmacologia
Instituto de Ciencias Biomedicas
Universidade Federal do Rio de Janeiro
Rio de Janeiro, Brazil

Haruo Sugi
Department of Physiology
Teikyo University
School of Medicine
Itabashi-ku, Tokyo 173, Japan

Jiro Suzuki
Division of Neurophysiology
Psychiatric Research Institute of Tokyo
2-1-8, Kamikitazawa
Setagaya-ku, Tokyo 156, Japan

Kimihisa Takeda
Laboratory of Physiology
Faculty of Education
Tottori University
Tottori, Japan

Susumu Terakawa
Department of Physiology
Tokyo Medical and Dental University
Yushima, Bunkyo-ku, Tokyo 113, Japan

P. N. R. Usherwood
Department of Zoology
University of Nottingham
Nottingham NG7 2RD, England

Akira Watanabe
Department of Physiology
Tokyo Medical and Dental University
Yushima, Bunkyo-ku, Tokyo 113, Japan

Robert Werman
Neurobiology Unit
Institute of Life Sciences
Hebrew University
Jerusalem, Israel

Jenny R. Zollman
Laboratory of Neurophysiology
Department of Neurology
College of Physicians and Surgeons
Columbia University
New York, New York 10032

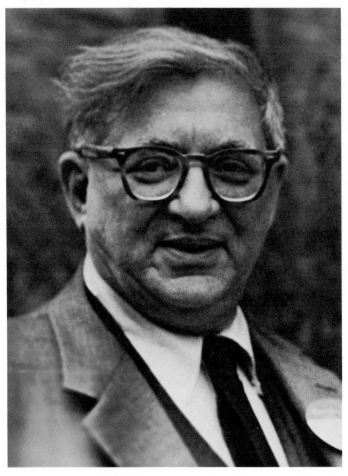

HARRY GRUNDFEST

Introduction

Dominick P. Purpura

Department of Neuroscience and Rose F. Kennedy Center for Research in Mental Retardation and Human Development, Albert Einstein College of Medicine, Bronx, New York 10461

By analysis of their specialized characteristics, electrophysiology relates the activity of excitable cells to the general physiology of cellular processes. In fact, electrophysiological techniques and concepts make a very important contribution to the study of that elusive yet nevertheless all-important and complex structure, the cell membrane. Appropriation of the data from general physiology and their elaboration, in terms of evolutionary and ecological concepts as adaptations to various functional specifications, are the commonly recognized vectors of comparative physiology. The study of bioelectric activity, however, makes the reciprocity of the symbiosis particularly clear. Comparative electrophysiology has provided general physiology with new information on the fundamental mechanisms of bioelectricity.

> Harry Grundfest
> ("Comparative Electrobiology of Excitable Membranes," *Advances in Comparative Physiology and Biochemistry,* O. Lowenstein, Ed. Academic Press, New York, 1966, pp. 1–116.)

This volume serves two related purposes. It expresses the respect and admiration of the contributors for Harry Grundfest, Scientist and Humanitarian, and it provides a format for detailing a variety of recent advances in the field of comparative electrobiology. Harry Grundfest's many contributions to studies of excitation and conduction in nerve, mechanisms of synaptic transmission, and excitation–contraction coupling in muscle constitute an appropriate base for elaboration of programmatic themes representative of the full spectrum of current research in electrobiology. The Editors' decision to restrict contributions from Harry's students, fellows, and colleagues to these specific themes was required by the necessity to publish a meaningful Festschrift of manageable proportions. From the overwhelming response to the Editors' invitations for chapters from Grundfest's former associates it is clear that additional volumes on neuropharmacology and the synaptic organization of the mammalian brain could have been readily generated.

The topics in this volume are grouped into three major subject areas that reflect three temporally overlapping "periods" of Grundfest's long and productive scientific career. For convenience, these may be defined as the "Nerve Period" (1932–1952), the "Synapse Period" (1950–1965), and the "Muscle Period" (1960 to the present). The reader should not conclude from this that Grundfest channeled his boundless energies into only *one* subject at a time! Examination of the more than 550 publications emerging from his Laboratory of Neurophysiology shows otherwise. Those privileged to have lunch with Harry during the "Great Pickle Period" (1954 to present) are well aware of his encyclopedic knowledge and voracious appetite for raw data and kosher pickles. What remains a mystery is his ability to write a new manuscript per week for decades on the energy derived solely from pickle power.

Appropriately, the first chapter in this volume, contributed by Keynes, is concerned with a topic on "Nerve" which represents one of the most exciting aspects of modern axonology, the analysis of gating currents. As is pointed out, these currents were suspected by Hodgkin and Huxley but could not be adequately demonstrated until recently when pharmacological agents became available for blocking voltage-sensitive sodium and potassium channels. With the many attempts now being made to develop molecular models of the sodium channel, Keynes' chapter is especially pertinent since it sets certain constraints on the nature of such models.

It is likely that macromolecular components of the excitable membrane are not the only elements that undergo conformational change during nerve activity, as judged from the report of Watanabe and Terakawa. Their demonstration of alterations in the physical properties of axoplasmic constituents due to calcium influx during excitation raises important issues concerning the relationship of impulse activity to axoplasmic transport processes, among other things. Whatever the ultimate significance may be of axoplasmic birefringence changes during excitation, there can be no question about the essential role of calcium activation in spike electrogenesis in crayfish giant axons, as shown by Yamagishi and Grundfest in 1971 and further detailed in the report by Suzuki.

The series of papers on "Nerve" concludes with a proposal for a new electronic membrane model of considerable complexity consisting of 10 independent "two-state" channels showing voltage-dependent conductance and current noise (Mauro and Rossetto).

Werman correctly points out in his chapter that Harry Grundfest's most important contributions to electrobiology have been in the general area of synaptic transmission, particularly in transmitter–receptor interactions. Werman credits his "Grundfestian training" for his present operational approaches to problems of synaptic pharmacology. What he really means is that the highly competitive and intellectually stimulating environment of the Laboratory of Neurophysiology in the early 1960s selected for those traits in research fellows that facilitated successful research. Werman's talents in mathematics provided the basis for a line of development which Grundfest nurtured and stimulated. Harry had long been expounding on the importance of conductance changes as essential measurements for quantitative studies of synaptic operations. The wisdom of this teaching is evident in Werman's successful development of mathematical models that utilize conductance changes to elucidate stoichiometric relations in transmitter–receptor interactions.

The pharmacological actions of aliphatic ω-amino acids and the dicarboxylic amino acids were examined on a variety of preparations by Harry Grundfest and his associates, beginning as early as 1957. The strong tradition in the use of pharmacological agents as methodological probes of membrane properties continues to be exploited in recent studies of former fellows, Freeman and Usherwood. Freeman's chapter is particularly relevant to an area of growing importance in neuropharmacology, namely the possible role of amino acids as "modulators" of neuronal and axonal excitability. It is of interest that Freeman has extended findings on nonsynaptic actions of glutamate on membranes of lobster muscle fibers to proposed actions of amino acid convulsants on CNS neurons. The provocative finding that glutamate acts on presynaptic terminals to enhance excitatory transmitter release may suggest a positive feedback mechanism in the excitatory actions of this ubiquitous amino acid. Usherwood's chapter, while clearly emphasizing the identity of action of glutamate and the natural transmitter on receptors at excitatory junctions on insect skeletal muscles, cautiously warns against dismissal of the bizarre effects of bath-applied glutamate on extrajunctional receptors. The chapters by Freeman and Usherwood thus serve to remind us of the remarkable *heterogeneity of excitable membranes,* which has been Grundfestian teaching for several decades.

The Laboratory of Neurophysiology pioneered in the use of biological preparations as well as developing research scientists and generating numerous publications. Electric organs of a variety of species, crayfish septate axons, electroreceptors, and the hatchetfish giant synapse are but a few of the preparations that have provided new insights into fundamental electrobiological principles. Bennett relates how, while a member of the Laboratory of Neurophysiology, he came upon the use of the hatchetfish to study structure-function relations at an identifiable synapse, i.e., the Mauthner fiber–giant fiber synapse. His chapter with Model and Highstein illustrates how the hatchetfish giant synapse has proved to be extraordinarily useful in permitting demonstration of synaptic vesicle depletion and recovery in association with alterations in transmission kinetics. Data have also been obtained that permit some inferences concerning the relationship between transmitter release and vesicle refilling time. The chapter by Bennett et al. exemplifies the perfect marriage of morphology with electrophysiology in continuing pursuit of the neurobiology of synaptic transmission. Suffice it to say that the courtship days of this union were spent in the Laboratory of Neurophysiology wherein Bennett and Pappas initiated a most productive series of collaborative studies on the morphophysiology of electrotonic junctional transmission.

Kandel had his first exposure to experimental neurophysiology in 1955 during a senior medical student elective with Grundfest and me. He was determined at that time to understand the neurophysiological basis of behavior and promptly set upon the task of mastering necessary skills in preparation for this mission. The rest is a matter of record, some of which is summarized in his contribution to this volume with Carew and Koester. Their report describes how four types of effector systems in *Aplysia* are regulated by the abdominal ganglia and how the analysis of these behaviors contributes to an understanding of the functional significance of a cell's biophysical properties. The classification of behaviors into graded and all-or-none responses and attempts to relate these in *Aplysia* to specific operations of neurons represent a bold and heuristically valuable approach to the cellular neurobiology of behavior.

In addition to his commitment to excellence in electrobiological investigations, Harry Grundfest has had a longtime interest in and appreciation for the continuing development of electronic instrumentation for electrophysiological studies. The lapel button identifying him as a senior member of the Institute of Electrical Engineers has always been worn with pride, and for good reason. For it was in Grundfest's Electronics Laboratory that microelectrodes, micromanipulators, and neutralized input capacity amplifiers were designed that made possible intracellular recording from a variety of cells. The brief chapter by Katz and Steinberg testifies to this continuing commitment to instrumentation for electrobiological research.

Crain recognizes the important role that Grundfest played in developing instrumentation that permitted him access to the functional activity of cultured dorsal root ganglion cells during his doctoral thesis research at Columbia in the early 1950s. Since then, Crain and his associates have gone on to develop a variety of nerve tissue culture model systems for analyzing some of the most complex and intriguing problems in developmental neurobiology. His contribution to this volume epitomizes this approach, particularly his recent demonstration that dorsal root axons seek out their specific target neurons in the medulla of brainstem explants. This provides the first *in vitro* model system for studying the development of *specific* synaptic connections in the mammalian CNS.

Harry Grundfest is currently in a "Muscle Period," the origins of which can be traced to the arrival of Girardier as a postdoctoral fellow to work with another postdoc, Reuben, in the Laboratory of Neurophysiology in the early 1960s. Girardier and Reuben hit it off so well and generated so many data that *even* Grundfest had difficulty assimilating the observations, to say nothing about understanding them. Reuben and his associates review the early history of the discovery of anion perm-selectivity of the transverse tubular system of crayfish muscle in a chapter that also introduces several more recent proposals on the mechanism of excitation–contraction coupling. The discovery that crayfish fibers in solutions causing KCl efflux become "scrambled" when viewed by light microscopy opened the door to an important interdisciplinary collaboration involving Reuben, Brandt, Grundfest, and a host of other associates over the past decade. A footnote to the story of the early years of this collaborative study may be noted in view of current operating budgets of most laboratories. Much of the early work on anion perm-selectivity involved gross examination of muscle fibers in various bathing solutions and observing "scrambled" or normal muscle fibers. The elegance in this study was in its simple yet dramatic and unequivocal end point. Never before (or again) have so many important data been collected so cheaply in the Laboratory of Neurophysiology . . . or perhaps anywhere.

Research productivity in the area of muscle electrobiology in the Laboratory of Neurophysiology has remained at a high level for the past 15 years as witnessed by the number of distinguished scientists, former associates in the Laboratory, who have contributed chapters in this area (Nakajima, Sugi, Kawai, Takeda, Chiarandini, and Suarez-Kurtz).

It is a sad commentary on the times when bureaucratic concerns about "cost-effectiveness" result in wanton destruction of training programs of the type that permitted scores of young men and women to receive training and guidance in neurobiological research in Grundfest's laboratory. How shortsighted not to appreciate the consequences of such a training program that are evident in part in the contributions to this volume. For they reflect current extensions of highly productive biological research in areas of increasing relevance to the health sciences. There can be no doubt that fundamental investigations of excitable membranes will provide important clues to disorders of nerve, synapse, and muscle that afflict many millions throughout the world.

Harry Grundfest has played a major role in shaping the attitudes, interests, and skills of many young scientists over the past four decades of his remarkable career. Werman (*this volume*) seeks a clue to Harry's motivation in a passage from an early autobiographical note, in which Harry writes, "My own . . . impulsion . . . toward biology . . . was not philosophical; my drive was essentially to find out what was on the other side of the mountain." This may be fine for mountain climbers but not for one who climbs the mountain to reach for the stars! No, Harry Grundfest has spent too many years in search of fundamental principles of electrobiology not to appreciate their significance for the ultimate understanding of the acme of the biological evolution, the human brain. Indeed nothing comes closer to the Inner-Space of Harry Grundfest than the passages *he* quoted for an introduction to his now classic chapter on the "Evolution of Conduction in the Nervous System" (*Evolution of Nervous Control*, edited by A. D. Bass, Amer. Assoc. Adv. Sci., Washington, D.C., 1959, pp. 43–86).

> *Don Juan:* . . . will you not agree with me . . . that it is inconceivable that Life having once produced them [birds], should, if love and beauty were her object, start off on another line and labor at the clumsy elephant and hideous ape, whose grandchildren we are?
>
> *The Devil:* . . . You conclude then, that Life was driving at clumsiness and ugliness?
>
> *Don Juan:* No, perverse devil that you are, a thousand times no. Life was driving at brains — at its darling object: an organ by which it can attain not only self-consciousness but self-awareness.

George Bernard Shaw
Man and Superman, Act III

Electrobiology of Nerve, Synapse, and Muscle,
edited by J. P. Reuben, D. P. Purpura, M. V. L. Bennett,
and E. R. Kandel. Raven Press, New York © 1976

On Gating Currents

R. D. Keynes

Physiological Laboratory, University of Cambridge, Cambridge, England

The principal landmark for axonologists in recent years has been Hodgkin and Huxley's (1952) description of the events at membrane level in the squid giant axon in terms of a sequence of time and voltage-dependent changes of the permeability of the membrane to Na^+ and K^+ ions. They demonstrated that the sodium conductance, g_{Na}, could be well described as a function of two dimensionless variables m and h, each of which obeyed a first-order differential equation, whereas the potassium conductance, g_K, was a function of a similar variable n. The five equations governing the cation conductances could be written as

$$g_{Na} = \bar{g}_{Na} m^3 h \tag{1}$$
$$dm/dt = \alpha_m(1 - m) - \beta_m m \tag{2}$$
$$dh/dt = \alpha_h(1 - h) - \beta_h h \tag{3}$$
$$g_K = \bar{g}_K n^4 \tag{4}$$
$$dn/dt = \alpha_n(1 - n) - \beta_n n \tag{5}$$

where $\bar{g}_{Na}$ and $\bar{g}_K$ were constants representing the peak conductances per unit area of membrane. The α's and β's are rate constants whose magnitude is determined by the instantaneous value of the membrane potential. Although under special conditions — for example, in voltage-clamp experiments with a greatly increased holding potential — these equations may need slight modification (Keynes and Rojas, 1976), over the normal physiological range they apply with remarkable fidelity, not only in squid axons but also (with some variation in the powers to which m and n are raised) in a wide variety of excitable tissues.

Since there are many different physical systems to which a pair of first-order equations like Eqs. (2) and (3) would apply equally well, the Hodgkin-Huxley formulation does not lead directly to a specific model for the sodium channels. However, as they pointed out, it does have one implication that cannot be evaded: any acceptable model must account properly for the voltage sensitivity of the rate constants. The conductance changes must somehow be coupled with a voltage-controlled movement within the membrane of a set of mobile charges or dipoles. I have presented elsewhere (Keynes, 1975) an example of the kind of molecular model that would be compatible with Eqs. (1) to (3), according to which the sodium channels are opened and closed by the rotation in the electric field of a group of three globular "*m*" particles and a single "*h*" particle. Since our new experimental evidence leads me increasingly to doubt whether it is correct to portray the inactivating "*h*" particles as separate entities, it would be misleading to perpetuate this particular picture. But however the mobile components of the gating system are arranged, an opening of the gate *must* involve an outward transfer of charge. Therefore, when the membrane is depolarized, the resulting flow of ionic current is preceded not only by the surge of capacity current but also by what has come to be called the "gating current." It is my intention to describe briefly the basic properties of the gating current in the squid giant axon, and to consider the value of gating current measurements for refining our views on what might be termed the molecular biology of nerve conduction.

The attempts of Hodgkin and Huxley (1952) and Chandler and Meves (1965) to measure the gating current in squid were frustrated by their inability to block the ionic currents completely enough to unmask the very small transfer of charge corresponding to the movement of the controlling particles. The secret of the recent successes in this field (see Armstrong and Bezanilla, 1974; Keynes and Rojas, 1974; Meves, 1974) is the availability of tetrodotoxin with which to cork up the sodium channels. Coupled with removal of sodium from both internal and external solutions, blockage of the potassium channels with cesium or a combination of rubidium and tetraethylammonium ions, and substitution of isethionate for chloride in the external medium, the presence of 300–1,000 nM TTX raises the membrane resistance of a branch-free stretch of axon to as much as 10,000 $\Omega \cdot cm^2$. Under these conditions, application of ± 120 mV voltage-clamp pulses reveals, as may be seen in Fig. 1, a substantial asymmetry of the displacement current, which is appreciably larger for depolarizing pulses than for hyperpolarizing ones. Elimination of the symmetrical capacity transient, either graphically as in Fig. 1 or with the aid of a signal averager as in Fig. 2, shows that the asymmetric component follows an exponential time course with a relaxation time of the order of a few hundred μsec. The typical family of records illustrated in Fig. 2 shows further that the gating current time constant varies with potential, decreasing steadily as the voltage during the pulse becomes increasingly positive, but remaining roughly constant for the restoration to a fixed holding potential at the end of the pulse. In this axon, as in many of the others, there was some rectification of the leakage current during the pulse, which resulted in the superimposition of a rectangular pedestal on the exponential tails.

The fundamental criteria for regarding the sharply rising and exponentially declining components of the asymmetric displacement current as due to the movement of mobile charged particles or dipoles that form an integral part of the membrane are that: (1) the total transfer of charge in one direction at the start of the pulse should be exactly equal to that in the opposite

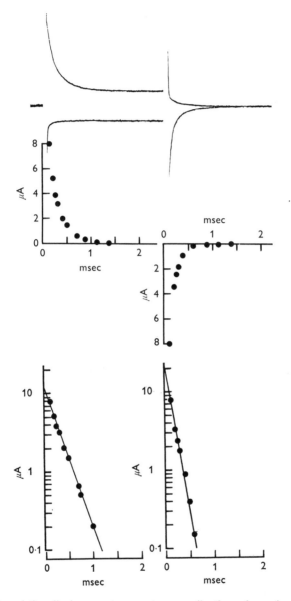

FIG. 1. Asymmetry of the displacement current on application of equal and opposite voltage-clamp pulses to a squid axon perfused with 300 mM CsF and bathed in Na- and K-free saline containing 1,000 nM tetrodotoxin. The top traces are single-sweep records of the membrane current for ±120 mV pulses. The difference between them is plotted beneath on linear and logarithmic scales. (From Keynes and Rojas, 1974.)

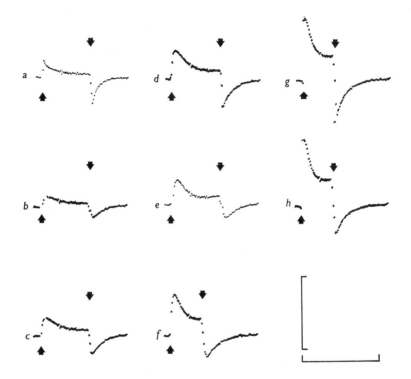

FIG. 2. A family of gating current records obtained by summation with a signal averager of the membrane currents for 60 positive and 60 negative pulses which started and finished at the arrows. The axon was perfused with 55 mM CsF, and bathed in Na- and K-free saline containing 300 nM saxitoxin. Pulse amplitude, a–h, increasing from 40 to 110 mV; holding potential −70 mV; vertical bar 5.56 μA; horizontal bar 2,500 μsec; membrane area 0.06 cm^2; temperature 7°C. (From Keynes and Rojas, 1974.)

direction at the finish, i.e., $Q_{on} = Q_{off}$; (2) the charge displacement should reach a definite saturation level Q_∞ when large enough pulses are applied to the membrane; (3) Q_∞ should be independent of temperature. All investigators are agreed (see, for example, Keynes and Rojas, 1974, Figs. 8, 9, and 14 therein) that for short pulses these conditions are met to within the accuracy of the measurements. However, when the period of depolarization is sufficiently lengthened, there is evidence both for squid (Bezanilla and Armstrong, 1975) and for the node of Ranvier (Nonner et al., 1975) that an appreciable fraction of the charges may return to their original position rather slowly on restoration of the holding potential, which gives rise to an apparent reduction in the ratio Q_{off}/Q_{on}. This change in the mobility of some of the charges appears to be related somehow to the process of inactivation of the sodium channels, but until its kinetics and voltage dependence have been examined in detail, little more can be said about it.

The next and crucial question, about which there has been some controversy, is whether these mobile charges can be identified with the sodium gating particles. Leaving aside the problem of inactivation, there are three ways of bringing about parallel reductions in the gating current and in the sodium conductance: perfusion with Zn^{2+} ions (Bezanilla and Armstrong, 1974) and treatment with either glutaraldehyde (Meves, 1974) or procaine (Keynes and Rojas, 1974). This certainly suggests a causal connection, but cannot provide final proof of it. The most convincing evidence is the close quantitative agreement between the kinetic and steady-state properties of the mobile charges on the one hand and of the sodium conductance system on the other. First, the time constant of the asymmetrical displacement current fits well, both in absolute magnitude and in voltage dependence, with the sodium conductance time constant $\tau_m = 1/(\alpha_m + \beta_m)$ (Keynes and Rojas, 1976). If the mobile charges had nothing to do with the sodium conductance, it seems most unlikely that both systems would have precisely the same relaxation time over a wide range of experimental conditions. It is true, as Armstrong and Bezanilla (1974) and we ourselves (Keynes and Rojas, 1974) originally reported, that there is some difficulty in reconciling with m^3 kinetics the values of the shutting-off time constants at the end of a pulse. However, our most recent measurements show that on repolarization of the membrane, τ_m is close to the predicted one-third of the gating current time constant as long as high holding potentials and large pulses are used (Keynes and Rojas, 1976). There is also a problem in explaining why the lengthening of the time constants of the gating current tails with increasing pulse size (Meves, 1974; Keynes and Rojas, 1974) is not apparently accompanied by a similar increase in τ_m, and why heavy water should slow down the conductance change but not the gating current (Meves, 1974). But it appears that an explanation can be found in terms of a process as yet unidentified that is interposed between the movements of the gating particles and the opening and closing of the sodium channels. Such a process might involve additional conformational changes within the gating particles or further stages of interaction between them before and after they take up new positions.

The next point to be considered is the agreement between the steady-state distribution of the mobile charges and the curves relating sodium conductance and the quantities m and h to membrane potential. From a number of measurements of the dependence of peak sodium conductance on membrane potential, made in intact axons at a holding potential in the neighborhood of -70 mV, we have found the midpoint of the curve for $(g_{Na}/\bar{g}_{Na})^{1/3}$ to fall at about -25 mV (Keynes and Rojas, 1975). This is satisfactorily close to the value of -35 mV for the midpoint of the m_∞ curve reported by Hodgkin and Huxley (1952), the difference possibly being due to the fact that our experiments were conducted in low external sodium in order to reduce errors arising from imperfect electric compensation for the resistance in series with the membrane. The midpoint for the steady-state charge distribution curve in comparable axons was -26 mV (Keynes and Rojas, 1976). When the conditions were altered, both curves were shifted to roughly the same extent along the voltage axis, the size of the shifts agreeing well with the data of Frankenhaeuser and Hodgkin (1957) for changes in external calcium concentration, and that of Chandler et al. (1965) for lowered internal ionic strength. Thus over quite a wide range of experimental conditions, the midpoints of the charge distribution curve and of the m_∞ curve agreed to within some 10 mV. The residual discrepancy may result from the difficulty of making the proper corrections for junction potential differences in the two sets of experiments, or it may be genuine, reflecting a further subtlety of the relationship between the distribution of the gating particles and the fraction of the sodium channels in a conducting state that has still to be unravelled. In either case, it is not great enough to cast serious doubt on the identification with the sodium gating particles of the mobile charges responsible for the asymmetrical displacement current.

An important characteristic of the steady-state charge distribution curve is its slope at the steepest point, which according both to Meves (1974) and ourselves (Keynes and Rojas, 1974) was 19 mV for an e-fold change. The corresponding figure for an e-fold change of the sodium conductance was 6.5 mV (Keynes and Rojas, 1976). We believe our estimate to be more reliable than Hodgkin and Huxley's (1952) value of 4–5 mV, because the measurements were again made with low external sodium to minimize trouble from incomplete series resistance compensation. Since for a singly charged particle displaced through the whole of the electric field the slope would be 25 mV for an e-fold change, it follows that the effective valency of the individual gating particles is $25/19 = 1.3$. By "effective valency" is meant the actual charge multiplied by the fraction of the electric field acting on the particle. At present, we have no way of distinguishing between the cases of a particle with a much larger total charge moving through a small part of the field and of a less highly charged particle moving through more of the field. All we can say is that the total charge cannot be less than 1.3. This uncertainty does not, however, prevent us from calculating the number of separate gating particles that have to make the transition to the "gate open" position at each channel, which is $19/6.5 = 3$. It is rather satisfactory that an argument thus based on a comparison of the steepness of the sodium conductance and charge distribution curves should yield precisely the same estimate of three controlling elements per channel as Hodgkin and Huxley's (1952) quite different approach. Their choice of a cube law in Eq. (1) depended on an examination of the time course of the initial rise of the sodium conductance on depolarization of the membrane, which was better fitted by an m^3 relation than m^2 or m^4. A least-squares curve fitting operation on our own data gave the same result (Keynes and Rojas, 1976).

The total quantity of mobile charge was estimated by Keynes and Rojas (1974) to be about 1,900 charges/μm^2, whereas Meves (1974) obtained a figure of 1,600 charges/μm^2. Armstrong and Bezanilla (1974) reported that they observed gating currents of similar magnitude, but did not give actual sizes. If there are three gating particles per channel, each with an effective valency of 1.3, the total number of channels in our experiments would be 1,900/3.9 = 490/μm^2. When we first produced it, this figure seemed disconcertingly high compared with counts of the sodium channels in rabbit vagus and crab nerve (Colquhoun et al., 1972), but subsequent measurements have given it satisfactory support. Thus counts of the TTX-binding sites made in squid axons with tritiated TTX by Levinson and Meves (1975) gave a value of 550/μm^2, and another method of measuring TTX-binding that depended on a study of the rate of blocking and unblocking of the sodium channels gave results of the same order of magnitude (Keynes et al., 1975). Although none of these estimates is sufficiently accurate to prove beyond doubt that each group of three gating particles can be equated with one sodium channel binding one molecule of TTX, the different figures are at least quite consistent with one another. Hodgkin (1975) has calculated that the achievement of maximum conduction velocity in a squid axon actually requires the provision of somewhat more than 500 sodium channels per μm^2.

Thus far, I have been able to argue without too much difficulty that on the evidence of the asymmetrical displacement current, the sodium gating particles behave much as would be expected from Hodgkin and Huxley's (1952) equations. I come finally to a consideration of the behavior of the gating current when the holding potential is lowered, and here the experimental facts are not as clear. The basic observation (Fig. 3; see also Fig. 7 in Meves, 1974) is that the records obtained by the technique of adding together the displacement currents for equal and opposite voltage-clamp pulses become inverted at a holding potential in the neighborhood of −50 mV. This does not mean, as was claimed at one time by Bezanilla and Armstrong (1974), that the gating currents are "almost completely eliminated" by prolonged depolarization of the membrane; and it is misleading to say as Meves (1974) does that there is a "reversal of the asymmetry current." It should be clear from the single-sweep records shown in Fig. 4 that the slow component of the displacement current is at all times outward for a depolarizing pulse and inward for a hyperpolarizing pulse, and even after several minutes at 0 mV it does not disappear. But with the recording technique used for Fig. 3, the "reversal" potential is merely that at which the mobile charges are equally distributed between their two positions, so that the unidirectional displacement currents are equal and opposite. What has happened, therefore, is that the midpoint of the steady-state charge distribution curve, which for a large holding potential lies at about −26 mV (Keynes and Rojas, 1976), has shifted in a negative direction. It is as yet far from

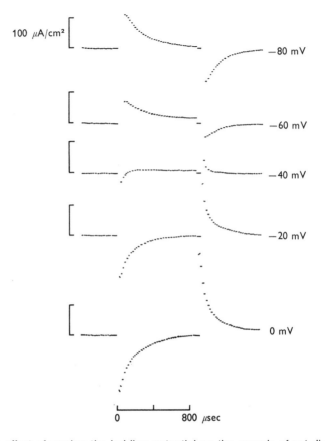

FIG. 3. The effect of varying the holding potential on the records of net displacement current obtained by summation of the membrane currents for equal and opposite voltage-clamp pulses. Axon perfused with a CsF solution of low ionic strength, and bathed in acetate saline containing 300 nM tetrodotoxin. Pulse size ±150 mV. The membrane potential was held for several minutes at the level indicated to the right of each record. (From Keynes, Rojas, and Rudy, 1974.)

clear what factors govern this shift, and in our experience its magnitude is somewhat variable; but there is no doubt of its reality. It is satisfactory to be able to add that Bezanilla and Armstrong (1975) have now revised their views on this issue, having recently reported that maintained depolarization reduces the size of the gating current rather than abolishing it, and at the same time alters the shape of the charge distribution curve; these views are in broad agreement with our own unpublished results.

An obvious question to ask is whether any "h" gating current is observed. It can readily be calculated from the data for h_∞ and τ_h given by Hodgkin and Huxley (1952) that if each channel incorporated a single independent h particle as well as the three m particles, then a pulse taking the membrane

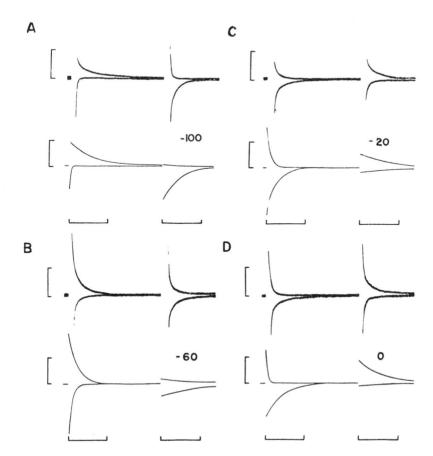

FIG. 4. The effect of varying the holding potential on single-sweep records of the unidirectional displacement current. The actual traces are shown above, and the calculated time course of the displacement current after subtraction of the capacity transient is shown below. Axon perfused with high ionic strength CsF solution and bathed in Na- and K-free isethionate saline containing 300 nM tetrodotoxin. Temperature 6.4°C. The holding potential in mV is given next to each group of records. Vertical calibration bars 100 μA/cm^2; horizontal bars 0.5 msec. (From Rojas and Keynes, 1975.)

potential to 0 mV would reveal a second component of the gating current about four times smaller and slower than the main one. Clearly no such component is to be seen in the record of Fig. 1, which is typical of the great majority of our gating current records in following an exponential time course with a single time constant. It would seem, therefore, that normally all the gating particles have identical relaxation times, and there is no evidence for the existence of another population of h particles that move more slowly. If this conclusion is accepted, how is inactivation brought about? This question can only be answered by entering into the realm of speculation, but my present feeling is that we may be dealing with the kind of three-state system discussed by Goldman (1975), and that inactivation is not to be regarded as an independent process. If the transition from the "gate open" to the "inactivated" state were primarily time rather than voltage dependent, then it would not necessarily be accompanied by an easily detectable passage of gating current. In a still more speculative vein, most of the facts that I have described would be compatible with the following sequence of events:

(1) The first event on depolarization of the membrane consists of a transfer of a number of the gating particles from state A (resting) to state B' (preconducting) with a time constant $\tau_{1 \, on}$ that is equated with the gating current time constant.

(2) At each channel for which all three particles are in state B', they now undergo a further transformation with a short time constant $\tau_{2 \, on}$ into state B (conducting). $\tau_m = \tau_{1 \, on} + \tau_{2 \, on}$. Unlike the initial movement of the particles in the electric field, this step involves hydrogen bonding and so is slowed by D_2O as observed by Meves (1974).

(3) In the conducting channels, there is next a slower conformational change that converts the particles to state C (inactivated) with a time constant τ_h, and closes the channels once more.

(4) In the channels where only one or two of the three particles have gotten into state B', the conformational change to state B and then to state C is modified so that it has the effect of preventing the remaining two or one particles from quitting state A even if the membrane is still further depolarized.

(5) Maintained depolarization blocks some of the channels in a related manner, and at the same time creates a second class of gating particle that is able to return only rather slowly to the resting state.

A scheme of this kind clearly involves too many ad hoc assumptions to be really satisfactory as a working hypothesis. However, the necessity for accommodating not only the experimental facts about the conductance changes [which include the complications on the inactivation front reported by Chandler and Meves (1970), and the slow effects of Narahashi (1964) and Adelman and Palti (1969)], but also the gating current data, should prevent the theorization from getting out of hand. One of the principal respects in which the gating current studies will certainly be valuable is indeed to provide a major new constraint for those engaged on the construction of molecular models of the sodium channels. As I am afraid will be all too apparent, there are numerous points, especially in relation to the mechanism of inactivation, where we do not yet have the basic information that we need on the behavior of the gating currents, and cannot even speculate constructively. But I hope that I have succeeded in conveying my conviction that the discovery of methods of examining them has opened a fresh and promising chapter in neurophysiology. It is a privilege to present this essay as a tribute to Harry Grundfest, who has made so many and varied contributions to earlier chapters.

REFERENCES

Adelman, W. J., and Palti, Y. (1969): The effects of external potassium and long duration voltage conditioning on the amplitude of sodium currents in the giant axon of the squid, *Loligo pealei. J. Gen. Physiol.,* 54:589–606.

Armstrong, C. M., and Bezanilla, F. (1974): Charge movement associated with the opening and closing of the activation gates of the Na channels. *J. Gen. Physiol.,* 63:533–552.

Bezanilla, F., and Armstrong, C. M. (1974): Gating currents of the sodium channels: Three ways to block them. *Science,* 183:753–754.

Bezanilla, F., and Armstrong, C. M. (1975): Inactivation of gating charge movement. *Biophys. J.,* 15:163a.

Chandler, W. K., Hodgkin, A. L., and Meves, H. (1965): The effect of changing the internal solution on sodium inactivation and related phenomena in giant axons. *J. Physiol. (Lond.),* 180:821–836.

Chandler, W. K., and Meves, H. (1965): Voltage clamp experiments on internally perfused giant axons. *J. Physiol. (Lond.),* 180:788–820.

Chandler, W. K., and Meves, H. (1970): Slow changes in membrane permeability and long-lasting action potentials in axons perfused with fluoride solutions. *J. Physiol. (Lond.),* 211:707–728.

Colquhoun, D., Henderson, R., and Ritchie, J. M. (1972): The binding of labelled tetrodotoxin to non-myelinated nerve fibres. *J. Physiol. (Lond.),* 227:95–126.

Frankenhaeuser, B. and Hodgkin, A. L. (1957): The action of calcium on the electrical properties of squid axons. *J. Physiol. (Lond.),* 137:218–244.

Goldman, L. (1975): Quantitative description of the sodium conductance of the giant axon of *Myxicola* in terms of a generalized second-order variable. *Biophys. J.,* 15:119–136.

Hodgkin, A. L. (1975): The optimum density of sodium channels in an unmyelinated nerve. *Philos. Trans. R. Soc. Lond. [Biol.],* 270:297–300.

Hodgkin, A. L., and Huxley, A. F. (1952): A quantitative description of membrane current and its application to conduction and excitation in nerve. *J. Physiol. (Lond.),* 117:500–544.

Keynes, R. D. (1975): The ionic channels in excitable membranes. In *Energy transformation in biological systems,* edited by G. E. W. Wolstenholme and D. FitzSimons. Ciba Foundation Symposium N.S.31.

Keynes, R. D., Bezanilla, F., Rojas, E. and Taylor, R. E. (1975): The rate of action of tetrodotoxin on sodium conductance in the squid giant axon. *Philos. Trans. R. Soc. Lond. [Biol.]* 270:365–375.

Keynes, R. D., and Rojas, E. (1974): Kinetics and steady-state properties of the charged system controlling sodium conductance in the squid giant axon. *J. Physiol. (Lond.),* 239:393–434.

Keynes, R. D., and Rojas, E. (1976): The temporal and steady state relationships between activation of the sodium conductance and movement of the gating particles in the squid giant axon. *J. Physiol. (Lond.),* 255:157–189.

Keynes, R. D., Rojas, E., and Rudy, B. (1974): Demonstration of a first-order voltage-dependent transition of the sodium activation gates. *J. Physiol. (Lond.),* 239:100–101P.

Levinson, S. R., and Meves, H. (1975): The binding of tritiated tetrodotoxin to squid giant axons. *Philos. Trans. R. Soc. Lond. [Biol.],* 270:349–352.

Meves, H. (1974): The effect of holding potential on the asymmetry currents in squid giant axons. *J. Physiol. (Lond.),* 243:847–867.

Narahashi, T. (1964): Restoration of action potential by anodal polarization in lobster giant axons. *J. Cell. Comp. Physiol.,* 64:73–96.

Nonner, W., Rojas, E., and Stampfli, R. (1975): Displacement currents in the node of Ranvier: Voltage and time dependence. *Pflügers Arch.,* 354:1–18.

Rojas, E., and Keynes, R. D. (1975). On the relation between displacement currents and activation of the sodium conductance in the squid giant axon. *Philos. Trans. R. Soc. Lond. [Biol.],* 270:459–482.

Electrobiology of Nerve, Synapse, and Muscle,
edited by J. P. Reuben, D. P. Purpura, M. V. L. Bennett,
and E. R. Kandel. Raven Press, New York © 1976

Delayed Birefringence Signals Observed in Nerve Fibers of Squid, Crayfish, and Crabs

Akira Watanabe and Susumu Terakawa

Department of Physiology, Tokyo Medical and Dental University, Yushima, Bunkyo-ku, Tokyo 113, Japan

Previous studies (Cohen et al., 1968, 1970) established that the nerve fiber changes its resting birefringence when the fiber is excited. It has further been shown that the birefringence change in squid giant axons is mostly dependent on the change in membrane potential. Thus the time course of the birefringence change associated with a conducted action potential is very similar to that of the change in membrane potential, and, when a square voltage pulse is imposed on the membrane with the aid of the voltage-clamp technique, the optical change can generally be regarded as a square pulse. To describe the time course of the optical signal accurately, however, several time constants with values that vary between 0.02 and 20 msec must be introduced (Cohen et al., 1971).

When repetitive stimulation is applied to the squid giant axon, a component with a much slower time course is found to follow the rapid component of the birefringence change. The total time course of the slow component depends, of course, on the number and frequency of the applied shocks; a train of five pulses with 10-msec intervals produces a slow signal of about 500-msec duration (Watanabe and Terakawa, 1976). Essentially similar slow optical changes can also be recorded from a crab nerve (Watanabe et al., 1973) and from a crayfish giant axon (Watanabe and Terakawa, 1974). The origin of the slow signal is still not entirely clear, but the phenomenon indicates the existence of processes with very long time constants at or near the membrane. Our tentative hypothesis is that the optical change is produced by a transient destruction of the orderly structure of the axoplasm following Ca invasion, which takes place during membrane excitation. An experimental basis for the hypothesis is that the optical signal is conspicuously influenced by several antimitotic drugs including colchicine. We hope this line of approach to the neuronal activity could serve to elucidate correlations between membrane excitation and processes taking place within the neuron (e.g., axoplasmic transport). It is further expected that the phenomenon might throw some light on the molecular mechanism of nerve excitation.

EXPERIMENTS ON SQUID AXONS

A squid giant axon was dissected from the mantle and mounted horizontally in an experimental chamber. The chamber, made of black and transparent lucite plates, was equipped with two holes sealed by pieces of coverslip to allow a light beam to pass through the mounted giant axon. A polarizer was placed between the light source and the axon, with its transmission axis at 45° to the longitudinal direction of the axon. An analyzer was placed between the axon and the detector. A photodiode (PIN 10, United Detector) was used as the detector. The analyzer was usually set in a crossed position. The light source was a quartz-halogen lamp. A heat-reflecting and a red-suppression filter were introduced between the lamp and the polarizer to eliminate infrared radiation, for which the polarizer and the analyzer (made from sheets of Polaroid film, HN22) did not work satisfactorily.

On stimulation with repetitive electric pulses applied at an end of the axon, an optical signal was detected as a transient change in intensity of light received by the photodiode (Fig. 1A). After each stimulating pulse, a brief signal with a shape similar to an upside-down action potential appeared. (The upward deflection indicates increase in light intensity at 0°.) This must be the signal that Cohen and his associates described. However, each brief response was followed by a slow phase of decreased light intensity. Stimulation with a single shock did not necessarily demonstrate the slow phase distinctly, because under the usual recording conditions of the birefringence signal some fluctuation of the base line was unavoidable. However, when we used repetitive shocks, the presence of such a slow signal was distinct (Fig. 1B). The slow phase summated and often formed a round peak after stimulation, and very gradually returned to the base line.

The slow decrease in light intensity probably indicates that there exists a slow phase in birefringence change following the rapid phase which is synchronous with the action potential. It is known, however, that axons change their turbidity slowly when they are stimulated repetitively (Hill and Keynes, 1949; Hill, 1950; Bryant and Tobias, 1952). The turbidity change

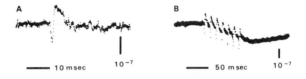

FIG. 1. Optical signals recorded from a squid giant axon under the cross-polar conditions. **A:** Response to a single shock. **B:** Response to a train of seven stimuli. An averaging computer was used to improve the signal-to-noise ratio; the number of sweeps was 2,000 in **A** and 1,000 in **B.** *Vertical bars,* calibration for the size of response expressed in its ratio to the total light intensity, i.e., the light intensity to be received by the detector on removal of the analyzer on the assumption that the analyzer is optically ideal. 16°C.

causes either an increase or a decrease of light intensity detected at 0°; the direction of the change depends on many factors including medium osmotic pressure and amount of tension applied to the mounted axon. Until turbidity change can be excluded as a contributing factor, one cannot conclude that the observed intensity change is due to a change in birefringence of the axon.

A method to differentiate the effect of birefringence from that of turbidity change is to use an optical compensator. In a transparent birefringent material placed between a polarizer and an analyzer — their polarizing axes crossed and set at 45° with the optical axis of the birefringent material — the light intensity of $I_0 \sin^2 (\gamma/2)$ emerges from the analyzer, where I_0 is the intensity of the incident light and γ the retardation of the material. When γ changes by a slight amount of $\Delta\gamma$, the change in emerging light intensity, ΔI, should be $I_0 \cdot \sin \gamma \cdot \Delta\gamma$, a quantity that depends on the resting retardation. With insertion of an optical compensator, one can change the value of γ. This procedure therefore changes the size of the response (ΔI).

We used a quarter-wave plate as the compensator, which has a retardation angle of $\pi/2$. When the slow axis of the quarter-wave plate is set parallel or perpendicular to the slow axis of the axon, the responses should have the equal amplitude with reversed polarity, since $\sin (\gamma + \frac{1}{2}\pi) = -\sin (\gamma - \frac{1}{2}\pi)$. Figure 2E and F shows an example of such experiments. The reversal of the signal was, if any, incomplete. It is hard to escape the conclusion that the observed change is contaminated by the intensity change caused by light scattering.

The amount of light intensity change due to light scattering could be assessed simply by removing the analyzer if the axon were isotropic. However, since we already know that the axon is birefringent, we cannot assume that the axon is isotropic in scattering the incident light. We must assume that the axon is dichroic, i.e., that the amount of scattering is different according to the azimuth of vibration direction of the incident light. The dichroic nature of the material can be described by two principal transmittances, k_1 and k_2 (see Shurcliff and Ballard, 1964, p. 65). As we define them, k_1 is the transmittance of the axon to a polarized light with its vibration direction perpendicular to the longitudinal direction of the axon, and k_2 is the transmittance of the axon to a polarized light with its vibration direction parallel to the longitudinal direction of the axon. It is possible to estimate k_1 and k_2 by a simple procedure. We fix the azimuth of the transmission axis of the polarizer at 45° to the longitudinal direction of the axon. When the azimuth of the transmission axis of the analyzer is perpendicular to the longitudinal direction of the axon, the emerging light intensity is proportional to k_1. When the azimuth of the transmission axis of the analyzer is parallel to the longitudinal direction of the axon, the emerging light intensity is proportional to k_2. A birefringence change of the axon does not influence the size of the scattering signal under these optical settings.

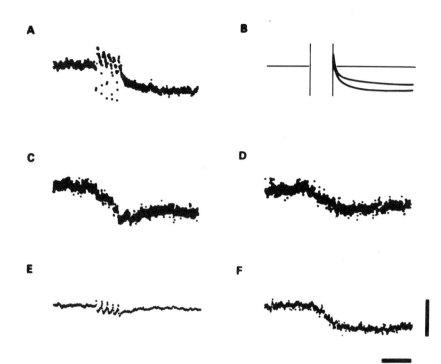

FIG. 2. The delayed birefringence change of a repetitively stimulated squid giant axon estimated from optical signals obtained under variable optical settings. Five successive stimuli were applied at an end of the axon with intervals of about 10 msec. **A:** Optical signal obtained under the cross-polar conditions. **B:** *Lower curve,* trace of the slow optical signal shown in **A;** *upper curve,* estimated delayed birefringence change based on records shown in **A, C,** and **D. C:** Optical signal obtained under the condition that the azimuth of the transmission axis of the analyzer was perpendicular to the longitudinal direction of the axon. **D:** Optical signal obtained under the condition that the azimuth of the transmission axis of the analyzer was parallel to the longitudinal direction of the axon. **E:** Optical signal obtained under the cross-polar conditions, but with a quarter-wave plate inserted between the axon and the analyzer with its slow axis perpendicular to the longitudinal direction of the axon. **F:** Optical signal obtained under similar conditions to **E,** but with the slow axis of the compensator parallel to the longitudinal direction of the axon. *Vertical bar,* 2×10^{-7} (in **A** and **B**), 10^{-6} (in **C** and **D**), and 2×10^{-6} (in **E** and **F**) of the total light intensity. *Horizontal bar,* 50 msec, applicable to all the records. 15°C.

Figure 2C and D shows results of one of the experiments to determine the changes of k_1 and k_2. In this particular example, the light intensity received at 0° decreased on excitation of the axon. In other axons, both increase and decrease of light intensity were observed, but as far as we have observed, k_1 and k_2 always changed to the same direction in one particular axon.

Having established that the effect of turbidity change could be recorded independently of the birefringence change, we next tried to assess their contribution to the observed signal under the cross-polar conditions. A calculation was made with the use of Jones' matrix (Shurcliff and Ballard, 1964, p. 80). It has been assumed that optical properties of the axon are represented by a model that is optically homogeneous, birefringent, and dichroically turbid. As a matter of fact, the axon is indeed birefringent and dichroically turbid, but it is never homogeneous. Instead, it has a form of cylinder surrounded by a plasma membrane that is associated by Schwann cell layers and connective tissue. The cytoplasm is also optically inhomogeneous. Fibrillar materials are densely populated in the ectoplasm and much less so in the endoplasm (Metuzals and Izzard, 1969). The assumption of homogeneity is made solely to simplify the system so that the calculation is feasible. Therefore, the result of the calculation is justified only when the experiment shows its usefulness within the range of our experimental accuracy.

The calculation yielded a simple formula:

$$I_X = \tfrac{1}{2}\,(I_I + I_{II}) - \cos\gamma\,(I_I \cdot I_{II})^{1/2} \tag{1}$$

where I_X is the light intensity obtained under the cross-polar conditions, I_I and I_{II} are the light intensities obtained with transmission axis of the analyzer perpendicular and parallel to the longitudinal direction of the axon, respectively, and γ is the retardation of the axon. In this formula I_X, I_I, and I_{II} can be measured experimentally, and γ can then be calculated from them.

We checked the applicability of the formula on several inanimate models, especially on stretched pieces of film made from polyvinyl alcohol and stained with iodine. The film was dichroic as well as birefringent. The polarizance P, defined as $(I_I - I_{II})/(I_I + I_{II})$, ranged between 0.05 and 0.43. The retardation calculated with the use of Eq. (1) agreed with that measured with the standard Sénarmont method (see Bennett, 1950) within a range of several percent. The results show that the material is represented quite well with the adopted model.

We also checked the applicability of Eq. (1) on the real squid axon; again there was a reasonable agreement between the calculated values and the values determined with the Sénarmont method. It was therefore felt that we could proceed further and calculate the changing part of the birefringence. The optical signal we could observe was very small in comparison with the light intensity observed from the resting axon. We therefore assumed, when the axon was excited, that I_I, I_{II}, and γ changed slightly and independently, and that only the first terms in the Taylor expansion would be sufficient for the calculation of the change in light intensity. Thus we obtained the formula that expresses the signal:

$$
\begin{aligned}
\Delta I_X = &\ \tfrac{1}{2}\,[1 - \cos\gamma\,(I_{II}/I_I)^{1/2}]\,\Delta I_I \\
&+ \tfrac{1}{2}\,[1 - \cos\gamma\,(I_I/I_{II})^{1/2}]\,\Delta I_{II} \\
&+ \sin\gamma\,(I_I \cdot I_{II})^{1/2} \cdot \Delta\gamma
\end{aligned} \tag{2}
$$

where Δ's indicate changes of the respective quantities during excitation. It will be seen that all the parameters except $\Delta\gamma$ can be obtained experimentally; $\Delta\gamma$ can then be calculated from them.

An example of this calculation is illustrated in Fig. 2B. Although the necessary correction for the turbidity change is significantly large, the major part of the signal, obtained under the cross-polar conditions, is ascribed to the birefringence change.

Another method to calculate the birefringence change is to start with records from experiments employing a quarter-wave plate (Fig. 2E and F). A formula similar to Eq. (2) was derived with the help of Jones' calculation. The method was less reliable because the experimental procedure was more complicated and because we used white light for the experiment, although the quarter-wave plate works accurately only at a prescribed wavelength. In spite of these difficulties, the values obtained with the latter method agreed reasonably well with those calculated by Eq. (2). We were thus convinced that the long-lasting optical change, recorded from the axon under the cross-polar conditions, originated primarily from a long-lasting birefringence change. We call it *the delayed birefringence change,* to distinguish it from the initial, rapid, spike-like change which we call *the initial birefringence change.*

EXPERIMENTS ON THE CRAB NERVE

The crab nerve gives a large birefringence signal. We started optical experiments with this material and were very much impressed with the slow time course of the response. The falling phase of the optical response lasted for more than 500 msec, although the main part of the action potential ended within 50 msec (Fig. 3). Because the nerve consists of many nerve fibers with variable diameters, one has to be very careful to draw a conclusion from the observed facts. Possible causes of the long-lasting optical response might be: (a) a dispersion of the compound action potential because of different conduction velocities of individual nerve fibers; (b) long-lasting action potentials of individual nerve fibers; or (c) the existence of some long-lasting aftereffects after passing of an excitation wave.

The first possibility can be tested experimentally. Erlanger and Gasser (1937) showed that individual fibers hold their own conduction velocities, and therefore the shape of the compound action potential becomes multi-peaked, smaller, and wider as it conducts along the nerve. The same should be the case for the optical signal if its long-lasting nature is due to the dispersion of the action potentials from individual fibers. The light signal was recorded at a part of the nerve, and stimuli were given at two places with different distances from the recorded region. As shown in Fig. 4, two responses were different only at their initial part; when the conduction distance was larger, the initial peak was smaller, wider, and multipeaked. The later phases of the two responses were almost identical in time course and amplitude. This is not compatible with the hypothesis that the long-lasting optical response is due to the existence of slowly conducting nerve fibers. Similar experiments were performed with some variations; for example,

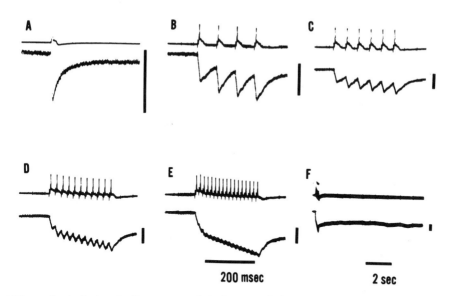

FIG. 3. Optical signals (*lower traces*) and extracellularly recorded action potentials (*upper traces*) recorded from a crab nerve. **A** to **E:** Optical and electrical responses to stimulation with variable numbers of shocks. The records are on the same time base. **F:** Responses to the same number of stimuli as that employed in **E,** with a slower time base. *Calibration bars,* 2.5×10^{-4} of the background light intensity. 20°C. (From Watanabe et al., 1973, with permission.)

stimuli were applied from both ends of a nerve with different delays. Action potentials from slowly conducted fibers should collide with those from the other end and a summation of the optical responses should not be observed. The experiment showed, in fact, that when the interval of two stimuli was 20 to 200 msec, the optical response was an approximate summation of the optical responses elicited by individual stimuli, except that the falling phase of the summated response was often slightly larger than the mathematical sum of the individual responses.

The second possibility cannot be tested rigorously because we cannot examine membrane potentials of all the fibers in the nerve. Intracellular recording of action potentials from the nerve fibers was carried out by M. Nagano (*personal communication*). She found that the action potential consists of a spike of approximately 80-mV amplitude followed by an after-potential. When outside Ca concentration is 60 mM (which we employed often since high-Ca physiological salines seemed to keep the excitability for a longer period after dissection), the after-potential was an after-depolarization that lasted as long as 50 msec. Although this is a rather long-lasting electrical activity, it is not long enough to explain the duration of the optical signal. It is possible, however, that there are smaller fibers with very long after-potentials.

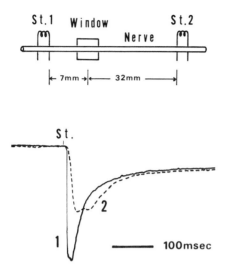

FIG. 4. A comparison of the optical responses of a crab nerve elicited by stimuli applied at sites with different conduction distances to the recorded region. **Upper:** Conditions of the experiment. **Lower:** Optical signals. *Solid curve* (marked as 1) and the *dotted curve* (marked as 2) are the traces of the optical records in response to stimulation applied through electrodes marked as St. 1 and St. 2, respectively. The amplitude of the response 1 was approximately 4.2×10^{-4} of the background light intensity. 20°C.

For us, however, the third possibility seems to be the most likely one because the optical activity was easily summated on repetitive stimulation (Fig. 3, B to E), and, when the number of stimuli was increased to 10 to 20, the optical responses persisted much longer than 10 sec (Fig. 3F). With 50 shocks, a response with a duration of approximately 1 min could be produced. Although we know very little about the electrophysiological properties of smaller fibers, it is difficult to believe that the membrane depolarization lasts for such long periods of time. Furthermore, we know that in other materials (giant axons of squid and crayfish) the optical responses last much longer than the electrical activity of nerve fibers. Probably in the crab nerve, too, the delayed birefringence change, unassociated with simultaneous membrane depolarization, is the major cause of the observed slow signal.

To elucidate the nature of the long-lasting optical signal, we first examined the possibility of the effects of a contraction during stimulation. One end of the crab nerve was fixed and the other end was tied to a glass rod extension of the stylus bar of an RCA 5734 mechanoelectrical transducer. The system was sensitive enough to record clearly the contraction of *Nitella* in response to a single stimulus (Kishimoto and Ohkawa, 1966). Its amplitude of contraction was approximately 0.2 μm. In the crab nerve, however, maximal stimulation did not produce any signal. In one experiment, the output of the transducer was fed to an averaging computer, and the responses to 3,000 stimuli were accumulated. No significant signal could be recorded. Assuming that no fatigue was taking place in this postulated mechanical response, the amplitude was calculated to be much less than 5 Å per stimulus. Because the length of the nerve was about 5 cm, the ratio was less than 10^{-8}. It is therefore unlikely that the contraction of the nerve is responsible for the optical response which is at least 10^{-4} of the background light intensity.

An alternative hypothesis would be that some birefringent structure inside the axoplasm is changing because of an increased influx of ions across the membrane following excitation. The resting axon is already birefringent; this birefringence is probably caused by the micelles being buried in axoplasm since the birefringence alters when the axon is immersed in media with different refractive indexes in a way similar to that predicted by Wiener's formula (Bear et al., 1937). Electron microscope studies have shown that axons are rich in microtubules, which seem to be rigid and probably play a role in maintaining solid structure of the axoplasm (see, for example, Tilney, 1968). Microtubules are known to be a major component of the mitotic spindle, a highly birefringent structure when observed under the polarizing microscope (Inoué and Sato, 1967). It is therefore probable that in axons, too, the amount of birefringence is correlated with microtubules in the axoplasm. For these reasons, we examined several agents that influence formation of microtubules.

Figure 5 shows the effect of colchicine on the axon birefringence. The resting birefringence and the size of the optical response were decreased on application of 10^{-4} M colchicine. The effect of colchicine was mostly irreversible; Fig. 5 shows one of the rare examples where partial recovery of the response was observed. Similar effects were also observed with 10^{-4} M vinblastine, although with this drug we sometimes observed a transient increase of the optical response. In one experiment we examined the effects of 10^{-5} M vincristine. A distinct decrease of the optical response,

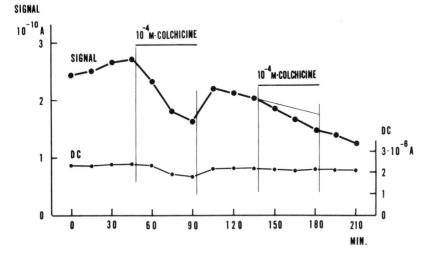

FIG. 5. The effect of colchicine on the time courses of the size of the optical signal (SIGNAL) and background light intensity (DC) recorded from a crab nerve. The two horizontal bars at the top indicate the periods of application of the colchicine (10^{-4} M). Following the first application of colchicine, the signal size started decreasing even in normal saline. With the second application of colchicine, an increase in the rate of decrease of the signal size was observed. Note the line of extrapolation from the previous three measurements. (From Watanabe et al., 1973, with permission.)

with a clear recovery on removing the agent, was observed. D_2O enhances birefringence of the mitotic spindle, probably by enhancing association of the protein molecules (Inoué and Sato, 1967). The effect of 40 to 50% D_2O on the birefringence response of the crab nerve was to increase the size of the response. The amount of change was variable, ranging from 15 to 93%. The resting birefringence was also increased by D_2O.

From these experiments it may be speculated that microtubules in the axoplasm have some effect on the production of the birefringence signal. Probably the excitation process at the membrane exerts some influence on the structure of the axoplasm. A reasonable assumption would be that the increased influx of Ca produces the effect. In 1972, Weissenberg showed that the process of polymerization of microtubules from the subunit protein (tubulin) is strongly inhibited by Ca. Under certain conditions, existence of Ca at a concentration of the order of 10^{-5} M reduces the flow birefringence of tubulin solution to half that at zero Ca (Abe and Kurokawa, *personal communication*). We can estimate the increase in concentration of Ca at the boundary between the membrane and the axoplasm with the formula:

$$c(o,t) = 2 \, \alpha(t/D \cdot \pi)^{1/2} \tag{3}$$

where c is the concentration of Ca as a function of distance from the membrane and time, α the rate of influx of Ca, and D the diffusion coefficient (see Crank, 1956, p. 31). In the squid axon, the amount of Ca influx per impulse is of the order of 10^{-14} mole/cm^2 (Hodgkin and Keynes, 1957; Tasaki et al., 1967). When repetitive stimulation is applied to an axon at a frequency of 100 Hz, the mean rate of influx is of the order of 10^{-12} mole/cm^2/sec. This can be taken as α. If we assume that the diffusion coefficient of Ca salt in the axoplasm is approximately the same as that of $CaCl_2$ in aqueous media, and take it as 10^{-5} mole/cm^2/sec (Harned and Owen, 1958), after 50-msec stimulation the concentration at the inner surface of the membrane goes up by approximately 10^{-7} M, which is probably enough to produce a detectable birefringence change. If the diffusion coefficient of Ca salt is lower, the concentration of Ca at the boundary should be increased according to Eq. (3).

When Ca was removed from the outside medium, the optical response was reduced significantly (Watanabe et al., 1973). In contrast with the effects of antimitotic drugs, the effect of Ca removal was rapid and reversible. The result supports the hypothesis that increased Ca influx produces the birefringence signal following excitation.

EXPERIMENTS ON CRAYFISH AXONS

In spite of the favorable size of the optical response obtainable from a crab nerve, a serious shortcoming of the material is that the correlation between optical change and membrane potential change cannot be rigidly established. Single axon preparations from the central nervous system of a crayfish proved to be suitable material for both optical and electrical studies. The crayfish giant axon is much smaller than the squid giant axon, but squid supply is highly seasonal and the animals do not survive for a long time in the aquarium. Crayfish can be kept alive in the aquarium for practically unlimited periods. Berestovsky et al. (1969) were the first to record the birefringence signal from a crayfish giant axon.

After dissection of one of the circumesophageal connectives or the abdominal cord, a giant axon was partially cleaned by removing smaller surrounding nerve fibers with a pair of needles; thus, when illuminated, the giant axon was clearly visible as a transparent tube-like structure. Glass capillary microelectrodes were used to record the membrane potential intracellularly. The axon was stimulated by an electric pulse applied at an end of the axon or by injecting current through a second intracellular electrode.

The optical responses associated with conducted action potentials were varied according to the axon and we classified them into four types. *Type A* did not show any clear spike-like response and its shape was approximately triangular (Fig. 6A); this type of response usually had a large signal-to-background ratio. *Type B* was similar to Type A in that it had a conspicuous tail, but it was preceded by a spike-like response (Fig. 6B). *Type C* had only the spike-like component with no tail (Fig. 6C). *Type D* had a spike but it was followed by a tail of reversed polarity to that of the spike (Fig. 6D). This type thus resembled that of the initial response obtained from a squid giant axon.

Individual axons showed different types of responses, and we could not control them. We sometimes had the impression that axons of a particular type appeared successively during a period of experiments, but no definite correlation with the season could be established. There was a loose correlation between the shape of the action potential and the type of the optical response. Thus, when the action potential had a prominent after-depolarization, the optical response was often of Type A; and when the action potential

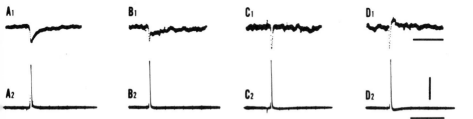

FIG. 6. Birefringence signals (*upper traces*) and intracellularly recorded action potentials (*lower traces*) from four different crayfish median axons. A_1, B_1, C_1 and D_1 are the examples of Types A thru D optical signals, respectively. The approximate spike amplitudes of the optical signals (per impulse, divided by background light intensity) were: A_1 5.8×10^{-5}, B_1: 2.2×10^{-5}, C_1: 1.3×10^{-5}, C_1: 1.2×10^{-5}. *Horizontal bars,* 50 msec. *Vertical bar,* 50 mV. 16 to 17°C. (From Watanabe and Terakawa, 1974, with permission.)

had a prominent after-hyperpolarization, the optical response was often of Type D. The correlation seemed reasonably clear in the median giant axon taken from circumesophageal connectives, but it was unclear in the lateral giant axon taken from the abdominal cord, which almost always showed a marked after-depolarization, but often with the Type D optical response.

With repetitive stimulation, optical responses usually summated. When the optical response was of Type A or B, the long-lasting tail (the after-response) was the part that summated (Fig. 7,A). When the optical response was of Type D, the pattern of summation was similar to that of squid giant axon; the light intensity was transiently increased, apparently due to summation of the phase of increased light intensity, but the direction of the response gradually changed and finally turned to the slow phase of decreased light intensity (Fig. 7B).

We have started examining the effect of colchicine on the birefringence signal of the crayfish giant axons and we found that the signal was often refractory to 10^{-4} M colchicine. With a higher concentration of colchicine, however, the expected decrease in signal was observed; the decrease was irreversible. The resistance of the birefringence signal to a lower concentration of colchicine might be due to a lower membrane permeability toward this agent. Ling and Thompson (1974) report that refractoriness to colchicine

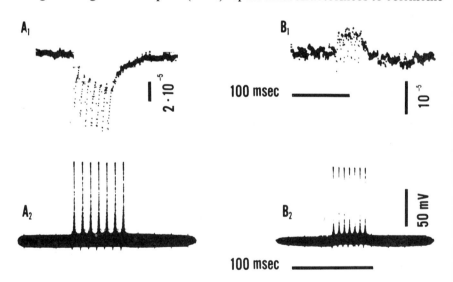

FIG. 7. Summation of optical signals of crayfish median giant axons elicited by tetanic stimulation (*upper traces*) and simultaneously recorded action potentials (*lower traces*). Trains of 7 shocks were applied repetitively with a period of 0.8 sec to accumulate the optical signal. A_1 and A_2: From the same axon as that shown in Fig. 4A; B_1 and B_2: from another axon that produced a Type D optical response and an action potential with an after-hyperpolarization in response to a single stimulus. During the initial stage of repetitive stimulation the after-potential was gradually changed to an after-depolarization as shown in B_2. 22°C. (From Watanabe and Terakawa, 1974, with permission.)

of some mammalian cells is attributable to the lower rate of colchicine up-take of the cells.

Hinkley and Samson (1974) found that 5 mM colchicine caused little obvious effect on the structure and number of microtubules, as examined by electron microscopy. We found, however, a definite decrease in resting birefringence in most of the axons treated with 5 mM colchicine, indicating that the drug was effective to some extent in disorganizing the axoplasmic structure of the crayfish giant axon.

CONCLUSIONS

It has been established that a slow change in birefringence could be pro-duced from the axons of squid, crab, and crayfish. At present, an exact mechanism for production of the slow signal cannot be decided, and the interpretation presented by us in connection with the experiments on the crab nerve should still be regarded as a hypothesis. We hope further experi-ments will reveal the place and mechanism for the production of the signal.

We feel, however, that the possibility that membrane excitation exerts some influence on the axoplasm should be carefully examined. If such an influence existed, it might have far-reaching implications in interpreting the integrative function of the nervous system. In a recent review, Ochs (1974) stated that a small but reproducible reduction of the rate of fast axoplasmic transport could be demonstrated in an axon stimulated repeti-tively. The problem of plasticity, which definitely occurs in many synapses, could equally be triggered by excitation of the cell membrane. Optical methods allow us to detect changes taking place in living axons and there-fore can supply information that is unavailable by many other methods in neurophysiology, simply because the axon is still alive while we are examin-ing it.

ACKNOWLEDGMENTS

The research has been supported by grants No. 744021 and 811005 from the Ministry of Education in Japan and by grant 73–123 from Naito Founda-tion.

REFERENCES

Bear, R. S., Schmitt, F. O., and Young, J. Z. (1937): The ultrastructure of nerve axoplasm. *Proc. R. Soc. Lond. [Biol.]*, 123:505–519.
Bennett, H. S. (1950): The microscopical investigation of biological materials with polarized light. In: *McClung's Handbook of Microscopical Technique*, 3rd ed., edited by R. M. Jones, pp. 591–677. Hafner, New York.
Berestovsky, G. N., Lunevsky, V. Z., Razhin, V. D., and Musienko, V. S. (1969): Rapid changes in birefringence of the nerve fiber membrane during excitation. *Dokl. Akad. Nauk. SSSR*, 189:203–206.

Bryant, S. H., and Tobias, J. M. (1952): Changes in light scattering accompanying activity in nerve. *J. Cell. Comp. Physiol.,* 40:199–219.

Cohen, L. B., Hille, B., and Keynes, R. D. (1970): Changes in axon birefringence during the action potential. *J. Physiol.,* 211:495–515.

Cohen, L. B., Hille, B., Keynes, R. D., Landowne, D., and Rojas, E. (1971): Analysis of the potential-dependent changes in optical retardation in the squid giant axon. *J. Physiol.,* 218:205–237.

Cohen, L. B., Keynes, R. D., and Hille, B. (1968): Light scattering and birefringence changes during nerve activity. *Nature,* 218:438–441.

Crank, J. (1956): *The Mathematics of Diffusion.* Oxford University Press, London.

Erlanger, J., and Gasser, H. S. (1937): *Electrical Signs of Nervous Activity.* University of Pennsylvania Press, Philadelphia.

Harned, H. S., and Owen, B. B. (1958): *The Physical Chemistry of Electrolytic Solutions,* 3rd ed. Reinhold, New York.

Hill, D. K. (1950): The effect of stimulation on the opacity of a crustacean nerve trunk and its relation to fibre diameter. *J. Physiol.,* 111:283–303.

Hill, D. K., and Keynes, R. D. (1949): Opacity changes in stimulated nerve. *J. Physiol.,* 108:278–281.

Hinkley, R. E., Jr., and Samson, F. E., Jr. (1974): The effects of an elevated temperature, colchicine, and vinblastine on axonal microtubules of the crayfish (*Procambarus clarkii*). *J. Exp. Zool.,* 188:321–336.

Hodgkin, A. L., and Keynes, R. D. (1957): Movements of labelled calcium in squid giant axons. *J. Physiol.,* 138:253–281.

Inoué, S., and Sato, H. (1967): Cell motility by labile association of molecules. The nature of mitotic spindle fibers and their role in chromosome movement. *J. Gen. Physiol.,* 50(6, Pt. 2): 259–292.

Kishimoto, U., and Ohkawa, T. (1966): Shortening of *Nitella* internode during excitation. *Plant Cell Physiol.,* 7:493–497.

Ling, V., and Thompson, L. H. (1974): Reduced permeability in CHO cells as a mechanism of resistance to colchicine. *J. Cell. Physiol.,* 83:103–116.

Metuzals, J., and Izzard, C. S. (1969): Spatial patterns of threadlike elements in the axoplasm of the giant nerve fiber of the squid (*Loligo pealii* L.) as disclosed by differential interference microscopy and by electron microscopy. *J. Cell Biol.,* 43:456–479.

Ochs, S. (1974): Energy metabolism and supply of ~P to the fast axoplasmic transport mechanism in nerve. *Fed. Proc.,* 33:1049–1058.

Shurcliff, W. A., and Ballard, S. S. (1964): *Polarized Light.* Van Nostrand, Princeton.

Tasaki, I., Watanabe, A., and Lerman, L. (1967): Role of divalent cations in excitation of squid giant axons. *Am. J. Physiol.,* 213:1465–1474.

Tilney, L. G. (1968): The assembly of microtubules and their role in the development of cell form. *Dev. Biol.,* Suppl. 2:63–102.

Watanabe, A., and Terakawa, S. (1974): Initial and delayed birefringence signals and membrane potential of a crayfish giant axon. *Proc. Japan Acad.,* 50:90–95.

Watanabe, A., and Terakawa, S. (1976): A long-lasting birefringence change recorded from a tetanically stimulated squid giant axon. *J. Neurobiol.,* Vol. 7.

Watanabe, A., Terakawa, S., and Nagano, M. (1973): Axoplasmic origin of the birefringence change associated with excitation of a crab nerve. *Proc. Japan Acad.,* 49:470–475.

Weisenberg, R. C. (1972): Microtubule formation in vitro in solutions containing low calcium concentrations. *Science,* 177:1104–1105.

Electrobiology of Nerve, Synapse, and Muscle,
edited by J. P. Reuben, D. P. Purpura, M. V. L. Bennett,
and E. R. Kandel. Raven Press, New York © 1976

Ca Activation in the Giant Axon of the Crayfish

Jiro Suzuki

*Division of Neurophysiology, Psychiatric Research Institute of Tokyo, Setagaya-ku,
Tokyo, 156, Japan*

The ionic mechanism of spike generation in the giant axon of the crayfish was studied by Yamagishi and Grundfest (1971). They showed that the afterdepolarization which followed the spike involved an increased conductance for Ca (depolarizing calcium activation). The amplitude of the overshoot in propagating spikes increased with the increase of the concentration of Ca in the external solution (Ca_0). However, in the absence of Na_0, or in the presence of tetrodotoxin (TTX), a propagating spike could not be elicited despite the presence of Ca in a high concentration.

In some crustacean muscle fibers including the giant barnacle muscle fiber, action potentials result from an initial increase in membrane permeability to Ca ions (Fatt and Ginsborg, 1958; Abbot and Parnas, 1965; Hagiwara and Naka, 1964). Action potentials of several kinds of ganglion cells are also produced by an increase of the conductance of the membrane to Ca ion (Geduldig and Junge, 1968; Koketsu and Nishi, 1969; Carpenter and Gunn, 1970; Iwasaki and Satow, 1971). In an amphioxus muscle cell, permeability changes for Na and Ca induce the action potential (Hagiwara and Kidokoro, 1971).

These Na–Ca or Ca systems are distinguished from the Na system, for example, the squid giant axon, in which the action potential is produced by the increase of the conductance to Na ion (Hodgkin and Huxley, 1952; Frankenhäuser and Hodgkin, 1958; Baker et al., 1971).

In the present paper, the Na–Ca system was studied in the giant axon of the crayfish. Intracellular stimuli were applied close to the site of intracellular recording so as to obtain depolarizing (decrementally propagating) responses by Ca activation in Ca saline or by an activation for Ba or Sr ion. Further investigations of the relation between Na and Ca activation were carried out with application of TTX, tetraethylammonium (TEA), Mn, or Co.

A preliminary paper has appeared (Suzuki and Grundfest, 1974).

METHODS

The circumesophageal nerve cord of the crayfish was used in the experiments. The giant axon was dissected carefully and placed in a trough. Its diameter ranged between 120 and 160 μm.

The axon was impaled with two KCl-filled microelectrodes, the resistance of which was about 20 MΩ. A pair of silver wire electrodes were used to stimulate the axon extracellularly.

The standard saline was van Harreveld's. The desired concentration of Ca, Ba, Sr, Mn, Co, and TEA was obtained by mixing appropriate amounts of Tris-Cl or Tris-propionate and Ca-, Ba-, Sr-, Mn-, Co-, and TEA saline. Every solution had almost equivalent osmolarity to the standard saline (469.1 mM). The pH of most solutions was 7.5.

Electrical properties of the axons in control saline were as follows in 30 fibers: the resting potential, -75.1 ± 5.5 mV, the overshoot of the action potential, 11.7 ± 7.7 mV, and the effective resistance, $12.5 \pm 3.7 \times 10^3$ Ω.

THE SPIKE-LIKE Ca RESPONSE

A depolarizing response could be obtained by a brief intracellular pulse in the axon bathed in Ca saline without Na, K, and Mg. The amplitude of the response was about 40 mV. As in the control spike, the response consisted of two components, the initial spike-like part and the afterdepolarization. The former had a brief duration and a relatively steep rate of rise, which was slower than the control (Fig. 1). The afterdepolarization lasted about 4 msec or longer, so that its duration was somewhat longer than that of the control.

This response may appear to exhibit a threshold (Fig. 1B) but not to propagate. No response was observed at a distance of 3 mm or more from the point of stimulation. This somewhat contradictory finding suggests that the axon was nonuniform. The amplitude of the response in Ca saline, evoked with stimulation by a long pulse, increased with a greater slope with increase of stimulus strength than did the passive electronic response. The change in response peak tended to flatten out finally, whereas the passive change still increased with stronger stimuli. The strength of the stimulus required to evoke a response in Ca saline was about 20 times that for the control response.

The amplitude of the depolarizing responses was maximal in a range of

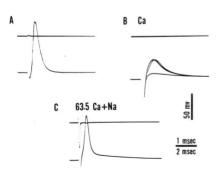

FIG. 1. Ca activation. **A:** Control. **B:** Response in Ca saline (40.5 mM CaCl₂, O-Na, O-K, O-Mg). **C:** Overshoot and afterdepolarization increased in high Ca solution (63.5 mM Ca, normal Na, K, and Mg). Time scale; 1 msec for **A** and **B**, 2 msec for **C**.

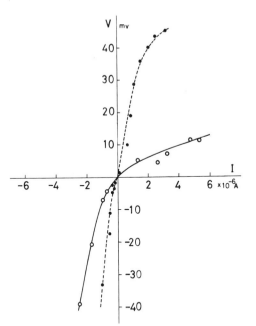

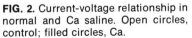

FIG. 2. Current-voltage relationship in normal and Ca saline. Open circles, control; filled circles, Ca.

concentration of 27.0 to 40.5 mM of Ca_0. In some experiments $CaCl_2$ was replaced with Ca propionate and osmolarity was adjusted with Tris-Cl or Tris-propionate. The membrane potential at the peak of the responses changed almost linearly with the logarithm of Ca_0 in the range of concentration up to 27 mM. The slope of the curve was 19.7 mV/decade Ca_0 for Ca propionate. In some other tissues, the amplitude of the Ca response is approximately linear with Ca_0 concentration (Hagiwara and Naka, 1964; Koketsu and Nishi, 1969).

The current voltage relation (Fig. 2) is similar to that of a squid giant axon (Cole, 1961). The effective resistance calculated is about $12.5 \times 10^3 \, \Omega$ for a hyperpolarizing current. In 40.5 mM $CaCl_2$, the resistance increased by about twofold or more. In another axon, the resistance increased by about 1.5 times in a saline including normal Na, K, Mg, and 63.5 mM Ca and Cl. In this saline, the spike showed a slower falling phase. These results suggest that an increasing Ca concentration reduced K activation.

THE EFFECT OF TTX

These Ca responses were neither depressed nor abolished when TTX was applied in the concentration of 2×10^{-8} g/ml, which was sufficient to block spikes in the control saline (Fig. 3); TTX also did not affect Ba response. TTX did not affect Ca or Ba responses in the presence or absence of Cl. When TTX was applied in the control saline, the normal spike was abolished

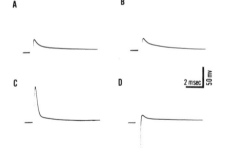

FIG. 3. Effect of TTX. **A:** Ca response. **B:** No effect of the application of TTX on Ca response. **C:** Normal spike. **D:** TTX almost depressed Na spike in the concentration of 2×10^{-8} g/ml.

as in other tissues (Narahashi et al., 1964; Nakamura et al., 1965; Yamagishi and Grundfest, 1971).

However, in detail, the initial spike component was abolished although the depolarizing (local) response and the afterdepolarization still remained (Fig. 3). These depolarizing responses did not propagate, so that they were not recorded in the preceding investigation. Onset and time course of this residual response were similar to those of the Ca response. In the giant axon of Loligo, only the early transient current is blocked by TTX and the late phase of Ca entry is insensitive to TTX (Baker et al., 1971). In the crayfish giant axon, the blocking effect of TTX may have a similar mechanism. Further investigation in this respect is required.

The results of the experiments with TTX confirm that the normal spike is composed of two parts, Na and Ca components, and also indicate that Na and Ca ions may have separate channels in the axonal membrane of the crayfish. TTX affected the resting potential of the axon (Yamagishi and Grundfest, 1971). Accordingly, the Ca response in the crayfish axon has similar properties to the spike of an *Aplysia* neuron (Geduldig and Junge, 1968). In Ca systems in other tissues, TTX does not affect Ca activation (Hagiwara and Nakajima, 1966; Katz and Miledi, 1969).

THE EFFECT OF Ba AND Sr

The depolarizing response was also observed in Ba or Sr saline when Ca as well as Na, K, and Mg were absent from the saline. The amplitude of these responses ranged 35 to 73 mV for Ba, higher than when Ca provided the ionic battery for the electrogenesis (Fig. 4). The amplitude of the responses was dependent on the concentration of Ba. The duration of the response was much longer than the Ca response, more than 9.1 msec for Ba. In the case of Sr, the response was smaller and shorter than in Ba (Fig. 4). In the barnacle muscle, the inward current in Ba is larger than that in Ca or Sr. Therefore, in this giant axon a similar mechanism is assumed to exist for a divalent cation flux (Hagiwara et al., 1974).

The *I-V* relationship in Ba or Sr saline is similar to that in Ca. The effec-

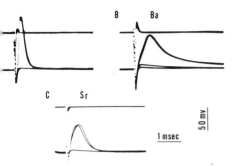

FIG. 4. Ba and Sr response. **A:** Control. **B:** Response in Ba saline (27 mM BaCl₂, O-Na, O-K, O-Mg). **C:** Response in Sr saline (27 mM SrCl₂, O-Na, O-K, O-Mg).

tive resistance of the axon in Ba or Sr saline is about three times the control. These divalent cations are assumed to depress K permeability (Hagiwara and Naka, 1964; Hagiwara et al., 1974).

The replacement of Ca with Ba or Sr in the normal saline sustained the propagating spike, which was smaller in amplitude than in the control saline. Furthermore, the addition of Ba or Sr (50 mM) to the control saline resulted in repetitive firing of spikes following a brief stimulus and an increase in the afterdepolarization. The repetitive discharge lasted for more than 50 msec at the longest. The overshoot and the afterdepolarization of each spike increased remarkably. In Ba solution of a lower concentration (30 mM), repetitive firing could not be observed but the overshoot and the afterdepolarization of the spike increased. Sr was less effective than Ba.

These results suggest Ba and Sr can provide the ionic battery for electrogenesis in the axon without Ca and also enhance the Na and Ca spike. In crustacean muscle fibers, the propagating action potential can be elicited in Ba or Sr solution without Ca (Fatt and Ginsborg, 1958; Werman and Grundfest, 1961). In those experiments the concentration of Ba or Sr was relatively low compared with the present results.

THE ABOLITION OF SPIKES BY Mn OR Co

The addition of Mn or Co (50 mM) to the control saline abolished spike generation (Fig. 5). In other words, the Na spike and the Ca component were blocked completely in the presence of Mn or Co ions at 50 mM. At a concentration of 30 mM of these ions, the spike was depressed and prolonged in the duration. The action potential recovered almost completely when the axon was bathed in the control saline again.

The current voltage relation in these cases was quite similar to those of Ba and Sr.

The propagated spike was depressed sooner than the direct spike. All the reports concerning the effect of Mn or Co on spike generation showed that these ions depressed the Ca spike or Ca permeability specifically, but

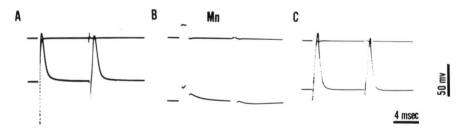

FIG. 5. Abolishment of spikes by Mn of 50 mM. **A:** Control (the preceding is a direct spike and the following is a propagating one). **B:** Complete abolishment of the spikes even with stronger stimuli. **C:** Complete recovery.

on the other hand, did not affect the Na spike (Hagiwara and Nakajima, 1966; Hagiwara and Takahashi, 1967; Geduldig and Junge, 1968).

However, in this axon a high concentration of Mn or Co blocks the Na component as well as the Ca component. One of the reasons for this difference may be the concentration of Mn or Co applied in these experiments.

THE ENHANCEMENT OF THE AFTERDEPOLARIZATION BY TEA

In the presence of TEA added to the control saline, the spike was followed by an enhanced afterdepolarization, whereas the peak amplitude of the spikes was not affected. In the Ca saline also the afterdepolarization was prolonged but the effect was not as remarkable as in the control saline. The concentration of TEA, which could prolong the duration of the spike and the afterdepolarization, was more than 10 mM. The slope of the falling phase of the spike was decreased (Fig. 6).

In 50 mM of TEA a single brief stimulus evoked repetitive and prolonged spikes. Each spike was followed by an enhanced afterdepolarization (Fig. 6).

In the *I-V* relationship in the presence of TEA, the effective resistance of the membrane was increased. TEA, in the external solution, affected the

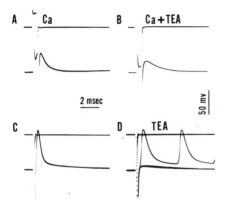

FIG. 6. Effect of TEA. **A:** Ca response. **B:** Slight prolongation of the afterdepolarization by TEA of 10 mM. **C:** Normal spike. **D:** Repetitive firing and prolongation of the afterdepolarization of the spike by TEA of 50 mM applied to the control saline.

K permeability of the axonal membrane as it affects that of the membrane of the crayfish and barnacle muscles (Fatt and Katz, 1953; Hagiwara et al., 1964; Hagiwara et al., 1969; Keynes et al., 1973); in the squid giant axon TEA affects the permeability of the membrane only when applied in the internal solution (Armstrong and Binstock, 1965; Hille, 1967).

DISCUSSION

Many data in this chapter indicate that Ca activation which is responsible for the afterdepolarization of the axon in the normal saline can arise sufficiently early so as to generate a spike-like response. However, this response is decrementally propagated, unlike the spike in the presence of Na. The failure to generate a propagating spike-like Na spike in the absence of Na indicates that the inward flux of Ca does not provide enough current to overcome the cable losses in the axon. In this respect, further investigations, for example, a space clamp technique, will give more useful results.

The influx of Ca can be replaced by Ba or Sr. Presumably Ba or Sr may pass the same channel as Ca like in the membrane of the barnacle muscle. The sequence of the amplitude of the responses in Ca, Ba, and Sr is Ba > Sr = Ca. This sequence seems to be similar to that of the current in the barnacle muscle (Hagiwara et al., 1974).

The results of the experiment with TTX suggest that Ca channel should be different and separate from that of Na. Moreover, Ca and Na do not compete with each other, whereas Ca depresses K activation (Adelman and Dalton, 1960). So, the Na–Ca system of activation can be proposed in this axonal membrane.

It is quite interesting that Mn or Co can abolish both Na and Ca activation. This result should be studied further from the point of view of the basic role of Ca ion in the excitation of the membrane.

SUMMARY

In the giant axon of the crayfish, depolarizing responses could be obtained by intracellular stimulation of a brief pulse in the Ca saline without Na, K, and Mg. The similar depolarizing responses with higher amplitude were seen in Ba or Sr saline in the absence of Na, K, Mg, and Ca. These spike-like responses were not affected by TTX in the presence or absence of Cl. In the presence of TEA, repetitive firing or enhanced afterdepolarization occurred. The addition of Co or Mn to the control saline only abolished the spike at high concentrations.

Ca activation, which is responsible for the afterdepolarization of the axonal membrane in the control saline, can arise sufficiently early so as to generate a spike-like response. Influx of Ca can be replaced by Ba or Sr.

The results with TTX suggested Ca channel may be different from that of Na.

REFERENCES

Abbott, B. C., and Parnas, I. (1965): Electrical and mechanical responses in deep abdominal extensor muscle of crayfish and lobster. *J. Gen. Physiol.*, 48:919–931.

Adelman, W. J., Jr., and Dalton, J. C. (1960): Interactions of calcium with sodium and potassium in membrane potentials of the lobster giant axon. *J. Gen. Physiol.*, 43:609–619.

Armstrong, C. M., and Binstock, L. (1965): Anomalous rectification in the squid giant axon injected with tetraethylammonium chloride. *J. Gen. Physiol.*, 48:859–872.

Baker, P. F., Hodgkin, A. L., and Ridgway, E. B. (1971): Depolarization and calcium entry in squid giant axons. *J. Physiol.*, 218:709–755.

Carpenter, D., and Gunn, R. (1970): The dependence of pacemaker discharge of Aplysia neurons upon Na+ and Ca2+. *J. Cell. Physiol.*, 75:121–128.

Cole, K. S. (1961): Non-linear current-potential relations in an axon membrane. *J. Gen. Physiol.*, 44:1055–1057.

Fatt, P., and Ginsborg, B. L. (1958): The ionic requirements for the production of action potentials in crustacean muscle fibers. *J. Physiol.*, 142:516–543.

Fatt, P., and Katz, B. (1953): The electrical properties of crustacean muscle fibers. *J. Physiol.*, 123:171–204.

Frankenhäuser, B., and Hodgkin, A. L. (1957): The action of calcium on the electrical properties of squid axons. *J. Physiol.*, 137:218–244.

Geduldig, D., and Junge, D. (1968): Sodium and calcium components of action potentials in the Aplysia giant neurons. *J. Physiol.*, 199:347–365.

Hagiwara, S., Chichibu, S., and Naka, K. (1964): The effects of various ions on resting and spike potentials of barnacle muscle fibers. *J. Gen. Physiol.*, 48:163–179.

Hagiwara, S., Fukuda, J., and Eaton, D. C. (1974): Membrane currents carried by Ca, Sr, and Ba in barnacle muscle fiber during voltage clamp. *J. Gen. Physiol.*, 63:564–578.

Hagiwara, S., and Kidokoro, Y. (1971): Na and Ca components of action potential in Amphioxus muscle cells. *J. Physiol.*, 219:217–232.

Hagiwara, S., and Naka, K. (1964): The initiation of spike potential in barnacle muscle fibers under low intracellular Ca2+. *J. Gen. Physiol.*, 48:141–162.

Hagiwara, S., and Nakajima, S. (1966): Differences in Na and Ca spikes as examined by application of tetrodotoxin, procaine and manganese ions. *J. Gen. Physiol.*, 49:793–806.

Hagiwara, S., and Takahashi, K. (1967): Surface density of calcium ions and calcium spikes in the barnacle muscle membrane. *J. Gen. Physiol.*, 50:583–601.

Hille, B. (1967): The selective inhibition of delayed potassium currents in nerve by tetraethylammonium ion. *J. Gen. Physiol.*, 50:1287–1302.

Hodgkin, A. L., and Huxley, A. F. (1952): Currents carried by sodium and potassium ions through the membrane of the giant axon of Loligo. *J. Physiol.*, 116:449–472.

Iwasaki, S., and Satow, Y. (1971): Sodium and calcium dependent spike potentials in the secretory neuron soma of the X-organ of the crayfish. *J. Gen. Physiol.*, 57:216–238.

Katz, B., and Miledi, R. (1969): Tetrodotoxin-resistant electric activity in presynaptic terminals. *J. Physiol.*, 203:459–487.

Keynes, R. D., Rojas, E., Taylor, R. E., and Vergara, J. (1973): Calcium and potassium systems of a giant barnacle muscle fibre under membrane potential control. *J. Physiol.*, 229:409–455.

Koketsu, K., and Nishi, S. (1969): Calcium and action potentials of Bullfrog sympathetic ganglion cells. *J. Gen. Physiol.*, 53:608–623.

Nakamura, Y., Nakajima, S., and Grundfest, H. (1965): The action of tetrodotoxin on electrogenic components of squid giant axons. *J. Gen. Physiol.*, 48:985–996.

Narahashi, T., Moore, J. W., and Scott, W. R. (1964): Tetrodotoxin blockage of sodium conductance increase in lobster giant axons. *J. Gen. Physiol.*, 47:965–974.

Suzuki, J., and Grundfest, H. (1974): The effect of divalent cations, TTX and TEA on the spike generation of crayfish giant axon. *Proc. XXVIth Int. Congr. Physiol. Sci.*, 11:151.

van Harreveld, A. (1936): A physiological solution for fresh water crustaceans. *Proc. Soc. Exp. Biol. Med.*, 34:428–432.

Werman, R., and Grundfest, H. (1961): Graded and all-or-none electrogenesis in arthropod muscle. II The effects of alkali-earth and onium ions on lobster muscle fibers. *J. Gen. Physiol.,* 44:997–1027.
Yamagishi, S., and Grundfest, H. (1971): Contribution of various ions to the resting and action potentials of crayfish medial giant axons. *J. Membr. Biol.,* 5:345–365.

Electrobiology of Nerve, Synapse, and Muscle,
edited by J. P. Reuben, D. P. Purpura, M. V. L. Bennett,
and E. R. Kandel. Raven Press, New York © 1976

An Electronic Model of a Membrane Consisting of Ten Independent "Two-State" Channels Showing Voltage-Dependent Conductance and Current Noise

Alexander Mauro and Michelangelo Rossetto

The Rockefeller University, New York, New York 10021

It is now well established from electrophysiological studies on a variety of cells that voltage-dependent conductance is a general property of electrically excitable membranes. However, the physical mechanism underlying this property remains to be elucidated.

The experimental demonstration that minute fluctuations in membrane potential occur in nodal preparations of medullated nerve fibers and in lobster and squid giant axons is good evidence that the membrane conductance in electrically excitable membranes undergoes fluctuations at a given level of membrane potential. These data in turn have given rise to several hypotheses concerning the behavior of "channels" (or "pores") in membranes, for example, the "multi-state" channel model and the "two-state" channel model [see a recent review pertaining to the measurements and theoretical interpretations of membrane "noise" (Verveen and De Felice, 1974)].

In the multi-state model the voltage dependence of membrane conductance occurs as a result of discontinuous levels ("jumps") of conductance which are available to each channel as the membrane potential is varied (the molecular mechanisms responsible for this behavior are not specified). In the two-state model the voltage dependence arises from the property that each channel is either "open" (conducting) or "closed" (nonconducting) with the average duration of the channel (or the average fraction of time the channel is open) being voltage dependent (again the molecular mechanisms are not specified). It should be emphasized that although the I,V characteristic of each channel is linear (ohmic), an ensemble of independently acting channels will give rise to a nonlinear I,V characteristic, i.e., a voltage-dependent conductance, with, of course, fluctuations in the total conductance.

Although unitary events supporting either type of channel behavior have not been observed in a biological membrane, they have been found and studied in bilayer model membranes which have been modified by minute amounts of "channel forming" agents, thereby forming single channels. For example, multi-state behavior of single channels has been reported by Bean et al. (1969), Bean (1972), and Bean (1973) in bilayers modified by EIM, an unidentified proteinaceous substance that acts to form channels; using different lipids in conjunction with EIM two-state behavior has been found by Ehrenstein et al. (1970) and Latorre et al. (1972).[1]

Although it is by no means clear whether one or the other mechanism applies to excitable membranes, we believe it is instructive — especially to students of excitability — to examine the behavior of a two-state model system which simulates by electronic circuits a membrane containing a number of two-state channels. We have chosen the simplest variant of the two-state channel model in that the channel turns on at a fixed rate, e.g., approxi-

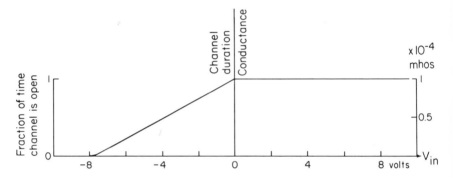

FIG. 1. Channel duration given in terms of the fraction of time a single two-state channel is open (*left scale*) and the average "membrane" conductance (*right scale*) versus V_{in}, the "membrane" potential. The duration in seconds is given by the product of the reciprocal of the switching frequency and the fraction of time a channel is open.

mately 100 cps, with a duration that varies linearly with the potential as shown in Fig. 1. (Note that the pulse duration is proportional to the fraction of time the channel is open.) Strict independence of the channels is ensured by the absence of synchronization between any of the channels. Since each channel-forming circuit is costly, we kept the total number to a minimum. We intuitively chose 10 as the appropriate number of channels that would give a reasonably "smooth" total current at a given membrane potential.

The main element of the model is a field effect switch (Fig. 2a) that is made to conduct by applying a train of voltage pulses to the control electrode. The switch in series with a resistance and a battery constitutes a single channel which is either "open" or "closed." A gating circuit (details are given in the Appendix) provides the gating pulses. The duration of each pulse is determined by the membrane potential V_{in}. As is shown in Fig. 2a, the membrane potential, V_{in}, controls both the pulse duration via the gating

---

[1] For evidence of channel formation by gramicidin and alamethicin see a recent review by Haydon and Hladky (1972).

circuit and the current flow through the channel. The magnitude of the current is given by $I = g(V_{in} - E)$, where E has a negative or positive value depending on whether a "K channel" or "Na channel" (without inactivation) is being simulated.

Figure 2b shows the parallel combination of 10 channels with a common EMF to all channels. The total current—the "membrane current"—is

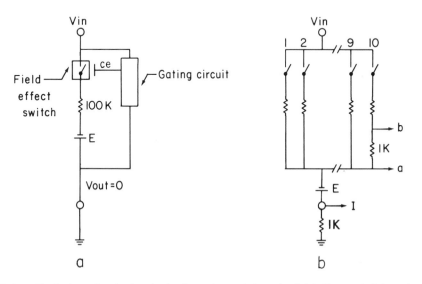

FIG. 2. a: Equivalent circuit of a single channel consisting of a field effect switch in series with the channel resistance (100 kΩ) and the channel EMF, *E*. The gating circuit generates a pulse train that is applied to the switch via a control electrode (ce). The switch is closed at a fixed rate of approximately 100 cps for a duration given by V_{in} according to Fig. 1. The membrane potential is given by the difference between the "inside" versus the "outside" (circuit ground), i.e., $V_{in} - V_{out}$, where $V_{out} = 0$. **b:** Circuit of 10 independent two-state channels in parallel. It should be understood that each field effect switch is controlled by its respective gating circuit, which is not shown in the diagram. The EMF is the same for all channels and thus is inserted as a single EMF, *E*, as shown. The total membrane current, I_y, is obtained by the voltage drop across the 1 kΩ resistor to the ground. Differential recording at a and b, across the 1 kΩ resistor in channel 10, gives the single-channel current.

recorded by measuring the potential drop across a small series resistance (1 kΩ). The current generated by a single channel (No. 10) is recorded by inserting a small resistance (1 kΩ) in series with the channel resistance (100 kΩ) and measuring the voltage drop across it with a differential amplifier, i.e., between the points a and b. Thus by employing a two-beam oscilloscope one can observe simultaneously both the current pulses of the single channel—the unitary event in this model membrane—and the summation of the currents contributed by the 10 channels—the "membrane current."

Figure 3a shows an oscillographic record of the single-channel current

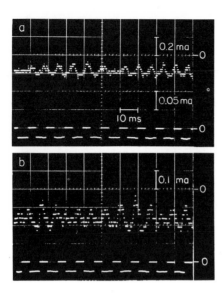

FIG. 3 a: Membrane current (*upper trace*) and a single-channel current (*lower trace*) for $E = 0$ and $V_{in} = -3$ V. Both currents are "inward" as indicated by the negative excursions with respect to zero (see Fig. 4 as to definition of "inward" and "outward"). **b:** Membrane current (*upper trace*) is shown at a higher amplification (0.1 mA/div.) to show more clearly the presence of discrete levels in the membrane current.

(lower) and the membrane current (upper) for $V_{in} = -3$ V and zero EMF ($E = 0$). Since V_{in} is less than zero, the current is inward. The duration of each pulse is given by the relationship between the fraction of time the channel is open and the membrane potential V_{in}, as given by Fig. 1. The membrane current is seen to have an average inward value with marked fluctuations, i.e., membrane current "noise." Indeed the current noise is an inevitable consequence of the stochastic summation of the separate channel currents acting independently. To emphasize this point the membrane current is shown at a higher amplification in Fig. 3b; the discrete levels in the current tracing are clearly evident. Recordings for $V_{in} > 0$ would show the absence of discrete levels because each channel would be conducting continuously.

Concurrent with the oscillographic recordings one can obtain an I,V plot under "voltage-clamp" conditions by applying V_{in} from a low-impedance voltage source (see Appendix). Such data, which were plotted with an X,Y recorder, are shown in Fig. 4. Considering first the condition $E = 0$, the current shows increasing values in the inward direction as the membrane potential V_{in} takes on values greater than $V_{in} = -8$ V. The resulting negative slope conductance is a direct consequence of the average conductance versus potential characteristic shown in Fig. 1.[2] Note this characteristic is a piece-wise linear approximation to the steady-state S-shaped curve of the conductance versus potential observed in biological membranes,

---

[2] The average conductance versus V_{in} was obtained by applying V_{in} solely to the gating circuits while the 10 channels in parallel were driven by a constant potential of 1 V. The resulting current in milliamperes thus gave the conductance in mmhos, i.e., $g = I \times 1$. Applying V_{in} and I_y to an X,Y recorder rendered the plots shown in Fig. 1.

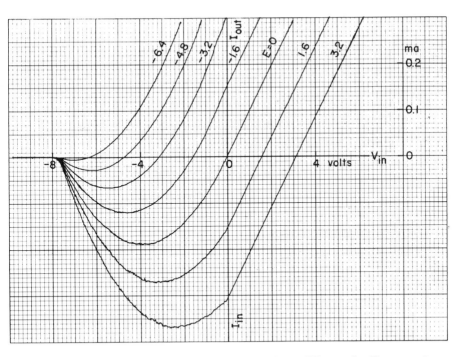

FIG. 4. The I,V plot for different values of E obtained with an X,Y recorder. The current recording in the range $V_{in} < 0$ gives the average current owing to the low-frequency response of the recorder relative to the channel-switching frequency of approximately 100 cps. I_{out} implies current flow in the direction of "inside" to "outside" ("outward current") and is plotted as positive values along the ordinate.

e.g., the K conductance and the Na conductance (without inactivation) in the squid axon. In the region $V_{in} = 0$ the I,V plot approaches a linear (ohmic) characteristic since the conductance is a constant for values $V_{in} > 0$. It should be emphasized that the noise component in the current tracing is barely perceptible because the low-frequency response of the X,Y recorder acts as a filter.

Let us now examine the consequences of the EMF taking on negative and positive values. As is shown in Fig. 4, as E takes on negative values, i.e., approaching the condition of the potassium system in biological membranes, the negative dI/dV characteristic becomes less steep. For the value $E = -6.4$ V the I,V plot is virtually monotonic. On the other hand when E takes on positive values the inward current values increase accordingly, resulting in a pronounced increase in the negative dI/dV values. In either case the behavior of any I,V plot is a direct consequence of the voltage dependence of the conductance as shown in Fig. 1. That is, each I,V plot is prescribed by the relation $I = g\,(V_{in} - E)$, where g is voltage dependent.

For a given value of E the membrane current reverses at the "reversal potential," i.e., $V_{in} = E$, as is shown in Fig. 4 for the various values of E

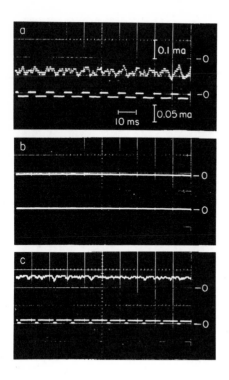

FIG. 5. Membrane current (*upper trace*) and a single-channel current (*lower trace*) near the reversal potential. **a:** $V_{in} < E$; **b:** $V_{in} = E$; **c:** $V_{in} > E$. $E = -1.6$ V. Note the reversal of the current from inward in **a** to outward in **c.**

indicated. It is interesting to observe simultaneously the behavior of the membrane current and the single-channel current in the vicinity of the reversal potential (in the range $V_{in} < 0$). In Fig. 5, for example, the oscillographic records are shown for $E = -1.6$ V. Note the reversal of the single channel current and the membrane current from inward at $V_{in} < E$ to outward at $V_{in} > E$ in Fig. 5a and c, respectively. Both tracings at the reversal potential, $V_{in} = E$, register zero current as shown in Fig. 5b. Also, as the current pulses change from inward to outward their durations increase as prescribed by Fig. 1 (compare Fig. 5a with c).

Since the gating circuit in this model responds instantaneously to changes in V_{in} to produce a change in the duration of the channel conductance, the voltage dependence of the average conductance of the 10 channels is accordingly time invariant. In order to demonstrate time-variant behavior of the conductance this membrane simulator would have to contain a delay circuit between V_{in} and the gating circuit. For example, an exponential delay would be needed to simulate the exponential kinetics observed in the conductance versus time with step changes in membrane potential in EIM treated bilayer membrane (Ehrenstein et al., 1974; Alvarez et al., 1975).

It is also relevant to emphasize that in the EIM-treated bilayer membrane the duration of a single channel at given membrane potential is not fixed but fluctuates in accordance with an exponential distribution of channel durations, which implies that the probability of termination of a channel is independent of the channel duration. As we stated at the outset, we chose a fixed duration as the simplest condition which at a minimal cost would allow the demonstration of both voltage-dependent conductance in a "two-state" multi-channel membrane and the associated membrane current "noise" which arises from the fluctuations in the membrane conductance.

APPENDIX

The gating circuit consists of three operational transconductance amplifiers (RCA CA 3060) as shown below. The two upper amplifiers form a triangle wave generator with a frequency of approximately 100 cps. The lower amplifier is used as a comparator between the triangular waveform and the

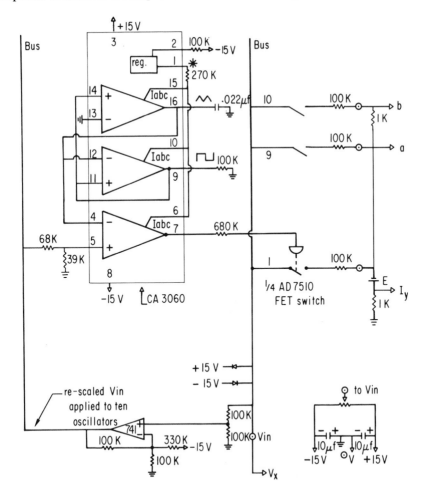

rescaled potential V_{in}. Thus, as V_{in} is varied, the duration of the pulse appearing at the output of the lower amplifier (terminal 7) varies linearly as shown in Fig. 1. This pulse is applied to the FET switch.

The operational amplifier 741 and its associated network of resistors serves to rescale V_{in} and to offset the conductance versus V_{in} characteristic to the left along the voltage axis as shown in Fig. 1.

The 270 kΩ resistor marked with an asterisk (*) is "trimmed" in each channel to make the amplitudes of the triangular waveforms equal in the 10 channels.

REFERENCES

Alvarez, O., Latorre, R., and Verdugo, P. (1975): Kinetic characteristics of the excitability-inducing material channel in oxidized cholesterol and brain lipid bilayer membranes. *J. Gen. Physiol.,* 65:421.

Bean, R. C., Shepherd, W. C., Chan, H., and Eichner, J. (1969): Discrete conductance fluctuations in lipid bilayer protein membranes. *J. Gen. Physiol.,* 53:741.

Bean, R. C. (1972): Multiple conductance states in single channels of variable resistance lipid bilayer membranes. *J. Membr. Biol.,* 7:15.

Bean, R. C. (1973): Protein-mediated mechanisms of variable ion conductance in thin lipid membranes. In: *Membranes,* edited by G. Eisenman, Vol. 2, p. 409. Marcel Dekker, New York.

Ehrenstein, G., Lecar, H., and Nossal, R. (1970): The nature of the negative resistance in bimolecular lipid membranes containing excitability-inducing material. *J. Gen. Physiol.,* 55:119.

Ehrenstein, G., Blumenthal, R., and Lecar, H. (1974): Kinetics of the opening and closing of individual excitability-inducing material channels in a lipid bilayer. *J. Gen. Physiol.,* 63:707.

Haydon, D. A., and Hladky, S. B. (1972): Ion transport across thin lipid membranes: A critical discussion of mechanisms in selected systems. *Q. Rev. Biophys.,* 5:187.

Latorre, R., Ehrenstein, G., and Lecar, H. (1972): Ion transport through excitability-inducing material (EIM) channels in lipid bilayer membranes. *J. Gen. Physiol.,* 60:72.

Verveen, A. A., and De Felice, L. J. (1974): Membrane noise. *Progr. Biophys. Mol. Biol.,* 28:189.

Electrobiology of Nerve, Synapse, and Muscle,
edited by J. P. Reuben, D. P. Purpura, M. V. L. Bennett,
and E. R. Kandel. Raven Press, New York © 1976

Desensitization and Stoichiometry of Transmitter–Receptor Interactions

Robert Werman

Neurobiology Unit, Institute of Life Sciences, Hebrew University, Jerusalem, Israel

The topic of this paper is the exploitation of electrophysiological data for understanding the fine structure of receptor function. The aspect of receptor fine structure that has most attracted me recently is the stoichiometry of the transmitter-receptor interaction (Werman, 1969). Harry Grundfest has been deeply involved in synaptic physiology at least since 1953 (Altimarino et al., 1953). Even though he has not directly worked with the question of stoichiometry, he has indicated that the Clark (1937) formulation of receptor kinetics as following the mass action principles of enzyme chemistry appears to be valid (Grundfest, 1957a, 1964a). This formulation has been one of the keystones of my approach to the problem of transmitter-receptor stoichiometry.

In this chapter, I will emphasize one of the main problems that we have encountered in our stoichiometric measurements, desensitization. Here, Grundfest was more directly involved, puzzling frequently about the possible significance of the phenomenon (Grundfest, 1957a,b, 1959, 1961, 1964b). He was also responsible for one of the major papers in the field (Epstein and Grundfest, 1970). Thus, there is little doubt that the seeds of my interest in the subjects were already largely sown during my apprenticeship. Even more important than these seeds, I think, was learning that conductance changes were indeed the key measurements to be made in any serious quantitative study of the synapse. With these debts in mind, I will describe our approach to the problem of desensitization in the stoichiometric analysis of transmitter-receptor interactions.

STOICHIOMETRY

The immediate electrical consequence of activation of a synaptic receptor is a change—usually an increase—in ionic conductance. This fact and the additive nature of conductances in parallel provide the electrophysiologist with a powerful tool for measuring the interaction between a transmitter and its receptor. If one assumes (Werman, 1969) that the activation of single receptors results in a mean conductance change that is normally distributed, the activation of n receptors should produce n times the unitary conductance change. Indeed, by an elegant technique, Katz and Miledi (1971) have demonstrated that activation of a single acetylcholine (ACh) receptor in the frog neuromuscular junction (NMJ) produces, at 22°C, an increase in conductance of 10^{-11} mhos, lasting 1 msec. This conductance is two orders of magnitude less than the maximal monovalent cation conductance through a simple channel 0.6 nm in diameter (Hille, 1970).

The conductance increases produced can be measured as a function of transmitter concentration and therefore treated the same way as the product of an enzyme-substrate reaction (Clark, 1937; Werman, 1969). Thus, in general,

$$\Delta g = n g_a = f(A) \tag{1}$$

where A is the concentration of transmitter, g the measured change in ionic conductance, n the number of receptors activated, and g_a the unitary conductance change. More specifically, assuming that n molecules of transmitter are needed to activate a receptor, that K_i is the association constant of the ith step and that g' is the change in conductance at steady state

$$g' = g'_{max} \cdot \frac{A^n}{A^n + K_n A^{n-1} + K_n K_{n-1} A^{n-2} + \ldots + K_n K_{n-1} \ldots K_2 K_1}. \tag{2}$$

It can be shown in general (Werman, 1969) for this function that

$$\lim_{A \to 0} \frac{d \log g'}{d \log A} = n. \tag{3}$$

Thus, the slope of the log-log plot of conductance as a function of concentration is a monotonically decreasing function of increasing concentration which decreases from n to 0 (Werman, 1969; Brookes and Werman, 1973).

Using this formulation, Brookes and I (Brookes and Werman, 1973) studied the stoichiometry of the GABA interaction with its receptors in the metathoracic flexor tibiae muscle of the locust. This preparation showed no apparent desensitization and the conductance increases appeared to increase monotonically with time to a maximum, steady-state value. Voltage changes in this preparation were minimal, usually showing a small, brief hyperpolarization and then a return of voltage to baseline (or even slight depolarization) as a result of redistribution of chloride ions, but without affecting the continually increasing conductance change. The lack of significant voltage/change ruled out serious membrane field effects (Magleby and Stevens, 1972).

The pooled data from 19 experiments are shown in a log-log plot in Fig. 1A where GABA concentration was varied from 4 to 10×10^{-5} M. The values obtained with increasing concentrations of GABA were fitted by a regression line with log-log slope of 3.15 ± 0.06 (SE of estimate). There is some hysteresis in the system and the curve obtained with descending

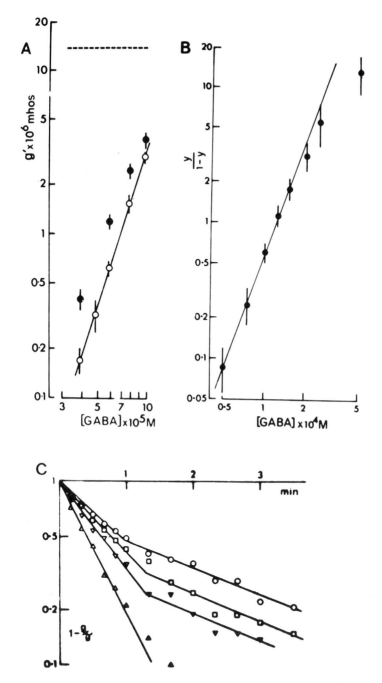

FIG. 1. The cooperativity and kinetics of GABA action on the membrane of locust muscle fibers. **A:** Experimental limiting slope of log-log plot of conductance increase at steady state, g', against GABA concentration. *Open circles,* means ($\pm$ SE, 9 experiments) on cumulative ascent of concentrations. *Closed circles,* means ($\pm$ SE, 10 experiments) on descent through concentrations. The slope of the regression line is 3.15 ± 0.06. *Dashed line,* estimated mean maximum response. **B:** Experimental Hill plot (mean $\pm$ SE, 9 experiments, propionate saline). The regression line was calculated from lower five points (slope $= 2.78 \pm 0.05$). (**A** and **B** from Brookes and Werman, 1973.) **C:** Kinetics of onset of GABA action (23°). The instantaneous conductance increase, g, was measured at multiples of 10 sec after GABA application until steady-state conductance, g', was obtained. The GABA concentrations applied were: 0, 100 μM; $\square$, 150 μM; $\triangledown$, 190 μM; $\triangle$, 240 μM. (From Brookes et al., 1973.)

concentrations is shifted to the left and the slope reduced to 2.45 ± 0.11. The absence of reduction of the slope, even at levels 1% of the extrapolated maximal conductance change, rules out the possibility that significant receptor activation can be produced by one or two molecules of GABA (Brookes and Werman, 1973; Werman, 1975). We thus conclude that at least three (and probably no more) molecules of GABA are needed to activate the inhibitory receptor in this system.

In order to examine the effect of higher doses of GABA on the system and at the same time avoid drastic changes in the membrane conductance and possible irreversible damage to the membrane, we replaced 75% of the external chloride ions with propionate ions. Such a change reduced the conductance to 18% of its control level on the average and GABA concentrations could be examined up to 50×10^{-5} M and beyond (Brookes and Werman, 1973). When a maximum conductance response is obtainable, a Hill plot can be constructed which provides further stoichiometric information (Fig. 1B). In this figure there is deviation of the experimental points from a straight line when more than 60% of receptors are activated. If the experimental points were all to fall in a straight line, the reaction would be one of infinite cooperativity described by the equation

$$g' = g'_{max}/(1 + K/A^n) \tag{4}$$

or, in the Hill form,

$$\frac{g'}{g'_{max} - g'} = \frac{A^n}{K}. \tag{5}$$

The location of the deviation from a straight line on the Hill plot indicates high positive cooperativity and the data of Fig. 1B can be well fitted by a curve with the formulation of Eq. (2) where $n = 3$ and $K_1^{-1} = 7.0 \times 10^{-4}$ M, $K_2^{-1} = 1.4 \times 10^{-4}$ M and $K_3^{-1} = 2.8 \times 10^{-5}$ M. That this reaction is of relatively great positive cooperativity can be seen from the fivefold increase of affinity in each reaction step; in addition, this curve deviates 10% from the straight line of 3 in the Hill plot when the Hill factor equals 0.033, whereas in the case of zero cooperativity, the 10% deviation is achieved at a much lower occupancy, with a Hill factor of 0.037×10^{-3}, a difference of almost three orders of magnitude (Brookes and Werman, 1973; Werman, 1975).

The high cooperativity of the reaction between GABA and its receptor allows the use of a simplifying assumption in order to calculate the thermodynamic parameters of the transmitter-receptor interaction. The limiting slope of the curve of Fig. 1B is seen to be 2.78 ± 0.05 (SE of estimate). Use of this slope as the cooperativity number in the infinite cooperativity reaction gives the following formulation:

$$\frac{1}{g'} = \frac{1}{g'_{max}} (1 + K/A^n) \tag{6}$$

TABLE 1. *Comparison of experimental and extrapolated values of maximum response* (g'_{max}), *concentration at half maximum response* ($A_{0.5}$) *and Hill slope* (*nH*) *in GABA produced conductance change in locust muscle* (*propionate saline, after Brookes and Werman, 1973*)

Data	g'_{max} (mhos × 10⁶)	$A_{0.5}$ (M × 10⁴)	*nH*
Experimental	5.76 ± 0.40 (SE)	1.18	2.78
Extrapolated	4.99 ± 0.43 (SE)	1.08 ± 0.10 (SE)	2.80 ± 0.24 (SE)

where $n = 2.78$. That this approximation is usable can be seen in Table 1. Extrapolated values were obtained by calculating the regression value of n which minimized the sum of the squares of deviation of the plot of $1/g'$ versus $1/A^n$. Values of g_{max} and $A_{0.5}$, the concentration giving half-maximal conductance change, were obtained from the intercepts. It can be seen that this approximation gives reasonably good estimates of the Hill slope and of $A_{0.5}$, but somewhat underestimates g'_{max}.

The use of this approximation allowed us to calculate the thermodynamic parameters of the interaction and these results are discussed elsewhere (Brookes et al., 1973). In addition, since we measure the development of the conductance change as a function of time, we were able to describe the kinetics of the reaction. The latter results are illustrated in Fig. 1C. It can be seen that the response is generally biphasic, and its slow phase appears to be exponential with a rate constant apparently independent of GABA concentration. With increasing GABA concentration (Fig. 1C) or with increasing temperature (Brookes et al., 1973), a faster process is seen to intervene. When the time constants are analyzed by a graphical peeling process, the values obtained are shown in Table 2. The equation assumed was:

$$1 - g/g' = a_0 e^{-k_a t} + b_0 e^{-k_b t} \qquad (7)$$

where g is the instantaneous conductance change at time t, g' is the steady-state conductance change, a_0 and b_0 are the initial fractions of the fast and

TABLE 2. *Time constants of fast and slow exponential components of response to GABA in locust muscle at 23°C* (*after Brookes and Werman, 1973*)

GABA (M × 10⁴)	g'/g_{max}	a_0	τ_a (sec)	b_0	τ_b (sec)
1.0	0.19	0.34	—[a]	0.66	182
1.5	0.51	0.49	32	0.51	169
1.9	0.78	0.62	32	0.38	180
2.4	0.92	>0.9[++]	33	<0.1[b]	—[b]

[a] Deviation from linearity prevents determination of a reliable value (see Fig. 1C).

[b] The slow process was not well defined at this concentration (see Fig. 1C).

slow components, respectively (their sum is one), and k_a and k_b are the rate constants of the fast and slow processes (Brookes et al., 1973). I will return to this figure and table later.

At this point it should be noted that the exponential onset of GABA action resembles that of a first-order reaction. Since the rate constant is independent of concentration, the kinetics cannot represent the effect of a macroscopic diffusion barrier. It would also appear that the rate constants described here are far too slow to represent the binding of GABA to receptor. Therefore the kinetic is most likely that of a conformational change of the receptor, the change permitting an increased chloride conductance (Brookes et al., 1973; Werman, 1975).

DESENSITIZATION

When we attempt to attack a cholinergic receptor in the same manner, we run into a new problem. Prolonged application of ACh introduces a new phenomenon, desensitization. The response to ACh reaches a maximum and then decreases with time, and no meaningful steady-state values appear to be obtainable. The method of determination of stoichiometry that we use cannot be applied under these circumstances. In order to analyze the process of desensitization, our first question is whether the process is accompanied by a change in the characteristics of the ionophore, the receptor, or both. A sensitive test of the characteristics of the ionophore is provided by measurement of the reversal potential of the ionophore conductance (Werman, 1965, 1966).

Manalis and I (*unpublished;* see also Manalis, 1969; Manalis and Werman, 1971; Werman and Manalis, 1970) examined the effects of brief iontophoretic pulses of ACh applied to the frog NMJ and found decreased sensitivity to an ACh pulse which was applied at intervals of 8 sec or less after a conditioning impulse. Katz and Thesleff (1957) showed that larger potentials are more readily desensitized than smaller ones and in the experiment of Fig. 2 we used large iontophoretic currents to accentuate the phenomenon. Four pulses were given at intervals of 0.5 sec. Increasing desensitization was seen and the fourth potential was reduced 25% in amplitude (Fig. 2A). When progressively stronger outward currents were given, the ACh potentials were reduced in size and inverted. The graph (Fig. 2B) shows the relation of the first (control) and fourth (most desensitized) ACh potentials to membrane potential in the region of the reversal potential. The regression lines show a difference in reversal potential of 0.3 mV which is both in the wrong direction and far less than the 11.7 mV which would account for desensitization. We therefore conclude that desensitization occurs at the level of the receptor and that the ionophore is not changed by desensitization.

It is of interest that very weak agonists of ACh action including edropho-

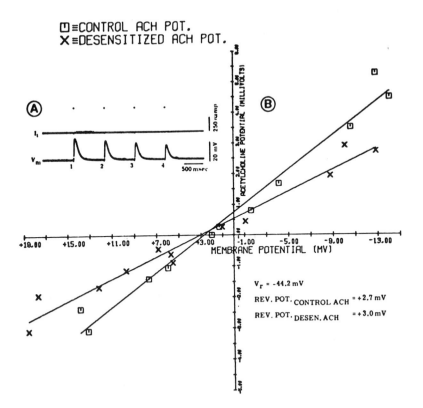

FIG. 2. Effect of desensitization on the ACh reversal potential. Desensitization does not affect ACh reversal potential at frog NMJ. **A:** Four pulses of ACh were given at 0.5-sec intervals (glycerol-treated muscle). The size of the fourth potential is reduced 25%. Resting potential = −44.2 mV. **B:** The size of the first (*tagged box*) and fourth (×) ACh potential are plotted against membrane potential in the region of the reversal potential and regression lines drawn (Manalis and Werman, *unpublished results*).

nium and heptyl-trimethylammonium ions produce only small responses at the frog NMJ even in large doses and actually block the action of ACh. When the substances were applied iontophoretically to the endplate and the reversal potentials of the conductance changes were compared with that of an ACh response at the same endplate, no significant differences were seen (Manalis, 1969; Manalis and Werman, 1971; Werman, 1975). We conclude that the cholinergic ionophore is not changed by the process of weak agonism. The results of these experiments are summarized in Table 3 where the results are expressed as the ratio of driving forces. The 5% reduction of driving force in the case of edrophonium cannot account for the more than sevenfold reduction in maximum response actually found. Thus, it is probable that only a small proportion of the receptors that are activated by the weak agonists produce the necessary conformational change for increased ionic conductance. The ionophores activated, however,

TABLE 3. *The ratio of driving forces for potentials produced by agonists of ACh to those produced by acetylcholine at the same frog neuromuscular junction*

Compound	Driving force ratio
ACh (2 doses)	0.99
ACh (desensitized to control)	1.01
Carbachol	1.01
Succinylcholine	1.02
Nicotine	1.00
Decamethonium (+ACh)	1.01
Heptyl-trimethylammonium	1.00
Edrophonium	0.95

do not appear to differ substantially in their properties from those activated by strong agonists (Werman, 1965, 1966, 1975). The similarity between desensitization and weak agonism appears to be strong, although the time constants of action appear to be substantially different.

It turns out that desensitization is dependent upon the ionic environment and in one cholinergic receptor, that of the molluscan neuron H response (hyperpolarization, chloride conductance increase); appropriate changes in the ionic environment can apparently eliminate desensitization entirely without affecting the transmitter-induced conductance increase (Ziskind and Werman, 1975a). When this is done, the necessary steady-state measurements can again be made (Ziskind and Werman, 1975b). In this preparation, bath-applied carbachol in doses of 2×10^{-5} to 2×10^{-4} M regularly produced mild hyperpolarization and an appreciable increase in ionic conductance of the H cell membrane. Continued (2 min or more) application of carbachol always resulted in a delayed reduction of the conductance increase which fell to a constant low level (0 to 75% of peak maximum). A typical response to carbachol (8×10^{-5} M) is illustrated in Fig. 3 (filled circles); the conductance increase rose to a maximum in about 1 min and then more slowly fell to a maintained level in the continued presence of carbachol. The relative degree of desensitization was also found to depend on carbachol concentration and the recovery from desensitization was long compared to either the wash-out time of the carbachol or restoration of the conductance to baseline values.

Replacement of the external Na^+ ions by equiosmolar concentrations of Mg^{2+}, Ca^{2+}, or $Tris^+$ (but not Li^+) eliminated desensitization in this preparation. An example of the elimination of desensitization is also shown in Fig. 3 (triangles) where the same dose of carbachol, now in the absence of Na^+ and Ca^{2+} ions, produced a larger conductance change with little change in the rising phase. The conductance increase was maintained throughout the period of carbachol presence, giving a well-defined steady-state value (Ziskind and Werman, 1975a).

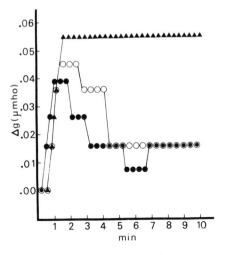

FIG. 3. Elimination of cholinergic desensitization by removal of sodium and calcium ions in molluscan H neuron. The response to 8×10^{-5} M carbachol is illustrated. When all external Na^+ and Ca^{2+} ions were replaced by Mg^{2+} ions (*triangles*), no desensitization was seen. After washing for 15 min in carbachol-free solution, the same concentration was applied in a solution in which only the external Ca^{2+} ions were replaced by Mg^{2+} ions (*open circles*) and desensitization was present. Finally, the response to 8×10^{-5} M carbachol in physiological solution (*filled circles*) was examined. (From Ziskind and Werman, 1975a).

Thus, through the elimination of desensitization, we now have the means of determining the cooperativity number of this ACh-receptor interaction and the various kinetic and thermodynamic properties. In Fig. 4 we see that the log-log slope measured from the peak responses of the ACh response in an H cell in the presence of desensitization was 1.75 whereas, after elimination of desensitization in the same cell, it increased to 2.88. It can be seen that the effects of desensitization, although present even at the lowest concentrations used in this experiment, increased with increasing carbachol concentration. In a series of seven cells, the mean slope of the log-log plots after elimination of desensitization was 2.91 ($\pm$ 0.18 SD). These observations indicate that at least three molecules of carbachol must interact with each receptor unit in order to activate it (Ziskind and Werman, 1975b).

In an attempt to quantify the phenomenon of desensitization, Katz and Thesleff (1957) studied the interaction of a prolonged pulse of ACh, iontophoresed onto the frog NMJ, with short test pulses of ACh delivered through

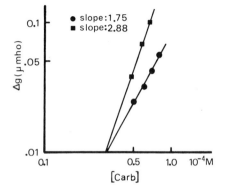

FIG. 4. Log-log plot of conductance as a function of carbachol concentration in the same molluscan H cell. When all external Na^+ and Ca^{2+} ions were replaced by Mg^{2+} ions (*squares*), a regression slope of 2.88 was obtained. In physiological solution, the slope (when the peak conductance change was measured) was only 1.75. (From Ziskind and Werman, 1975b.)

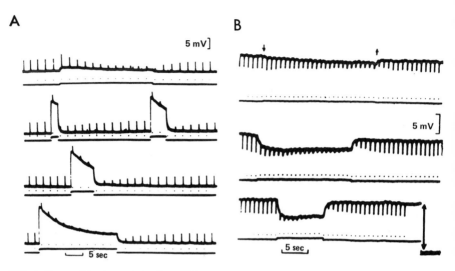

FIG. 5. Desensitization of the frog NMJ by substained iontophoretic application of ACh. The prolonged currents are seen as step function changes in the lower traces and brief test pulses of ACh from a second, nearby pipette are marked as dots. The responses are seen on upper traces. **A:** In normal Ringers. Different durations and strengths of conditioning application are illustrated. Note that recovery of test pulse response is not accompanied by a change in membrane potential (see Fig. 2). **B:** As in **A** but muscle in isotonic potassium sulfate and the fiber was made about 15 mV inside position by outward current applied intracellularly. The sign of response is now inverted. The conditioning pulse exhibits little evidence of desensitization but the test pulses are diminished by both a reduction in driving force and progressive desensitization. At the end of the lower record, the intracellular recording electrode was withdrawn (*arrow*). (From Katz and Thesleff, 1957, as modified by Grundfest, 1959.)

a second microelectrode (Fig. 5A). Assuming that the desensitization takes place at the receptor (Fig. 2), they discuss two simple models for receptor inactivation, a serial model:

$$A + R \underset{}{\rightleftharpoons} AR \underset{k_2}{\overset{k_1}{\rightleftharpoons}} AR' \tag{8}$$

and a parallel model:

$$A + R \overset{a}{\underset{k_2}{\overset{}{\rightleftharpoons}}} \begin{matrix} AR \\ \\ AR' \end{matrix} \tag{9}$$

where A is transmitter concentration, R, the number of free receptors, AR, active receptors, AR', desensitized receptors; a is an affinity constant and k_1 and k_2 forward and backward rate constants for desensitization, respectively. They claim that desensitization is a simple exponential process and its rate constant is given by the relationship

$$1/\tau = k_2 + (k_1 aA)/(1 + aA) \tag{10}$$

in the case of the series model, and by

$$1/\tau = k_2 + k_1 A/(1 + aA) \tag{11}$$

in the case of the parallel model. Examination of Eqs. (10) and (11) shows that in both cases, recovery from desensitization ($A = 0$) should always be slower than its development ($A > 0$). When examining the behavior of weak conditioning pulses in experiments like those shown in Fig. 5A (upper trace), they found that the development of desensitization was no faster than or even slower than recovery from desensitization. They therefore rejected both models.

We have shown (Armon et al., *unpublished results*) that formulas (10) and (11) are not in general correct. I will outline the results of dealing with a single model, the serial-parallel model which includes as special cases Eqs. (8) and (9) of Katz and Thesleff (1957). The model also includes the measurement of the cooperativity number of the reaction and is given by the relationships:

$$
nA + R \underset{k_2}{\overset{k_1}{\rightleftharpoons}} A_n R
$$
$$
{\scriptstyle k_6}\big\Vert{\scriptstyle k_5} \qquad {\scriptstyle k_3}\big/\big/{\scriptstyle k_4}
$$
$$
A_n R' \tag{12}
$$

It can be seen that if $n = 1$, the serial model of Eq. (8) is obtained when k_5 and k_6 are both zero and the parallel model of Eq. (9) is given when k_3 and k_4 are both zero. The equations describing this system are:

$$
\begin{cases}
dR/dt = -A^n R(k_1 + k_6) + k_2 A_n R + k_5 A_n R' \\
dA_n R/dt = k_1 A^n R - (k_2 + k_3) A_n R + k_4 A_n R' \\
R + A_n R + A_n R' = R_T
\end{cases} \tag{13}
$$

where R_T is the total receptor population. The steady-state solution of this series of equations is given by:

$$
\begin{cases}
(R/R_T)_{ss} = c/[c + (a + b)A^n] \\
(A_n R/R_T)_{ss} = aA^n/[c + (a + b)A^n] \\
(A_n R'/R_T)_{ss} = bA^n/[c + (a + b)A^n]
\end{cases} \tag{14}
$$

where

$$
\begin{cases}
a = k_1 k_4 + k_6 k_4 + k_1 k_5 \\
b = k_2 k_6 + k_3 k_6 + k_1 k_3 \\
c = k_2 k_5 + k_3 k_5 + k_2 k_4
\end{cases} \tag{15}
$$

The maximum response, as A is increased, will be given by $Ka/(a + b)$ where $K = g_a R_T$, the conductance increase produced by activation of all receptors, and $A_{0.5} = \left(\dfrac{c}{a + b}\right)^{1/n}$. Since

$$\frac{\Delta g_{ss}}{\Delta g_{max}} = \frac{K(AnR/R_T)_{ss}}{Ka/(a+b)} = \frac{A^n}{A^n + c/(a+b)} \tag{16}$$

it can be seen that the log-log representation of $\Delta g(=KA_nR)$ against concentration will approach n with lowering concentrations and that the Hill plot will also give n as a slope.

It can also be shown that if desensitization were to result from receptor polymerization, i.e.,

$$A_nR + mA \rightleftharpoons A_{(n+m)}R' \tag{17}$$

the log-log plot would still give n (Armon et al., *unpublished*). In addition, it can be shown that the time solution of development of conductance change is given by:

$$A_nR/R_T = \beta_1 e^{\lambda_1 t} + \beta_2 e^{\lambda_2 t} + (A_nR/R_T)_{ss} \tag{18}$$

and that desensitization is described by the relationship,

$$A_nR'/R_T = \gamma_1 e^{\lambda_1 t} + \gamma_2 e^{\lambda_2 t} + (A_nR'/R_T)_{ss} \tag{19}$$

where λ_1 and λ_2 are negative and β_1, β_2, γ_1, and γ_2 are all functions of concentration and various k's. Neither λ_1 nor λ_2 become zero nor are they equal at more than two concentrations when the assumptions necessary to give the serial or parallel reactions are invoked. Nor, in general, do either γ_1 or γ_2 become zero.[1] Thus, we find no justification for rejecting either the serial or parallel models.

In Fig. 6A, a calculated solution of the kinetic equations for the development of a conductance change with step-function concentrations is given, when the cooperativity number is taken as three. With the reaction constants chosen, in the presence of low transmitter agonist concentrations, there appears to be no desensitization, but the latter becomes apparent with increasing agonist concentrations. Thus, it is possible that if only a given range of concentrations is examined, one may not see desensitization that is actually present. In fact, we can find specific examples where, in the presence of desensitization, all concentrations will give monotonically increasing changes in conductance with time (Fig. 6B). An example of this

---

[1] Actually another set of solutions is also possible with a single time constant (Armon et al., *unpublished results*), but this solution has an oscillatory form:

$$AR/R_T = e^{-\gamma t}\left[\left(\left(\frac{AR}{R_T}\right)_0 - \left(\frac{AR}{R_T}\right)_{ss}\right)\cos(\delta t) - \theta_1 \sin(\delta t)\right] + \left(\frac{AR}{R_T}\right)_{ss} \tag{20}$$

and

$$AR'/R_T \equiv e^{-\gamma t}\left[\left(\left(\frac{AR'}{R_T}\right)_0 - \left(\frac{AR'}{R_T}\right)_{ss}\right)\cos(\delta t) - \theta_2 \sin(\delta t)\right] + \left(\frac{AR'}{R_T}\right)_{ss} \tag{21}$$

It is not likely that this is the exponential solution which Katz and Thesleff (1957) had in mind.

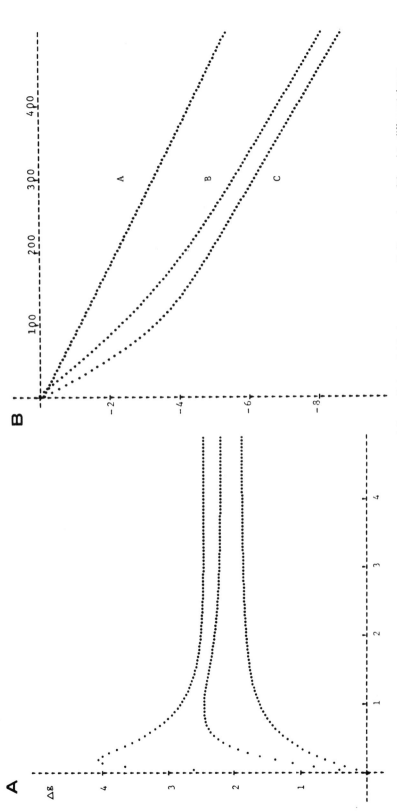

FIG. 6. Calculated conductance responses of receptors from the serial-parallel model (using a cooperativity number of three) to different doses of transmitter. **A:** Abscissa is time in units of 10 sec and ordinate units are 0.1 $R_T g_a$ (mho). Reaction constants chosen were: $k_1 = k_6 = 1 \times 10^{11}$ sec^{-1} M^{-3}; $k_2 = k_3 = 0.1$ sec^{-1}; $k_4 = 0.05$ sec^{-1}; $k_5 = 0$. The concentrations are in ascending order: 0.75, 1.00, and 2.00×10^{-4} M. **B:** Kinetics of a reaction of the parallel formulation which shows only monotonic conductance increases with time. In $(1 - g/g')$ is plotted against time; the units are 0.1 and seconds, respectively. The constants chosen were: $k_1 = 1.15 \times 10^9$ sec^{-1} M^{-3}; $k_2 = 6.68 \times 10^{-3}$ sec^{-1}; $k_3 = k_4 = 0$; $k_5 = 1.3 \times 10^{-2}$ sec^{-1}; $k_6 = 1.5 \times 10^8$ sec^{-1} M^{-3}. The concentrations were: $A = 1.5 \times 10^{-4}$ M; $B = 2.5 \times 10^{-4}$ M; $C = 3 \times 10^{-4}$ M (see Table 4).

TABLE 4. *Simulated monotonic responses in parallel reaction (see Fig. 6B). Time constants of fast and slow components of the conductance response*

A $(M \times 10^4)$	g'/g_{max}	a'_0	τ_a (sec)	b'_0	τ_b (sec)
1.5	0.66	0.20	(71.1)	0.80	100.0
2.5	0.78	0.87	35.7	0.13	83.3
3.0	0.88	0.91	23.5	0.09	82.4

is found in the parallel model [Eq. (9)], where, if $k_2 < k_5$, we can demonstrate that the response is always monotonic (Armon et al., *unpublished*). The presence of a monotonically increasing response cannot, therefore, be considered sufficient evidence of the absence of desensitization. An examination of Fig. 5B (from Katz and Thesleff, 1957) shows that when frog muscle is immersed in isotonic potassium sulfate, conditioning pulses of ACh show little evidence of desensitization. On the other hand, the test pulses show evidence of great desensitization. Without the test pulse, one would be little inclined to postulate the presence of desensitization.[2]

The results obtained from locust muscle GABA receptors (Fig. 1C; Table 2) now gain a new significance. The two time constant kinetic is predicted by our formulation. The lack of sensitivity to concentration of the time constants would appear, at first glance, however, to negate application of the kinetic formation. It turns out that appropriate choice of kinetic constants can lead to a relative insensitivity of the time constants to concentration. Thus, in Fig. 6B we see that, without excessive effort, one can choose parameters that roughly mimic the results of Brookes et al. (1973). Analysis of the data in Fig. 6B by the methods of Brookes et al. (1973) provides the data of Table 4. The slow component is seen to be relatively insensitive to concentration changes and the fast component (whose contribution is not seen at the lowest concentration) shows progressive development with higher concentration. These results suggest that occult desensitization could possibly explain the two time constant system described by Brookes et al. (1973).

CONCLUSIONS

The problem of receptor desensitization is important for anyone who studies the fine structure of transmitter-receptor interactions. It is not clear

---

[2] It is of interest that the treatment here, replacement of external Na^+ ions (by K^+ ions), is similar to that used in the molluscan cholinergic receptor to eliminate desensitization (Fig. 3). Replacement of Na^+ ions by K^+ ions has not been tried in that preparation yet; comparison is therefore limited. Our treatment demonstrates, however, that the measurement of cooperativity from steady-state values is not invalidated even in the presence of occult desensitization.

that the phenomenon plays any significant physiological role and the possible roles assigned to it appear, on analysis, to be doubtful. Despite the absence of a clear function for desensitization, the phenomenon must be understood in order to gain deeper insight into the workings of the chemoreceptor – and more specifically, the synaptic receptor.

A parsimonious quantitative formulation of the desensitization problem is provided by the serial-parallel model and the results of analysis of this model appear compatible with all existing data (Armon et al., *unpublished*). Several unexpected corollaries of the model are of great interest. Thus, the model predicts a two time constant kinetic in general. In addition, monotonically increasing responses with time for all transmitter concentrations are not incompatible with desensitization. Thus, we no longer possess an unequivocal electrophysiological criterion for the absence of desensitization.

It is of interest that manipulation of the ionic environment can greatly reduce and perhaps even eliminate desensitization (Ziskind and Werman, 1975*a*). It is reassuring that validity of the model guarantees the determination of the cooperativity of the reaction from measurements made at steady state even in the presence of desensitization. Thus, even if occult desensitization were present in several cases where the cooperativity has been determined from steady-state measurements – locust GABA receptors (Brookes and Werman, 1973); molluscan H cells (Ziskind and Werman, 1975*b*) and GABA and glycine receptors in the Mauthner cell of fish (Werman and Mazliah, 1974) – the conclusions do not appear to be invalidated.

If it appears that this presentation has raised problems rather than offered solutions, perhaps this, too, is the result of a Grundfestian training. It was Harry who said, "My own . . . impulsion . . . toward biology . . . was not philosophical; my drive was essentially to find out what was on the other side of the mountain" (Grundfest, 1954). I feel that I have described another mountain or at least a ground swell, and it may offer a challenge to those who, like Harry and myself, are curious about the other side.

ACKNOWLEDGMENTS

I thank my colleagues, M. Spira, E. Armon, L. Ziskind, and R. S. Manalis, for permission to use unpublished materials.

REFERENCES

Altimarino, M., Coates, C. W., Grundfest, H., and Nachmansohn, D. (1953): Mechanisms of bioelectric activity in electric tissue. I. The response to indirect and direct stimulation of electroplaques of *Electrophorus electricus. J. Gen. Physiol.,* 37:91–110.

Brookes, N., Blank, M., and Werman, R. (1973): The kinetics of the conductance increase produced by γ-aminobutyric acid at the membrane of locust muscle fibers. *Mol. Pharmacol.,* 9:580–589.

Brookes, N., and Werman, R. (1973): The cooperativity of γ-aminobutyric acid action on the membrane of locust muscle fibers. *Mol. Pharmacol.*, 9:571–579.

Clark, A. J. (1937): General Pharmacology. In: *Handbuch der Experimentallen Pharmakologie*, edited by A. Haffter and H. Heubner. Vol. 4. Springer, Berlin.

Epstein, R., and Grundfest, H. (1970): Desensitization of gamma aminobutyric acid (GABA) receptors in muscle fibers of the crab *Cancer borealis*. *J. Gen. Physiol.*, 56:33–45.

Grundfest, H. (1954): Appendix – Autobiographical sketches of participants. In: *Nerve Impulse – Transactions of the Fourth Conference*, edited by D. Nachmansohn, pp. 223–224. Josiah Macy, Jr. Foundation, New York.

Grundfest, H. (1957a): General problems of drug actions on bioelectric phenomena. *Ann. NY Acad. Sci.*, 66:537–591.

Grundfest, H. (1957b): The mechanisms of discharge of the electric organs in relation to general and comparative electrophysiology. *Progr. Biophys.*, 7:1–85.

Grundfest, H. (1959): Synaptic and ephaptic transmission. In: *Handbook of Physiology-Neurophysiology*, edited by J. Field. Vol. I, Chap. 5, pp. 147–197. American Physiological Society, Washington.

Grundfest, H. (1961): General physiology and pharmacology of junctional transmission. In: *Biophysics of Physiological and Pharmacological Actions*, edited by A. M. Shanes, pp. 329–389. American Association for the Advancement of Science, Washington.

Grundfest, H. (1964a): Effects of drugs on the central nervous system. *Ann. Rev. Pharmacol.*, 4:341–364.

Grundfest, H. (1964b): Chemical determinants of behavior: The chemical mediators. In: *Unfinished Tasks in the Behavioral Sciences*, edited by A. Abrams, H. H. Garner, and J. E. P. Toman, pp. 67–110. Williams and Wilkins, Baltimore.

Grundfest, H. (1969): Synaptic and ephaptic transmission. In: *The Structure and Function of Nervous Tissue*, edited by G. H. Bourne, Vol. II, chap. 8, pp. 463–491. Academic Press, New York.

Hille, B. (1970): Ionic channels in nerve membranes. *Progr. Biophys. Mol. Biol.*, 21:1–32.

Katz, B., and Miledi, R. (1971): Further observations on acetylcholine noise. *Nature*, 232:124–126.

Katz, B., and Thesleff, S. (1957): A study of the desensitization produced by acetylcholine at the motor end-plate. *J. Physiol.*, 138:63–80.

Magleby, K. L., and Stevens, C. F. (1972): The effect of voltage on the time course of end-plate currents. *J. Physiol.*, 223:151–171.

Manalis, R. S. (1969): Reversal potential measurements for potentials produced by a group of cholinergic compounds iontophoretically applied to the frog endplate. Doctoral thesis, Indiana University, Bloomington, 142 pp. 1969.

Manalis, R. S., and Werman, R. (1971): Relationship between endplate membrane potential and iontophoretic potentials produced by different doses of acetylcholine. *Fed. Proc.*, 30:617.

Werman, R. (1965): The specificity of molecular processes involved in neural transmission. *J. Theoret. Biol.*, 9:471–477.

Werman, R. (1966): Criteria for identification of a central nervous system transmitter. *Comp. Biochem. Physiol.*, 18:745–766.

Werman, R. (1969): An electrophysiological approach to drug-receptor mechanisms. *Comp. Biochem. Physiol.*, 30:997–1017.

Werman, R. (1975): The transduction of chemical signals into electrical information at synapses. In: *Stability and Origin of Biological Information*, edited by I. R. Miller, pp. 226–244. Wiley, New York.

Werman, R., and Manalis, R. S. (1970): Reversal potential measurements for strong and weak agonists of acetylcholine at the frog neuromuscular junction. *Israel J. Med. Sci.*, 6:320–321.

Werman, R., and Mazliah, J. (1974): The actions of glycine and GABA compared on the Mauthner cell. *Proc. I.U.P.S.* 11:149.

Ziskind, L., and Werman, R. (1975a): Sodium ions are necessary for cholinergic desensitization in molluscan neurons. *Brain Res.*, 88:171–176.

Ziskind, L., and Werman, R. (1975b): At least three molecules of carbamylcholine are needed to activate a cholinergic receptor. *Brain Res.*, 88:177–180.

Electrobiology of Nerve, Synapse, and Muscle,
edited by J. P. Reuben, D. P. Purpura, M. V. L. Bennett,
and E. R. Kandel. Raven Press, New York © 1976

Studies of an Excitatory Neurotransmitter: Synaptic and Nonsynaptic Interactions of L-Glutamic Acid*

Alan R. Freeman

*Department of Physiology, Temple University School of Medicine,
Philadelphia, Pennsylvania 19140*

It is widely recognized that the amino acid L-glutamate manifests in many regions of the vertebrate (central nervous system) CNS, activity which is consistent with a role as an excitatory neurotransmitter. Since this compound is also the major candidate for the excitatory transmitter in arthropods (Gerschenfeld, 1973), the latter preparations serve as a useful model in the study of vertebrate excitatory transmission.

The invertebrate neuromuscular synapse permits the execution of investigative procedures that are difficult to carry out in vertebrates. The application of the voltage-clamp procedure to neuromuscular functions has yielded important information demonstrating the electrophysiological similarity between iontophoretically applied glutamate and the naturally occurring excitatory transmitter in both the crayfish (Takeuchi and Onodera, 1973) and the locust (Anwyl and Usherwood, 1974).

Some controversy has existed concerning the mechanism of action of the glutamate induced depolarization observed in a wide variety of cells in the vertebrate CNS. It seems reasonable to accept the notion that a specific transmitter action takes place at numerous synaptic sites (Krnjević, 1970) in which case considerable understanding regarding the physiological mechanism is gained through comparison with the above-mentioned arthropod investigations. On the other hand, when one considers the enormous complexity of the central nervous system, it appears inappropriate to reject entirely the possibility that excitatory amino acids may also exert an influence by effects manifested on nonsynaptic zones of neuronal plasma membranes (Curtis and Watkins, 1963). Indeed, it is our view that L-glutamic acid may exhibit, under certain conditions, activity at some synaptic sites which is identical to that of the endogenous neurotransmitter. In addition we feel this compound may, in some instances, cause cellular depolarization by an action on nonsynaptic loci of a variety of CNS cell types. This notion has a basis of considerable support (Grundfest, 1966, 1972). In other words, when applied by external perfusion methods, both actions take place to a greater or lesser extent dependent upon the specific cellular sensitivity and geometric factors of a given region of the CNS. With this viewpoint in mind, we have chosen the excitatory neuromuscular synapse of the lobster as the test object. Evidence exists in this preparation that L-glutamic acid has powerful and distinctly different activity on both synaptic and nonsynaptic membranes; both of which may interact to alter the system function in the normal physiological state (Colton and Freeman, 1972, 1973a,b,c, 1975a,b). Furthermore, the electrophysiological interaction of electrically and chemically excitable membranes has been established convincingly in this preparation (Ozeki et al., 1966a,b).

This chapter brings together studies, using the lobster neuromuscular synapse, directed both toward exploring the identity and character of L-glutamate as a neurotransmitter and also toward further investigating the nature of its action on nonsynaptic membranes.

METHODS

Tissue Preparation

Walking limbs of 1-kg lobsters were severed and the stretcher muscle in the carpopodite was partially exposed. In some instances, the excitor axon innervating the muscle was exposed by dissection of the meropodite segment. Detailed procedures for this preparation can be found elsewhere (Grundfest et al., 1959).

In some experiments, contraction of the muscle was reduced by increasing osmotic pressure with sucrose. In those instances, specific controls were carried out to account for possible complication of the findings (Colton and Freeman, 1975a,b).

Application of Amino Acids to the Tissue

Artificial sea water at pH 7.4 was superfused over the muscle fibers at a temperature of 8° to 10°C and the amino acids to be tested were included in the medium at specified concentrations.

For dose-response studies, glutamate or aspartate or combinations of the two, were administered usually for 2 to 4 min, then washed out for a similar time period. The amino acids were applied beginning with the lowest concentrations, then sequentially advancing to the highest concentrations (Shank and Freeman, 1975a,b; Shank et al., 1975c).

Electrophysiological Measurements

Superficial muscle fibers were impaled with two standard KCl-filled glass microelectrodes positioned approximately 100 μm apart. The membrane potential was measured with one electrode and constant currents were passed through the other for the purpose of determining the input resistance of the muscle fibers (Freeman and Fingerman, 1970). When required, precise, potentiometric measurements of absolute resting potentials were carried out with appropriate corrections for liquid junction potentials encountered during ion substitution experiments (Freeman, 1971, 1973). Specific resistance was not calculated due to the fact that this computation requires, for a distributed system, a thorough knowledge of the muscle fiber geometry and the nature of the spatial decay of current from the origin (Bennett et al., 1966). Such information for each cell cannot be obtained readily. Thus, "effective" or "input" resistance is employed here.

When excitatory postsynaptic potentials (EPSPs) were to be studied, the excitor axon innervating the muscle fibers was stimulated with a bipolar pair of surface electrodes. Membrane potentials and current amplitudes were monitored on a dual channel oscilloscope and, in some instances a Gould 220 brush pen recorder (Shank and Freeman, 1975a). In some cases reversal potentials were determined (Colton and Freeman, 1975a).

Chemical Methods

Chemical analyses of single, isolated, excitatory, and inhibitory nerve fibers were carried out using the formerly described dissection procedures. Gas chromatographic analyses were performed according to the method of McBride et al. (1974).

RESULTS

Temperature Dependency of Applied Glutamate Effect

Figure 1 portrays simultaneously the action of bath applied L-glutamic acid on both membrane potential and relative effective resistance. At a temperature of 17°C, a depolarization is observed with a minimal response at about 5×10^{-5} M. The limit of the depolarization is about 20 mV at approximately 5×10^{-4} M with a half-maximum for the effect of 1.5×10^{-4} M. Significant here is the fact that the glutamate response is accompanied by an increase in input resistance which is proportional to the magnitude of the membrane potential change. Thus, the maximum depolarization is associated with nearly a 1.5-fold increase in resistance. This observation would appear inconsistent with the expected result for a putative excitatory neurotransmitter; that of a depolarization and a conductance increase. A possible explanation for these findings might be to suggest that glutamate causes potassium inactivation of the nonsynaptic membrane; an effect separate and distinct from its action at the synapse. This argument implies that the rise in resistance manifest as a result of K-channel inactivation, is of a greater

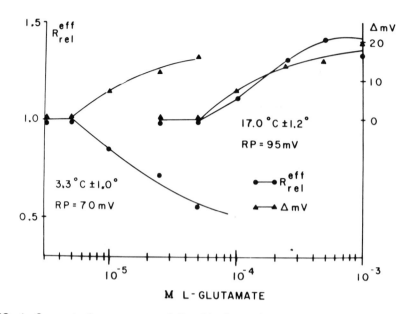

FIG. 1. Concentration-response relationship for L-glutamate applied to the bathing medium perfusing the stretcher muscle. *Abscissa,* concentration of L-glutamate in moles per liter; *ordinates,* relative effective resistance (R_{eff} induced/R_{eff} control) — *closed circles;* and voltage (change in potential from control) — *closed triangles.* Data points represent average values of at least six experiments.

magnitude than the presumed decrease arising at the synaptic loci; the overall effect being an increase in input resistance.

In separate studies, Colton and Freeman (1972, 1973*a,b,c,* 1975*a*), demonstrated that the potassium conductance of the lobster muscle membrane is highly temperature sensitive, showing a dramatic decrease at low temperatures. They further showed that low temperature did not alter the ionic selectivity of the synaptic membrane. This finding is consistent with that already reported for a crustacean muscle membrane (Fischbarg, 1972).

If the above argument holds, it should be possible to reveal the synaptic response of glutamate by removing the complication of its action on parallel K channels of the electrically excitable membrane. (The use of the terms electrical and chemical excitability are as outlined by Grundfest (1961), pertaining to nonsynaptic and synaptic membranes, respectively.)

The left-hand portion of Fig. 1 demonstrates this point. At 3.3°C, where K channels are thermally inactivated, glutamate causes a depolarization, now accompanied by a fall in input resistance. Exposure of relatively pure synaptic activity also allows for a marked increase in sensitivity. In this respect, the limits of the recorded depolarization are about the same as 17°C but the half-maximum point is seen to shift to about 1.5×10^{-5}; an order of magnitude more sensitive. Under these conditions, minimum responses appear at glutamate concentrations lower than 3×10^{-6} M.

Ionic Basis of the Dual Glutamate Response

Exploration of the mechanism of the proposed nonsynaptic effect is outlined in Figs. 2 and 3. In these studies, membrane selectivity is investigated by classical methods of ionic alteration in the bathing medium. Figure 2 shows that the resting, control membrane is predominantly K selective (60 mV slope), whereas the low slope of 5 for the control response of Fig. 3 demonstrates a low Na selectivity. These results are those familiar to the resting condition of many cell membranes and are consistent with established figures for lobster muscle fibers (Grundfest, 1966).

In the presence of glutamate, K selectivity falls, as evidenced by the 40 mV slope in Fig. 2, and shifts toward sodium as seen by the increase in slope for this ion in Fig. 3. These findings are compatible with the notion that L-glutamate causes potassium inactivation and thereby shifts the membrane selectivity towards sodium. This would account for both the observed resistance rise and also the depolarization recorded at 17°C.

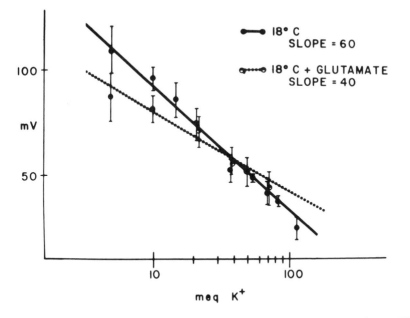

FIG. 2. Relationship between membrane potential and external K^+ concentration at 18°C with and without 5×10^{-4} M glutamate added to each K^+ concentration. *Abscissa*, external concentration of K^+; *ordinate*, membrane potential. Data points represent average potentials ± SD of the observation.

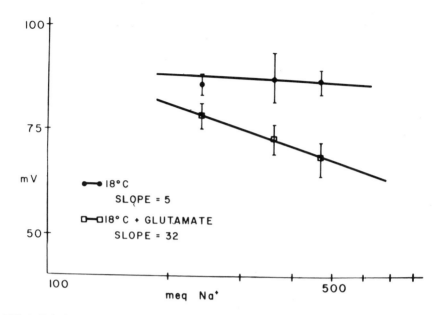

FIG. 3. Relationship between membrane potential and external Na^+ concentration at 18°C with and without 5×10^{-4} M glutamate added to each Na^+ concentration used. *Abscissa,* concentration of Na^+; *ordinate,* membrane potential. Data points represent average potentials $\pm$ SD of the observation.

Additional confirmation for this idea is obtained from experiments carried out in a medium in which all the sodium is replaced by an impermeant species such as Tris. Separate experiments indicated that the glutamate induced depolarization was abolished in Tris as would be predicted if the original glutamate induced depolarization was based on the shift in membrane selectivity discussed above.

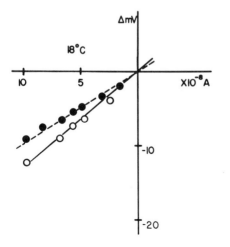

FIG. 4. Current-voltage relationships from a single fiber equilibrated in a Na^+-substituted medium (Tris$^+$, 465 mM, ASW) with (*open circles*) and without (*filled circles*) 2×10^{-4} M glutamate added to the bath. *Abscissa,* current; *ordinate,* voltage (change in potential from control). Temperature = 18°C. Resistance values are: control Tris$^+$ ASW, $R_{eff} \times 1.4 \times 10^5$ Ω; Tris$^+$ ASW + glutamate, $R_{eff} = 1.6 \times 10^{-5}$ Ω.

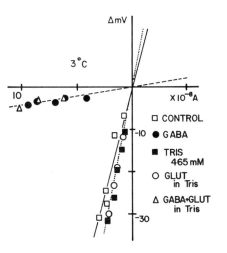

FIG. 5. Current-voltage relationships of the lobster muscle membrane at 3°C in control medium and in a Na$^+$-substituted (Tris$^+$ ASW) medium. *Abscissa*, current; *ordinate*, voltage (change in potential from control). Concentration of GABA used in both the normal medium and with glutamate in the Tris$^+$-substituted medium was 5×10^{-5} M. Values of resistance are: control, $R_{eff} = 20 \times 10^5$ Ω; GABA, $R_{eff} = 0.66 \times 10^5$ Ω; Tris$^+$-substituted medium, $R_{eff} = 25 \times 10^5$ Ω; glutamate in Tris$^+$, $R_{eff} = 25 \times 10^5$ Ω; glutamate plus GABA in Tris$^+$, $R_{eff} = 0.77 \times 10^5$ Ω.

In principle this ion substitution should not alter the ability of glutamate to inactivate K channels even though the potential change is removed. Figure 4 demonstrates that this amino acid still causes a resistance increase in a Tris-substituted bathing medium, tending to support the notion developed here that the basis for the effect is inactivation of potassium channels in the nonsynaptic, electrically excitable membrane.

This line of reasoning may be extended a step further to test the nature of the synaptic action revealed at low temperature.

Figure 5 shows data from experiments carried out at 3°C in a Tris-substituted bathing medium.

Similar to the findings at 18°C, separate studies revealed that the glutamate-induced depolarization is abolished as would be the case if synaptic activation were to involve, as in other arthropods, a substantial permeability increase towards sodium (Ozeki and Grundfest, 1967; Takeuchi and Onodera, 1973; Anwyl and Usherwood, 1974; Gerschenfeld, 1973).

Separate studies (Colton and Freeman, 1972, 1973a,b,c, 1975a,b) revealed that the neurally evoked EPSP behaves similarly to applied glutamate with respect to potential and resistance changes when sodium is replaced in the medium. This leads to the suggestion as in the case for crayfish (Takeuchi and Takeuchi, 1964) that applied glutamate interacts with the endogenous neuroreceptors at synaptic sites.

Linearization of the Voltage-Current Relationship

One of the problems encountered in studying "open-circuited" phenomena in muscle tissue is the nonlinearity of the voltage-current relationship. Observed in the lobster preparation (Ozeki et al., 1966a,b) this property is troublesome in interpreting findings whose voltage excursions extend

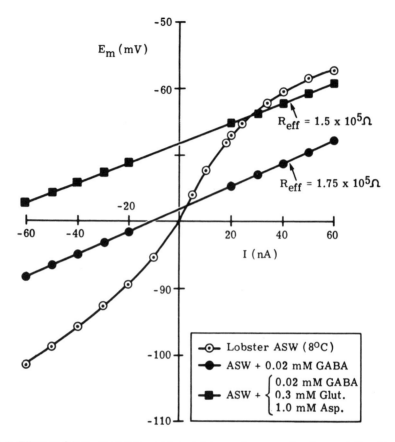

FIG. 6. Effect of GABA, glutamate, and aspartate on the current-voltage relationship of a lobster muscle fiber. The resting membrane potential was −80 mV; GABA (0.02 mM) depolarized the cell 2 mV and glutamate (0.3 mM) + aspartate (1.0 mM) depolarized the cell 10 mV further. The effective resistance (R_{eff}) of the cell in the presence of GABA was 1.75×10^5 Ω and was reduced to 1.5×10^5 Ω by the excitatory amino acids.

beyond the nearly linear zone of the curve. Figure 6 demonstrates this point. The control display recorded in normal saline is roughly linear to about 15 mV depolarizing from the origin. It should be mentioned here that the studies presented to this point were carried out, for the most part, within this limit.

Since it is desired to investigate the interaction of applied amino acids with receptors occupied by endogenous transmitter, neuronally evoked EPSPs must be studied and thus, some method must be employed to ensure that the findings are not occluded by high-amplitude excursions to regions of non-linearity. An attempt at point voltage clamping proved unfeasible and was attributable to the long fiber space constant. Therefore an alternative method was chosen, that of linearizing the basic curve.

The premise for this approach was based on adding to the system a parallel conductance large enough to shunt the high-resistance zone of the curve. It was additionally required that the parallel conductance should not be associated with an internal EMF which could result in a depolarization of the membrane. Addition of GABA, the inhibitory transmitter, accomplished this end. Including 0.02 mM of this compound in the medium completely linearized the display while holding the resting potential close to the original value. The potential moves closer to E_{Cl} which is slightly depolarizing to the resting potential in ASW containing 5 mM potassium (Grundfest, 1966; Motokizawa et al., 1969). Figure 6 also shows clearly the effect of adding aspartate and glutamate in a 3-to-1 ratio; a depolarization and conductance increase.

It is recognized here that the most desirable criterion to be employed as an index of receptor occupancy is the postsynaptic conductance change (Werman, 1969). However, the glutamate-induced depolarization, recorded under conditions of a linearized voltage-current relationship is directly proportional to the conductance change and thus may be taken under these circumstances as a reliable and more easily quantitated index of receptor saturation.

Characterization of the Glutamate Receptor

The following data are representative of in-depth studies undertaken to explore the nature of the interaction of L-glutamic acid and its synaptic receptor site (Shank et al., 1973; Shank and Freeman, 1974a,b,c; 1975a,b; Shank et al., 1975c).

Figure 7 depicts a family of concentration-response curves. The curve to the far right (open circles) represents the action of glutamate alone, and demonstrates the familiar sigmoid relationship typical of drug receptor interaction as displayed in response versus log concentration format (Colquhoun, 1973). Under the conditions reported here, the amino-acid L-aspartate exhibits virtually no activity of its own, i.e., no depolarization or resistance change. However, the presence in the bathing medium of this compound dramatically alters the effect of L-glutamate. This point is evidenced by the shift to the left of the glutamate response with increasing levels of aspartate. It should be pointed out that aspartate causes this shift without appreciably altering the contour or maximum of the glutamate curve. Thus, aspartic acid potentiates the effect of glutamate while showing no agonistic activity itself. The potentiative action of aspartate has been noted qualitatively by Kravitz and co-workers (Kravitz et al., 1970).

In an effort to ascertain the number of subunits partaking in the glutamate-receptor interaction, the data of Fig. 7 are plotted in log-log coordinates as presented in Fig. 8. The limiting slope of such a display may be equated to the number of involved receptor subunits or, in more general terms, the

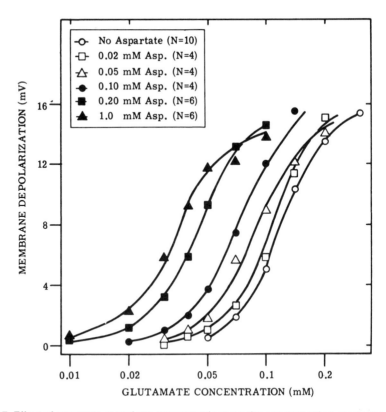

FIG. 7. Effect of aspartate at various concentrations on the concentration-response curve for glutamate. At concentrations of 0.2 mM and less, aspartate has no excitatory action by itself. At 1.0 mM aspartate by itself depolarizes the fibers an average of approximately 0.5 mV. Each point is the average of the number given in the parentheses. GABA was included in the bathing medium at a concentration of 0.02 mM.

molecularity of the reaction (Werman, 1969). As shown, the slope for glutamate alone is about 3 and is approximately the same in the presence of low levels of aspartate. This slope is seen to fall somewhat in concentrations of 0.2 and 1.0 mM aspartate. The basic slope of 3 necessitates that the reaction of glutamate with receptor is cooperative in nature (Werman, 1969; Colquhoun, 1973) in which the occupancy by three molecules of the agonist is necessary for the receptor to be in the activated or conductive state. Thus the receptor may be considered to be composed of three subunits.

This point is emphasized in the display shown in Fig. 9. Using the idea developed by Werman (1969), three theoretical curves have been calculated. The solid lines represent a classical monomolecular interaction (lowest slope), a trimolecular interaction showing independent subunit cooperativity (next highest slope), and a trimolecular reaction showing allosteric cooperativity (highest slope). Clearly, the actual data (dotted lines) fit very closely

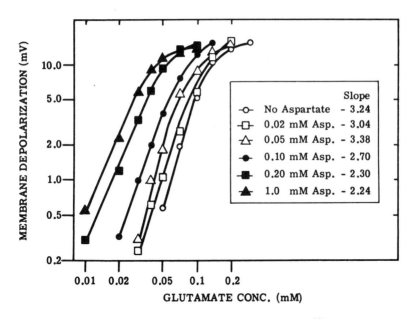

FIG. 8. Log-log plots of dose-response curves for glutamate and glutamate plus aspartate. The data are replotted from that given in Fig. 7. The lines were drawn as estimated by eye.

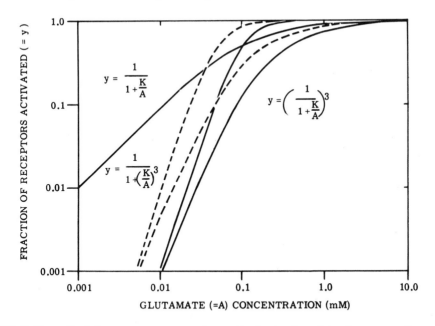

FIG. 9. Theoretical dose-response curves formed by the log-log plots where one or three glutamate molecules activate one receptor. *Solid lines,* calculated theoretically from the equation indicated. *Lowest slope line,* for a unimolecular interaction without cooperativity. *Highest slope line,* for a trimolecular interaction with allosteric cooperativity. *In-between slope,* for a trimolecular interaction with independent subunit cooperativity. *Dashed lines,* actual data curves calculated from Fig. 7. K is the mass action constant taken as 1×10^{-4}. A is the agonist concentration. Notation is that developed in principle by Werman (1969).

the curves showing 3 subunit cooperativity. It is beyond the scope of this investigation to suggest further that the specific nature of this three-molecule complex is of the independent subunit type or of the allosteric variety (Colquhoun, 1973; Karlin, 1967). At this time the simplest interpretation of the potentiation by aspartate is that this substance acts at an independent site to enhance the affinity of glutamate for the receptor ("affinity site") but is not involved directly in the receptor-ionophore coupling mechanism. The drop in slope observed in highest aspartate levels indicates a partial ability to competitively block glutamate sites and does not appear to be important at lower amounts of this compound.

The Potentiative Ability of Aspartate

A simple quantitative index of the ability of aspartate to potentiate glutamate may be calculated from the data presented in Fig. 7. A half-maximum response of 6 mV is chosen and a line drawn across the family of curves. The amount of glutamate necessary to evoke this magnitude is noted on the abscissa for each aspartate concentration. With the glutamate alone effect taken as unity, the ratio of this to each lower effective concentration of glutamate may be taken as an index of potency. The relative potency is displayed in semilog format in Fig. 10. This sigmoid relationship favors the idea that aspartate interacts with a separate receptor site ("affinity site") obeying standard kinetics. It is noteworthy here that the limiting log-log slope calculated from these data is precisely unity. This finding strongly

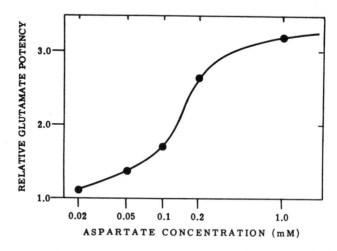

FIG. 10. Concentration-response curve for L-aspartate (lobster muscle fibers). The "relative glutamate potency" for each concentration of aspartate was obtained by dividing (a) the concentration of glutamate in the presence of a given concentration of aspartate which caused a depolarization of 6 mV and (b) the concentration of glutamate which caused a 6 mV depolarization when aspartate was not present. The curve was derived from the data shown in Fig. 7.

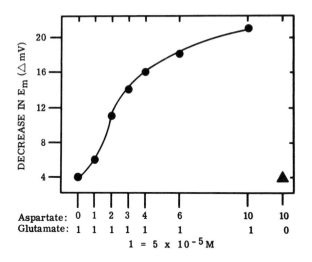

FIG. 11. Glutamate-aspartate responses: Enhancement of aspartate at various concentration ratios. *Abscissa,* glutamate concentration is held constant at 5×10^{-5} M. Aspartate level is increased from zero to 10-fold multiples of the glutamate levels, thus, directly indicating the molar ratio. *Ordinate,* depolarization in millivolts. *Triangle* indicates level of depolarization with 5×10^{-4} M aspartate alone. Curve optimum is taken at the greatest magnitude of y at which d^2y/dx^2 exhibits a maximum. This zone occurs at a molar ratio of about 3 or 4 to 1.

favors the idea that the "affinity site" involves a classic one to one aspartate-receptor complex as opposed to the trimolecular cooperativity demonstrated at the glutamate receptor.

In a separate study directed toward revealing an optimal potentiation ratio, the glutamate concentration of the bathing medium was held constant at 5×10^{-5} M whereas the aspartate level was raised from zero to 10-fold multiples of the glutamate concentration. The results are presented in Fig. 11. The solid triangle to the right indicates that aspartate alone at 5×10^{-4} M shows no significant depolarizing ability. However, its property of potentiating the action of glutamate is dramatically demonstrated by the fact that this amount of aspartate enhances the depolarizing ability of 10×10^{-5} M glutamate, fivefold (from 4 to 20 mV). On inspection of the figure it is evident that the attainment of the maximal effect slope begins at about a 3 or 4 to 1 aspartate to glutamate ratio. This functional transition zone might be construed as a phenomenological optimum (the greatest value of y at which d^2y/dx^2 exhibits a maximum). Accordingly, a molar ratio of 3 aspartate to 1 glutamate is selected for the following studies.

Stereospecificity of Glutamate and Aspartate Sites

The upper trace of Fig. 12 shows the effect of ASP/GLUT (3/1) on three parameters: membrane potential, membrane resistance, and summated

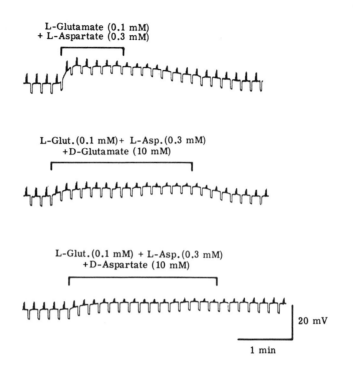

FIG. 12. Comparison of the effects of D-glutamate and D-aspartate on the synergistic action of L-glutamate and L-aspartate together. The amino acids were applied at the specified concentrations for the time periods indicated. The periodic upward deflections represent a train of 4 EPSPs evoked at a frequency of 2/sec, and the downward deflections represent the hyperpolarization response of the muscle fiber to a negative electrical current of 20 nA passed into the cell for 2 sec; these EPSPs and input resistance responses were generated at 10-sec intervals. GABA was included in bathing medium at a concentration of 0.02 mM.

EPSP amplitude. Notable are a simultaneous depolarization, resistance decrease and diminution of EPSP amplitude. These findings are all expected if it is presumed that L-glutamate is acting at receptors identical to those of released excitatory transmitter. It might be mentioned here that nonsynaptic actions of glutamate outlined earlier are shunted by the GABA-induced conductance increase; an additional advantage of this technique. The middle and bottom traces indicate that the D form of glutamate and aspartate tend to block the action of the corresponding L compounds. Specificity for this phenomenon is supported by the data depicted in Fig. 13. The upper trace shows the predicted action of a high level of L-glutamic acid alone (without the potentiative effect of L-aspartate). The middle trace indicates that D-glutamate blocks the L-response whereas the bottom trace shows that D-aspartate has little action. This finding is consistent with the idea that glutamate and aspartate sites are spatially separate and specific for the L form of the amino acid. The observed attenuation of EPSP magnitude in

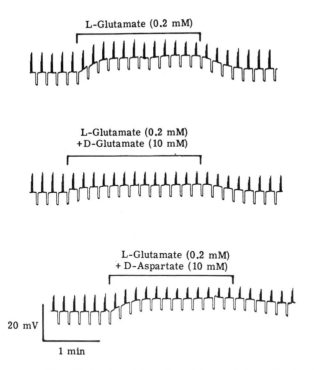

FIG. 13. Comparison of the effects of D-glutamate and D-aspartate on the depolarizing action of L-glutamate alone. Experimental conditions are the same as in Fig. 12.

the middle and lower traces is supportive of the concept that both types of sites are also playing a role in the neurally evoked EPSP. Furthermore, the sites of action of both applied amino acids appear to be the same as those responding during endogenous transmitter release. Additional evidence favoring site specificity is offered by the results shown in Fig. 14. Part A shows that D-glutamate induces a moderate shift to the right of the L-glutamate curve. This finding indicates competitiveness of D-aspartate for the L-glutamate site and is not entirely unexpected since, as discussed for Fig. 7, high levels of L-aspartate also showed competition for the L-glutamate site. Part B shows the anticipated action of D-aspartate on the ASP-GLUT shift. The curve containing D-aspartate shows that the potentiation effect of L-aspartate is entirely blocked, confirming the findings of Figs. 12 and 13 indicating separation and specificity of the aspartate and glutamate sites.

Amino Acid Content of the Excitor Axon

Experiments using gas chromatographic techniques applied to single, isolated excitatory axons yielded data generally consistent with those of Kravitz et al. (1963).

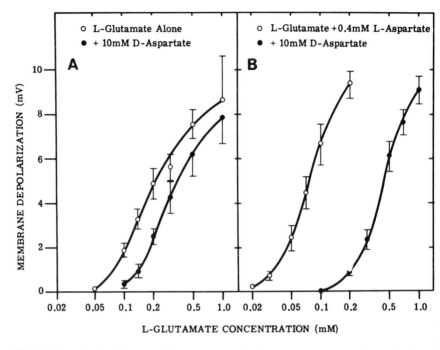

FIG. 14. The effects of D-aspartate on concentration-response curves for L-glutamate alone **(A)** and in combination with L-aspartate **(B)**. The points on each curve represent the mean ± SEM of 4 or 5 experiments. GABA was included in the bathing medium. Under the conditions employed L-aspartate at 0.4 mM does not elicit any membrane depolarization

Data abstracted from McBride et al. (1974) are presented in Table 1

It is interesting to note that the relative content of aspartate to glutamate appears in the same ratio as was found optimal as an enhancement ratio (Fig. 11).

Though this result may be entirely coincidental, one cannot overlook the compelling possibility that a combination of aspartate and glutamate might be released together in the proper ratio, during the process of neurotransmission. This possibility is particularly relevant in light of the foregoing argument favoring the involvement of both aspartate and glutamate sites during transmitter release.

TABLE 1. *Concentration of free aspartic and glutamic acid in singly dissected excitor axons of lobster walking limbs*

Acid	mmoles/liter tissue	Relative content
Aspartic	132	3.2
Glutamic	42	1.0

Figures are abstracted from McBride et al., 1974.

Possible Model for Excitatory Synaptic Transmission in the Lobster

The findings presented in this chapter might be summarized in terms of the model diagrammed in Fig. 15. The sequence of neurotransmission correcting to this model might be outlined as follows:

L-aspartate and L-glutamate are released from the excitatory nerve terminal in a 3-to-1 ratio. Three glutamate molecules react cooperatively with three receptor subunits resulting in coupling of the ionophore. The presence of a single aspartate molecule on an adjacent site governs the affinity of the glutamate receptor; high affinity with aspartate and low affinity without aspartate. The former might be termed the three subunit agonist receptor, while the latter could be called a unitary "affinity site."

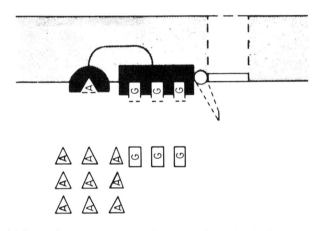

FIG. 15. Model for excitatory neuromuscular transmission in the lobster neuromuscular synapse. Aspartate (A) and glutamate (G) are released in a 3-to-1 ratio. Three glutamate molecules interact cooperatively at the agonist receptor whereas one molecule of aspartate interacts with the affinity site. The presence of aspartate at its site increases the affinity of agonist receptor for glutamate.

DISCUSSION

The findings outlined here point out that L-glutamic acid has two distinct actions on the membranes of lobster muscle fibers. On the nonsynaptic, electrically excitable membrane, this agent causes K inactivation and a shift in selectivity towards sodium accompanied by an increase in membrane resistance. Thus, when superfused at appropriate temperatures, glutamate induces a depolarization based on this shift in selectivity. If this property were to exist in nonsynaptic zones of neurons within the vertebrate CNS, the resulting high resistance and depolarization could partially account for the powerful excitatory influence of certain amino acids applied to CNS preparations (Curtis and Watkins, 1963). This line of reasoning has been implicated in the mechanism of centrally acting convulsant drugs (Freeman, 1973).

In a physiologic sense, this phenomenon may have value in that circulating amino acids could alter dramatically both the threshold of excitability and the cable properties of central neurones thereby subserving a role as "modulators" of neurotransmission.

Under experimental conditions in which pure synaptic activity is revealed bath applied L-glutamic acid appears to act in a manner identical to that of the natural excitatory neurotransmitter. The common mechanism is related to a transmitter-induced increase in sodium selectivity at the synaptic membrane resulting in a conductance increase and accompanying depolarization. This finding confirms evidence reported in arthropod systems (Takeuchi and Onodera, 1973; Anwyl and Usherwood, 1974; Ozeki and Grundfest 1967; Gerschenfeld, 1973; Kravitz et al., 1970). Also notable is the increase in sensitivity yielding perceptible effects at glutamate levels lower than 3×10^{-6} M.

Though not explored in this presentation, still another action of applied glutamate cannot be overlooked. In this respect, this compound has the ability to act at the presynaptic terminals to enhance release of endogenous excitatory transmitter (Colton and Freeman, 1975b). This could indicate the presence of positive feedback if released glutamate were to act partially presynaptically to enhance further the release of successive amounts of this transmitter.

Analysis of concentration-response curves of L-glutamate with respect to the post synaptic receptor, leads to the suggestion that the agonist receptor site is composed of three subunits showing cooperative interaction in coupling to the ionophore. L-aspartic acid, having no agonistic action itself, appears to interact in a unimolecular fashion with a spatially separate receptor. The effect of this interaction is to increase the affinity of agonist sites for glutamate. The optimum molar ratio for the enhancement of glutamate activity appears to be about 3 to 1 aspartate to glutamate.

The D forms of the amino acids block specifically the sites for their corresponding L forms. Neurally evoked EPSPs respond similarly to D amino acids. This point favors the idea that both aspartate and glutamate receptor sites play a role in excitatory neurotransmission. The responses of EPSPs to both L and D forms of the amino acids, as outlined earlier, support the notion that the receptors interacting with bath applied compounds are the same as those combining with endogenous neurotransmitter. It is worth mentioning that the levels of D amino acids are relatively high and may in part explain the lack of effect of these compounds when applied at lower concentration in other systems (Takeuchi and Takeuchi, 1964).

The excitor axon supplying the muscle under investigation contains both aspartate and glutamate in the same molar ratio as that found optimal for the potentiation of glutamate responses, i.e., about 3 to 1.

It is suggested that aspartate and glutamate are both released during excitatory synaptic transmission in the lobster. Glutamate serves as the agonist while aspartate functions as a modulator indirectly controlling the magnitude of the glutamate-induced depolarization.

Ongoing investigations in this laboratory are being directed toward further exploring the glutamate-aspartate synergism and the direct demonstration of release of these agents during neurotransmission.

ACKNOWLEDGMENT

This work has been supported in part by NIMH Grant #MH 10695 and NIH Grant #RR-054-17.

REFERENCES

Anwyl, R., and Usherwood, P. N. R. (1974): Voltage clamp studies of glutamate synapse. *Nature*, 252:591.

Bennett, M. V. L., Freeman, A. R., and Thaddeus, P. (1966): "Reversal" of postsynaptic potentials in non-isopotential systems. *Biophys. J.*, 6:122a.

Colton, C., and Freeman, A. R. (1972): Observations on the neurotransmitter characteristics of glutamate on the lobster neuromuscular junction. *The Physiologist*, 15:145.

Colton, C. A., and Freeman, A. R. (1973a): Temperature induced changes in the physiological response of lobster neuromuscular junction to glutamate. *Biophys. J.*, 13:72a.

Colton, C. A., and Freeman, A. R. (1973b): Dual effect of glutamate at the lobster neuromuscular junction. *Fed. Proc.*, 32:334a.

Colton, C., and Freeman, A. R. (1973c): Evidence for a synaptic and non-synaptic response to L-glutamate in lobster. *The Physiologist*, 16:287.

Colton, C. K., and Freeman, A. R. (1975a): Dual response of lobster muscle fibers to L-glutamate. *Comp. Biochem. Physiol.*, 51C:175.

Colton, C. K., and Freeman, A. R. (1975b): La^{3+} blockade of glutamate action at the lobster neuromuscular junction. *Comp. Biochem. Physiol.*, 51C:285.

Colquhoun, D. (1973): The relation between classical and cooperative models for drug action. In: *Drug Receptors, A Symposium*, edited by H. P. Rang, pp. 149–182. University Park Press, Baltimore.

Curtis, D. R., and Watkins, J. C. (1963): Acidic amino acids with strong excitatory actions on mammalian neurones. *J. Physiol.*, 166:1.

Fischbarg, J. (1972): Ionic permeability changes as the basis of the thermal dependence of the resting potential in barnacle muscle fibers. *J. Physiol.*, 224:149.

Freeman, A. R., and Fingerman, M. (1970): Experiments on the transmembrane potential of chromatophores. In: *Experiments in Physiology and Biochemistry*, Vol. 3, edited by G. A. Kerkut, Chap. 5, p. 161. Academic Press, New York.

Freeman, A. R. (1971): Electrophysiological activity of tetrodotoxin on the resting membrane of the squid giant axon. *Comp. Biochem. Physiol.*, 40:71.

Freeman, A. R. (1973): Electrophysiological analysis of the actions of strychnine, bicuculline and picrotoxin on the axonal membrane. *J. Neurobiol.*, 4:567.

Gerschenfeld, H. M. (1973): Chemical transmission in invertebrate central nervous systems and neuromuscular junctions. *Physiol. Rev.*, 53:1.

Grundfest, H., Reuben, J., and Rickles, W. H. (1959): The electrophysiology and pharmacology of lobster neuromuscular synapses. *J. Gen. Physiol.*, 42:1301.

Grundfest, H. (1961): Ionic mechanisms in electrogenesis. *Ann. NY Acad. Sci.*, 94:405.

Grundfest, H. (1966): Comparative electrobiology of excitable membranes. In: *Advances in Comparative Physiology and Biochemistry*, Vol. 2, pp. 1–116, Academic Press, New York.

Grundfest, H. (1972): Neuromuscular transmission in arthropods. *I.E.P.T.*, Sect. 14, Vol. 2:621.

Karlin, A. (1967): On the application of "a plausible model" of allosteric proteins to the receptor for acetylcholine. *J. Theoret. Biol.,* 16:306.

Kravitz, E. A., Kuffler, S. W., Potter, D. D., and Van Gelder, N. M. (1963): Gamma-aminobutyric acid and other blocking compounds in crustacea. II. Peripheral nervous system. *J. Neurophysiol.,* 26:729.

Kravitz, E. A., Slater, C. R., Takahashi, K., Bownds, M. D., and Grossfeld, R. M. (1970): Excitatory transmission in invertebrates—glutamate as a potential neuromuscular transmitter compound. In: *Excitatory Synaptic Mechanisms.* Edited by P. Anderson and J. K. S. Jansen, pp. 85–93. Scandinavian University Books, Oslo.

Krnjević, K. (1970): Glutamate and γ-aminobutyric acid in brain. *Nature,* 228:119.

McBride, W. J., Shank, R. P., Freeman, A. R., and Aprison, M. H. (1974): Levels of free amino acids in excitatory, inhibitory and sensory axons of the walking limbs of the lobster. *Life Sci.,* 14:1109.

Motokizawa, F., Reuben, J. P., and Grundfest, H. (1969): Ionic permeability of the inhibitory post synaptic membrane of lobster muscle fibers. *J. Gen. Physiol.,* 54:437.

Ozeki, M., Freeman, A. R., and Grundfest, H. (1966a): Immunity of different electrogenic components of crustacean nerve-muscle preparations to tetrodotoxin and saxitoxin. *J. Gen. Physiol.,* 49:1319.

Ozeki, M., Freeman, A. R., and Grundfest, H. (1966b): Analysis of interactions among the electrogenic components of crustacean muscle fibers. *J. Gen. Physiol.,* 49:1335.

Ozeki, M., and Grundfest, H. (1967): Crayfish muscle fiber: Ionic requirements for depolarizing synaptic electrogenesis. *Science,* 155:478.

Shank, R. P., Freeman, A. R., Colton, C. A., McBride, W. J., and Aprison, M. H. (1973): Role of aspartate in neuromuscular excitation in the lobster. *The Physiologist,* 16:448.

Shank, R. P., and Freeman, A. R. (1974a): Interaction of glutamate and aspartate with receptors on the neuromuscular excitatory membrane in the walking limb of the lobster. *Fed. Proc.,* 33:449.

Shank, R. P., and Freeman, A. R. (1974b): Action of glutamate analogs on muscle fibers in lobster walking limbs. *The Physiologist,* 17:329.

Shank, R. P., and Freeman, A. R. (1974c): Effect of glutamate analogs on neuromuscular excitation in the walking limb of the lobster. Neuroscience Society 4th Annual Meeting.

Shank, R. P., and Freeman, A. R. (1975a): Cooperative interaction of glutamate and aspartate with receptors in the neuromuscular excitatory membrane in walking limbs of the lobster. *J. Neurobiol. (in press).*

Shank, R. P., and Freeman, A. R. (1975b): Agonistic and antagonistic activity of glutamate analogs on neuromuscular excitation in the walking limbs of lobsters. *J. Neurobiol. (in press).*

Shank, R. P., Freeman, A. R., McBride, W. J., and Aprison, M. H. (1975c): Glutamate and aspartate as mediators of neuromuscular excitation in the lobster. *Comp. Biochem. Physiol., (in press).*

Takeuchi, A., and Onodera, K. (1973): Reversal potentials of the excitatory transmitter and L-glutamate at the crayfish neuromuscular junction. *Nature,* 242:124.

Takeuchi, A., and Takeuchi, N. (1964): The effect on crayfish muscle of iontophoretically applied glutamate. *J. Physiol.,* 170:296.

Werman, R. (1969): An electrophysiological approach to drug-receptor mechanisms. *Comp. Biochem. Physiol.,* 30:997.

Electrobiology of Nerve, Synapse, and Muscle,
edited by J. P. Reuben, D. P. Purpura, M. V. L. Bennett,
and E. R. Kandel. Raven Press, New York © 1976

Amino Acid Receptors on Insect Muscle

P. N. R. Usherwood

Department of Zoology, University of Nottingham, Nottingham NG7 2RD, England

The day is long since past when suggestions that amino acids might be neurotransmitters are summarily dismissed. Indeed, the evidence that L-glutamate is the transmitter at excitatory junctions on insect skeletal muscle grows almost weekly and is received so enthusiastically that we are in grave danger of ignoring observations which seemingly fail to support a transmitter role for this amino acid. Although one would have to be very brave and perhaps somewhat foolish to refute completely the "glutamate-transmitter" hypothesis for insect skeletal muscle one should recognize that much remains to be done before it can receive unequivocal acceptance. A role for GABA as a peripheral inhibitory transmitter in insects seems much more assured, which is somewhat surprising since on balance its action on insect muscle has not received the same attention as that of L-glutamate.

I first studied amino acids as putative transmitters in 1963 when, as a Research Associate in Professor H. Grundfest's laboratory, I investigated the effects of GABA and, in passing, L-glutamate on the skeletal muscles of various insect species. After demonstrating peripheral inhibitory synapses in insects, Grundfest and I went on to show that GABA mimicked the transmitter at these synapses (Grundfest and Usherwood, 1965; Usherwood and Grundfest, 1964, 1965). We also found that insect muscle fibers could be depolarized by L-glutamate, suggesting that it might be worthwhile studying the possible transmitter role of this amino acid at excitatory synapses on insect muscle fibers. Since 1965 the putative transmitter roles of L-glutamate and GABA in insects have been greatly substantiated. In this chapter I will review the latest findings to emanate from my laboratory.

L-GLUTAMATE—BATH APPLICATION

When L-glutamate is added at concentrations greater than 10^{-5} M to the medium bathing a locust skeletal muscle the muscle undergoes either a transient contraction (phasic muscle) or a prolonged, sustained contracture (tonic muscle). It would be incorrect, however, to assume from these observations that the excitatory synapse is the only site of action of L-glutamate on insect muscle. For example, it has been found that the membrane potential (E_m) changes in response to bath-applied glutamate are frequently biphasic with a hyperpolarization of 2 to 10 mV preceding a depolarization. The threshold for the hyperpolarization is somewhat lower than that for the depolarization. These changes in E_m are accompanied by an increase in effective membrane conductance (G_{eff}) although it is not yet certain whether this conductance increase is associated with both of the potential changes. The G_{eff} of a locust muscle fiber slowly returns to normal when the glutamate is removed from the bath, but even short ($\simeq 5$ min) periods of application are often followed by a variable period of subnormal G_{eff}.

One of the major problems accompanying any study of the possible transmitter role of L-glutamate is that this ubiquitous amino acid is rapidly sequestered by most tissues. Active uptake of L-glutamate by insect muscle fibers cannot, therefore, be discounted, and might be accompanied by a change in E_m without a concomitant increase in G_{eff}. Hironaka (1974) found that the depolarization of lobster leg muscle fibers by bath-applied L-glutamate was blocked in chloride-free saline. He proposed that L-glutamate activates an outward chloride pump located in the surface membrane of these muscle fibers. There seems little doubt that the disparity between E_m and the chloride equilibrium potential for locust muscle fibers (Usherwood and Grundfest, 1965; Usherwood, 1968, 1969a) indicates the presence of a chloride pump in the surface membrane of these fibers. However, evidence that chloride is implicated in the hyperpolarization of locust muscle fibers by bath-applied glutamate — either by an increase in chloride permeability or by inactivation of an electrogenic outward chloride pump — is equivocal since when chloride is excluded from the bathing medium and replaced by the impermeant anion sulfate and time is allowed for equilibration, the hyperpolarizing component of the biphasic glutamate potential is reduced but not lost completely. Similar observations to those obtained from locust muscle have been obtained from flight muscles of the fly, *Sarcophaga*. With 10^{-4} M glutamate a slight hyperpolarization was seen, which reached a maximum value after 30 min in L-glutamate, and then slowly declined, sometimes reversing to a depolarization (Neal and Usherwood, *unpublished*). During the period of glutamate treatment there was a slight decrease in G_{eff}. In the trochanteral depressor muscle of *Sarcophaga* bath-applied glutamate caused a monophasic (depolarization) change in E_m which subsided during long-term treatment and was always accompanied by an increase in G_{eff}. Perhaps the type of response obtained from insect muscle with bath-applied glutamate depends upon the relative areas of synaptic and nonsynaptic membrane, i.e., on the relative magnitudes of the junctional and extrajunctional responses and on the accessibility of the excitatory junctions. The results of prolonged application of L-glutamate to flight, trochanteral, and retractor unguis muscles of *Sarcophaga* lend some support to this idea. The concentrations of L-glutamate required to change E_m, G_{eff}, and the amplitude of the excitatory postsynaptic potential

(EPSP) was much higher for flight muscle than for trochanteral muscle. Abolition of the EPSP of flight muscle was seen with 10^{-2} wt/vol glutamate but only after protracted (> 1 hr) periods of application. The loss of the EPSP was accompanied by a decrease in G_{eff} of about 10%. The EPSP of trochanteral muscle was abolished by slightly lower concentrations of glutamate, i.e., 10^{-3} to 10^{-2} wt/vol, but again the loss of the EPSP was accompanied by a decrease of G_{eff}. The EPSP of retractor unguis muscle was abolished by 10^{-5} to 10^{-4} wt/vol glutamate and here there was an increase in G_{eff}. The excitatory junctions on the large flight muscle fibers are located deep down in clefts in the fibers: those on the smaller but tightly packed trochanteral depressor muscle fibers are found more superficially although on the inner faces of the fibers. The junctions on the very small retractor unguis muscle fibers are the most superficial and presumably the most readily accessible to bath-applied glutamate.

When L-glutamate is injected from a micropipette into a locust muscle fiber there is a rapid decrease in G_{eff} of that fiber (Daoud and Usherwood, *unpublished*). This observation suggests that the period of subnormal G_{eff} which follows bath application of glutamate could be due to entry of this amino acid. When small quantities of Ca^{2+} are injected into *Aplysia* neurons, the surface membrane is hyperpolarized because of a specific increase in potassium conductance (Meech, 1974). Perhaps glutamate binds free Ca^{2+} when it enters the myoplasm of locust muscle fibers either from the bathing medium or via iontophoresis. Such activity could lead to a fall in G_{eff} due to K^+ inactivation. It remains to be seen whether G_{eff} of locust muscle fibers is affected by a change in intracellular Ca^{2+}. A depolarization accompanied by a decrease in G_{eff} occurs during topical application of L-glutamate to lobster muscle at room temperature (ca. 18°C) (Colton and Freeman, 1973). At temperatures below 3°C an increase in G_{eff} was observed during glutamate application. Colton and Freeman (1973) suggested that as well as acting on the excitatory junctional membrane of lobster muscle fibers, L-glutamate also exerts an influence over the properties of the extrajunctional membrane of these fibers, at temperature above 3°C, by inactivating potassium.

The idea of L-glutamate influx into arthropod muscle fibers is supported by work in this laboratory by Miller and Usherwood (*unpublished*). We found that when crab legs are perfused in saline in which all sodium is replaced by Tris-chloride, the rate of uptake by the leg muscles is reduced dramatically to a few percent of normal. In other words the glutamate uptake by these muscles is typical of a large number of other uptake processes in a wide variety of cells and tissues, involving most of the common amino acids, many sugars as well as certain other substances such as transmitter norepinephrine (Iversen and Kravitz, 1966). Sodium-linked transport of organic molecules has been extensively studied in other preparations and these studies have led to the formulation of the sodium gradient hypothesis (Schultz and Curran, 1970). This proposes that a major part of the energy necessary for accumulation of these molecules within the cytoplasm is supplied by the sodium ion concentration difference which exists between the external medium and the cytoplasm. The results obtained for crab muscle indicate that in addition to the major sodium-dependent flux of L-glutamate there is a small flux of glutamate into tissues of the crab leg which is not inhibited in sodium-free saline.

EXTRAJUNCTIONAL DEPOLARIZATIONS AND HYPERPOLARIZATIONS TO L-GLUTAMATE IONTOPHORESIS

In 1968 Beránek and Miller and Usherwood and Machili demonstrated the occurrence of L-glutamate sensitive sites on the membrane of locust muscle fibers which were identified as excitatory junctional regions. However, Beránek and Miller (1968) and, later, Usherwood (1969*b*) showed that although the greatest area of sensitivity to L-glutamate was to be found at the excitatory junctions, nevertheless measurable but slight sensitivity could be demonstrated also for the extrajunctional regions. However, in

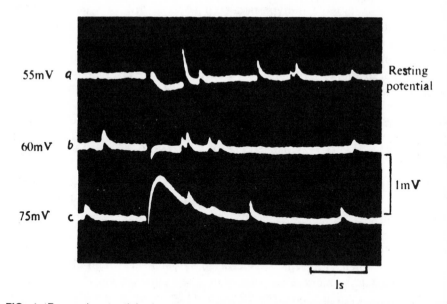

FIG. 1. Reversal potential of response obtained during activation of extrajunctional glutamate receptors on extensor tibiae muscle fibers of the locust *Schistocerca gregaria*. *a:* A small hyperpolarizing potential produced at an extrajunctional site at the resting potential of 55 mV in response to the iontophoretic application of L-glutamate. *b,c:* Reversal of this potential by increasing (hyperpolarization) the membrane potential of the muscle fiber with a current passing electrode. The population density of extrajunctional D-receptors must have been much lower than that for the H-receptors on this particular fiber. (From Cull-Candy and Usherwood, 1973.)

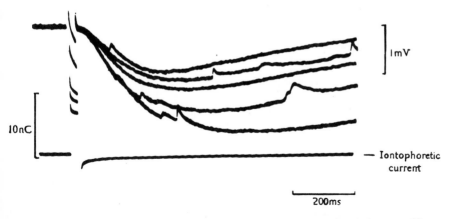

FIG. 2. Superimposed potential generated by iontophoresis of L-glutamate every 60 sec at a single extrajunctional site on a locust extensor tibiae muscle fiber. Larger currents of L-glutamate resulted in hyperpolarizations of a greater amplitude and increased rise time. The population density of extrajunctional D-receptors must have been much lower than that for the H-receptors on this particular fiber. (From Cull-Candy and Usherwood, 1973.)

the preparations used by these workers the ratio of junctional to extra-junctional membrane was large and therefore did not enable them to com-pletely exclude the possibility that their so-called extrajunctional responses were really junctional responses produced by diffusion of L-glutamate to junctional sites distant from the glutamate electrode. It was not until the work of Lea and Usherwood (1970, 1973*a,b*) that unequivocal evidence for extrajunctional amino acid receptors on locust muscle fibers came to light. Working with the isoxazole ibotenic acid they confirmed earlier findings of Usherwood (*unpublished*) that this substance increased the chloride per-meability of locust muscle fibers without acting on the excitatory post-synaptic membrane. They also found that when ibotenic acid was applied iontophoretically to the extrajunctional membrane of these fibers transient hyperpolarizations were observed. Perhaps more significantly, L-glutamate and ibotenic acid were shown to compete for the extrajunctional sites. Cull-Candy and Usherwood (1973, 1974) later confirmed these findings and further demonstrated the presence of two populations of extrajunctional glutamate receptors. One population (H-receptors) activates chloride ionophores (Figs. 1 and 2) and interacts with both L-glutamate and ibotenic acid; the other population (D-receptors) activates sodium and potassium ionophores and interacts with L-glutamate but not ibotenic acid. Picrotoxin blocks the response which follows activation of the H-receptors but not the D-receptors (Fig. 3). We also found that the reversal potential for the depolarizations which result from activation of the D-receptors was more negative than the reversal potential for either the junctional glutamate potential or for the EPSP. This suggests that the permeability changes

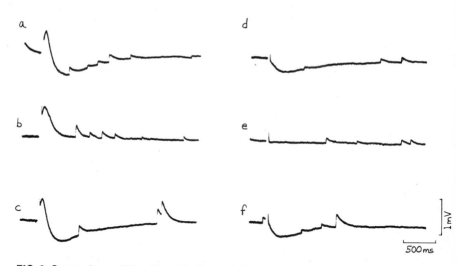

FIG. 3. Comparison of the effect of bath-applied picrotoxin (10^{-3} M), on the extrajunctional responses of a locust extensor tibiae muscle fiber to both L-glutamate and D,L-ibotenate (applied iontophoretically from a double barrel micropipette); *a,d:* The biphasic response to glutamate and the hyperpolarizing response to ibotenate respectively in normal saline. *b,e:* The glutamate and ibotenate responses after a 20-min period in 10^{-3} M picrotoxin. The hyperpolarizing component of both responses is blocked, so only a depolarizing response to glutamate remains; *c,f:* The action of picrotoxin on the glutamate and ibotenate hyperpolarizing responses is reversible on washing in normal saline for 20 min. (From Cull-Candy and Usherwood, *unpublished data.*)

associated with the extrajunctional D-receptors and the junctional receptors for L-glutamate are not exactly identical. Most of the information on extrajunctional receptors has been obtained by Cull-Candy and Usherwood (1973, 1974) using the locust extensor tibiae nerve-muscle preparation where the ratio of extrajunctional to junctional membrane is very high. This makes it possible to apply drugs by micropipettes to extrajunctional sites while excluding the possibility of diffusion of drug to excitatory and inhibitory junctions. The use of very high resistance (>150 MΩ) drug ejection electrodes which prevent significant background leakage of drug from the micropipettes has also proven profitable since the extrajunctional receptors are rapidly desensitized. Extrajunctional D-receptors have been found on the retractor unguis nerve-muscle preparation of the locust but they are difficult to study here because of the small diameter of the muscle fibers and the rich innervation of these fibers.

JUNCTIONAL RECEPTORS

Many laboratories have been engaged in gaining an understanding of the properties of the postsynaptic receptors at excitatory junctions on insect skeletal muscle, and much evidence has been obtained which supports the suggested role of L-glutamate as the transmitter at these sites. It is now quite clear that these receptors have an unusually high degree of specificity for this amino acid. Of the many different substances examined so far only L-aspartate approaches L-glutamate in its ability to react with the junctional receptors and then only at a threshold concentration about one hundred times greater than that for L-glutamate. One of the major difficulties of investigating the sensitivity of the glutamate junctional receptors is that inactivation of transmitter at the insect excitatory synapse appears to involve sequestration of L-glutamate by glial cells, muscle fibers and nerve terminals (Faeder and Salpeter, 1970). Therefore the effectiveness of a substance in altering the postsynaptic response to iontophoretically applied L-glutamate or to the natural transmitter might be due to its action on the glutamate uptake system, which indirectly influences postsynaptic responsiveness, rather than on the postsynaptic membrane itself. Some of the recent reports on the synergistic behaviour of L-glutamate and aspartate at arthropod nerve-muscle junctions could also be explained in this way.

Kainic acid is a pyrrolidine derivative isolated from the sea-weed *Digenia simplex* (Ueno et al., 1955; Murayama et al., 1965), and has certain structural features in common with L-glutamate (Johnston et al., 1974). In a short article published in 1972, Shinozaki and Shibuya presented results of studies on the action of this substance on a crayfish nerve-muscle preparation which cast some doubt upon the possible role of L-glutamate as a transmitter at excitatory synapses on crustacean muscle fibers. They found that kainic acid potentiated the depolarizing action of bath-applied glutamate but did not affect the amplitude of the EPSP. They found also that application of kainic acid to a muscle desensitized to L-glutamate following prolonged bath application of this pyrrolidine restored the glutamate-induced depolarization without affecting the size of the EPSP. In contrast to its action on the crayfish nerve-muscle preparation kainic acid reversibly potentiated both the glutamate potential and the excitatory junction potential of the crab walking leg (Wheal and Kerkut, 1976). Wheal and Kerkut suggested that kainic acid is a glutamate agonist and is at least twice as potent as this putative transmitter. Kainic acid (10^{-4} to 10^{-3} M) depolarizes lobster walking leg muscle, but is less effective than glutamate in this respect. Concentrations of kainic acid, which produce little or no depolarization alone, potentiate the depolarizations to L-glutamate. These findings suggest that kainic acid is less potent than glutamate on lobster muscle fibers (Constanti and Nistri, 1975). Daoud and Usherwood (1975) found that kainic acid increased the amplitude of the EPSP of locust extensor tibiae nerve-muscle preparations at a threshold concentration of 5×10^{-5} M. At 10^{-5} M it potentiated the glutamate potential and increased the miniature EPSP frequency. At 10^{-3} M the EPSP and junctional glutamate response were depressed and the miniature frequency fell. These results indicate that kainic acid acts both presynaptically and postsynaptically at the locust excitatory nerve-muscle junction.

The reversal potentials for the EPSP and junctional glutamate potential

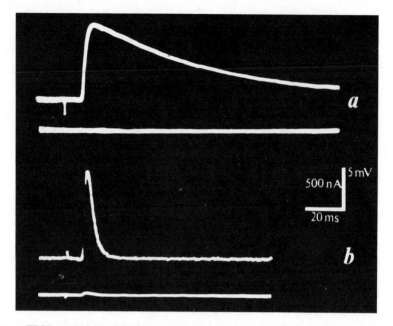

FIG. 4. *a:* EPSP recorded intracellularly from an extensor tibiae muscle fiber of the locust *Schistocerca gregaria. b: Upper record,* synaptic current recorded from the same muscle fiber with the membrane potential held at the resting level using voltage clamping; *lower record,* clamped membrane potential. Only a small deviation of 0.1 to 0.2 mV is seen after nerve stimulation. (From Anwyl and Usherwood, 1974.)

recorded from locust extensor tibiae muscle fibers are almost identical and close to zero membrane potential. Using a voltage-clamp technique it has been possible to study synaptic or junctional currents (Fig. 4) and glutamate currents (Anwyl and Usherwood, 1974*a,b,* 1975). The reversal potentials for these currents (Fig. 5) are almost identical with those for the EPSP and glutamate potential. The nature of the ion fluxes responsible for these potentials remains to be established firmly. A reversal potential close to zero suggests inward cationic and possibly anionic currents and outward cationic currents, i.e., involving sodium, and chloride and/or potassium. Removal of all extracellular chloride and its replacement by sulfate, however, has no effect on the reversal value for either the glutamate potential or the EPSP and it seems unlikely, therefore, that this ion is involved in generating these potentials. However, changes in external sodium and external potassium do produce changes in response amplitude and reversal potential, suggesting that these ions contribute to both the junctional glutamate potential and the EPSP. To a limited extent the changes in reversal potential can be predicted using the Goldman–Katz–Huxley equation (Anwyl and Usherwood, 1975). In 1960, Takeuchi and Takeuchi demonstrated that the postsynaptic membrane of the frog nerve-muscle junction is selectively permeable to Na^+ and K^+ and that the ratio of the conductance

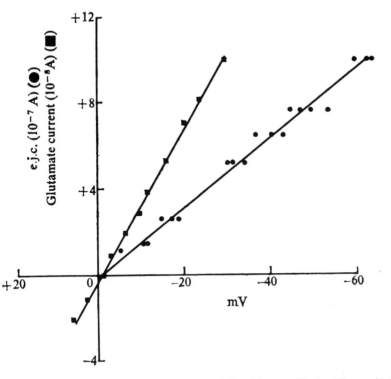

FIG. 5. Relationship between the membrane potential and the amplitude of the excitatory junctional current (e.j.c.) and glutamate current recorded from a junction on an extensor tibiae muscle fiber of *Schistocerca gregaria*. (From Anwyl and Usherwood, 1974.)

increase to Na^+ and K^+ during acetylcholine action remains constant when the extracellular concentrations of Na^+ and K^+ are changed. This does not hold for insect excitatory junctions when extracellular K^+ and Na^+ are altered. Since the membrane conductance of an ion might be expected to vary with its concentration in and on either side of the postjunctional membrane it is perhaps not surprising that the ratio of conductances for K^+ and Na^+ changes when the extracellular concentrations of these ions are altered.

DENERVATED MUSCLE

Usherwood (1963a,b) showed that locust leg muscles can be completely denervated by cutting their motor axons and allowing time for the nerve terminals to degenerate, the rate of degeneration of the peripheral ends of the cut motoneurons being temperature dependent (Rees and Usherwood, 1972). Following the degeneration of the motor nerve terminals a gradual atrophy of the muscle fibers ensues, signaled by a rapid fall in the resting potential to about -50 mV, i.e., about 10 mV below normal. Associated with muscle atrophy there is a rapid change in the responsiveness of the extrajunctional membrane to iontophoretically applied L-glutamate. This gives the impression of a spread of junctional L-glutamate receptors to embrace the entire extrajunctional membrane (Usherwood, 1969b). This observation was made before the extrajunctional L-glutamate receptors on innervated muscle fibers were discovered and although it supports the idea that L-glutamate is the excitatory transmitter by analogy with the changes which take place in the distribution of cholinergic receptors of frog muscle following denervation, the changes in glutamate sensitivity following denervation of insect muscle obviously require further investigation. Recent studies in this laboratory support early conclusions that junctional type L-glutamate receptors appear on the extrajunctional membrane of denervated muscle (Mathers and Usherwood, *unpublished*). We have also observed a concomitant decline in the population density of extrajunctional L- and D-receptors: there is no evidence to date that the L- and D-receptors are transformed into junctional-type receptors following denervation. The extrajunctional receptors also disappear following partial pharmacological denervation (i.e., loss of the neurally evoked response but maintenance of spontaneous transmitter release) for 5 days (Cull-Candy et al., 1973) with black widow spider venom (Mathers and Usherwood, *unpublished*).

PRESYNAPTIC PHARMACOLOGY

Usherwood and Machili (1968) found that low concentrations of L-glutamate enhance the rate of spontaneous release of transmitter from terminals of locust excitatory motoneurons, and Dowson and Usherwood (1970) subsequently showed that this increase in miniature EPSP frequency is accompanied by an increase in EPSP amplitude. Dowson and Usherwood (1970) also found that aspartate diminished both the miniature frequency and the amplitude of the EPSP. One of my students, Miss B. Fulton, has recently confirmed these findings. She has also established that the terminals are very sensitive to acetylcholine, which increases the miniature EPSP frequency and EPSP amplitude, and adrenalin, glycine, and GABA, which diminish the miniature EPSP frequency. It seems likely that these changes result from a variety of sites of action involving receptors on the presynaptic membrane, transmitter inactivation and transmitter recycling and release. Nevertheless, there is evidently much to be learned about the presynaptic pharmacology of chemical synapses, not only in arthropods but also in vertebrates.

CONCLUSIONS

One of the major criteria for establishing whether a substance is a neurotransmitter is that of identical postsynaptic action with the natural transmitter. Studies of excitatory junctions on skeletal muscles of a variety of insects have clearly demonstrated that L-glutamate and the natural transmitter interact in an identical fashion with receptors on the postsynaptic membrane of these sites. Other criteria, such as storage in and release of glutamate from terminals of insect excitatory motoneurons, remain to be established. Although there is good evidence for a glutamate-uptake system at these junctions one cannot be sure that such a system plays a role in determining the time course of the EPSP. The bizarre effects of bath-applied glutamate and the occurrence of two populations of extrajunctional receptors for L-glutamate remain unexplained, but do not detract from the putative transmitter role suggested for this amino acid.

REFERENCES

Anwyl, R., and Usherwood, P. N. R. (1974a): Voltage-clamp studies of the glutamate response at the insect neuromuscular junction. *J. Physiol.,* 242:86–87.

Anwyl, R., and Usherwood, P. N. R. (1974b): Voltage-clamp studies of a glutamate synapse. *Nature,* 252:591–593.

Anwyl, R., and Usherwood, P. N. R. (1975): The ionic permeability changes caused by the excitatory transmitter at the insect neuromuscular junction. *J. Physiol.,* 249:24–25P.

Beránek, R., and Miller, P. L. (1968): The action of iontophoretically applied glutamate on insect muscle fibres. *J. Exp. Biol.,* 49:83–93.

Colton, C., and Freeman, A. R. (1973): Evidence for a synaptic and non-synaptic response to L-glutamate in lobster. *The Physiologist,* 16(3):287.

Constanti, A., and Nistri, A. (1975): Actions of glutamate and kainic acid on the lobster muscle fibre and the frog spinal cord. *Br. J. Pharm.,* 53(3):437.

Cull-Candy, S. G., Neal, H., and Usherwood, P. N. R. (1973): Action of black widow spider venom on an aminergic synapse. *Nature,* 246:353–354.

Cull-Candy, S. G., and Usherwood, P. N. R. (1973): Two populations of L-glutamate receptors on locust muscle fibres. *Nature New Biol.,* 246:62–64.

Cull-Candy, S. G., and Usherwood, P. N. R. (1974): Distribution of glutamate sensitivity on insect muscle fibres. *Neuropharmacology,* 13:455–461.

Daoud, A., and Usherwood, P. N. R. (1975): Action of kainic acid on a glutamatergic synapse. *Comp. Biochem. Physiol.,* 52C:51–53.

Dowson, R. J., and Usherwood, P. N. R. (1972): The effect of low concentrations of L-glutamate and L-aspartate on transmitter release at the locust excitatory nerve-muscle synapse. *J. Physiol.,* 229:13–14.

Faeder, I. R., and Salpeter, M. (1970): Glutamate uptake by a stimulated insect nerve-muscle preparation. *J. Cell Biol.,* 46:300–307.

Grundfest, H., and Usherwood, P. N. R. (1965): Peripheral inhibition in skeletal muscle of insects. *J. Physiol.,* 178:14.

Hironaka, T. (1974): Chloride-related depolarization of crayfish muscle membrane induced by L-glutamate. *Nature,* 248:251–253.

Iversen, L. L., and Kravitz, E. A. (1966): Sodium dependence of transmitter uptake at adrenergic nerve terminals. *Mol. Pharmacol.,* 2:360–362.

Johnston, G. A. R., Curtis, D. R., Davies, J., and McCulloch, R. M. (1974): Spinal interneurone excitation by conformationally restricted analogues of L-glutamic acid. *Nature,* 248:804–805.

Lea, T., and Usherwood, P. N. R. (1970): Increased chloride permeability of insect muscle fibres on exposure to ibotenic acid. *J. Physiol.,* 211:32P.

Lea, T., and Usherwood, P. N. R. (1973a): Effect of ibotenic acid on chloride permeability of insect muscle-fibres. *Comp. Gen. Pharmacol.,* 4:351–363.

Lea, T., and Usherwood, P. N. R. (1973b): The site of action of ibotenic acid and the identification of two populations of glutamate receptors on insect muscle fibres. *Comp. Gen. Pharmacol.*, 4:333–350.

Meech, R. W. (1974): The sensitivity of *Helix aspersa* neurones to injected calcium ions. *J. Physiol.*, 237:259–277.

Murayama, K., Morimura, S., Nakamura, Y., and Sunagawa, G. (1965): Synthesis of pyrrolidine derivatives — II. Synthesis of kainic acid and its derivatives by Wittig reaction. *J. Pharm. Soc. Japan*, 85:757–765.

Rees, D., and Usherwood, P. N. R. (1972): Fine structure of normal and degenerating motor axons and nerve-muscle synapses in the locust, *Schistocerca gregaria*. *Comp. Biochem. Physiol.*, 43A:83–101.

Schultz, S. G., and Curran, P. F. (1970): Coupled transport of sodium and organic solutes. *Physiol. Rev.*, 50:637–718.

Shinozaki, H., and Shibuya, I. (1972): Effects of kainic acid on crayfish neuromuscular junction. *Jap. J. Pharmacol.*, 22:100.

Takeuchi, A., and Takeuchi, N. (1960): On the permeability of end-plate membrane during the action of transmitter. *J. Physiol.*, 154:52–67.

Ueno, Y., Nawa, H., Ueyanagi, J., Morimoto, H., Nakamori, R., and Matsuoka, T. (1955): Studies on the active components of *Digenea simplex* Ag., and related compounds — I. Studies on the structure of kainic acid. *J. Pharm. Soc. Japan*, 75:807.

Usherwood, P. N. R. (1963a): Response of insect muscle to denervation. I. Resting potential changes. *J. Insect Physiol.*, 9:247–255.

Usherwood, P. N. R. (1963b): Response of insect muscle to denervation. II. Changes in neuromuscular transmission. *J. Insect Physiol.*, 9:811–825.

Usherwood, P. N. R. (1968): A critical study of the evidence for peripheral inhibitory axons in insects. *J. Exp. Biol.*, 49:201–222.

Usherwood, P. N. R. (1969a): Electrochemistry of insect muscle. *Adv. Insect Physiol.*, 6:205–278.

Usherwood, P. N. R. (1969b): Glutamate sensitivity of denervated insect muscle fibres. *Nature*, 223:411–413.

Usherwood, P. N. R., and Grundfest, H. (1964): Inhibitory postsynaptic potentials in grasshopper muscle. *Science*, 143:817–818.

Usherwood, P. N. R., and Grundfest, H. (1965): Peripheral inhibition in skeletal muscle of insects. *J. Neurophysiol.*, 28:497–518.

Usherwood, P. N. R., and Machili, P. (1968): Pharmacological properties of excitatory neuromuscular synapses in the locust. *J. Exp. Biol.*, 49:341–361.

Wheal, H. V., and Kerkut, G. A. (1976): Structure activity studies on the excitatory receptor of the crustacean neuromuscular junction. *Comp. Biochem. Physiol.*, 53C:51–55.

Electrobiology of Nerve, Synapse, and Muscle,
edited by J. P. Reuben, D. P. Purpura, M. V. L. Bennett,
and E. R. Kandel. Raven Press, New York © 1976

Neuromuscular Transmission in Mealworm Larvae (Tenebrio molitor)

K. Kusano and L. Janiszewski*

Department of Biology, Illinois Institute of Technology, Chicago, Illinois 60616; and
*Department of Animal Physiology, Institute of Biology, N. Copernicus University,
Toruń, Poland

The osmolarity of mealworm hemolymph is known to be about 720 mosmoles per liter. Chemical analysis indicates that approximately one-third of the total osmotic concentration consists of inorganic salts (75.5 mM Na^+, 36.5 mM K^+, 130 to 160 mM Cl^-) and that the remainder is mainly the disaccharide, trehalose, with some amino acids (Buck, 1953; Wyatt and Kalf, 1957; Belton and Grundfest, 1962); Ca^{2+} and Mg^{2+} are also present in the hemolymph, but their exact amounts are not known. Thus the ratio of Na^+ and K^+ in the hemolymph of mealworm larvae is quite different from that of the body fluid of vertebrates. Such peculiar ionic distribution is commonly known in the phytophagous insects. An extreme example can be found in the Lepidoptera, such as the silkworm, *Bombyx mori,* in which the hemolymph contains an unusually low concentration of Na^+ but very high concentration of K^+ and Mg^{2+}. In this animal the Na^+ gradient across the muscle fiber membrane (Na^+_o/Na^+_i) is known to be less than unity. Unfortunately, data on the intracellular ionic composition of mealworm muscle fiber is very incomplete as it is in general for insects due to the difficulty involved in isolating the tissue. Nevertheless such an ionic environment of insect excitable tissues has attracted a number of neurobiologists to examine the ionic mechanisms involved in their excitation processes (Usherwood, 1969). Belton and Grundfest (1962) first studied the electrical characteristics of mealworm muscle fibers. They found several very unusual characteristics of the muscle fibers: (1) the membrane potential can be changed from about −30 to −90 mV by altering the anionic concentration; (2) membrane potential is remarkably insensitive to very large changes in extracellular K^+. In this paper we describe electrophysiological properties of mealworm neuromuscular junctions. The detailed analysis of electrically excitable membrane characteristics of muscle fibers will be published elsewhere. The foregoing data was obtained while we were in post doctoral training during the years 1961 to 1963 in the Laboratory of Neurophysiology at Columbia University and has never been published except in abstract form (Kusano and Grundfest, 1966).

METHODS

Larvae of the mealworm (*Tenebrio molitor*) were cultured in the laboratory. The larva was decapitated, slit open along the dorsal midline, and pinned out flat on a paraffin block. The coelomic contents were removed. The abdominal muscle fibers, *mm. ventrali interni,* run from the thoracic region to the posterior end. Most of them are elliptical in cross section (ca. 500×50 μm), but others are nearly circular (ca. 150 μm in diameter). They are segmented at each body segment. The length of these segments is about 2 mm. Except for differences due to different cross-sectional areas the two types of fibers appear to have essentially identical properties. All experiments were carried out *in situ.* The standard saline had a composition (in mmoles) of 70 NaCl, 30 KCl, 5 $CaCl_2$, 10 $MgCl_2$, and 475 glucose or sucrose. The pH of the standard saline and of modified salines were adjusted to 7.2 with tris(hydroxymethyl)aminomethane. The modification of the standard saline could be made in two ways, by replacing all or part of the various ionic species already present with some other salt or with sucrose, or by replacing some or all of the sucrose with a salt, keeping osmotic relations approximately constant. External stimulation was applied at a low frequency (ca. 0.5/sec) to the connectives of the segmental ganglion by a pair of silver wire electrodes which were insulated with "Teflon" except at the tips. An intracellular glass microelectrode filled with 3 M KCl was used to measure membrane potentials. The electrode was connected to a high impedance amplifier through a Ag–AgCl junction. The external reference electrode was also a Ag–AgCl junction. Therefore, zero-level changes due to the tip potentials in the various solutions were corrected for, after measurements were done on the excitatory postsynaptic potential (EPSP) and on the equilibrium potential of the EPSP (E_{EPSP}). When the solution was changed, the preparation was allowed to adapt for 20 min, then the recording electrode was reinserted to the same position and another set of measurements was made. The experiments were carried out at room temperature (18° to 22°C).

RESULTS

General Remarks

Each segment of an anatomical fiber functionally acts as a single fiber, and it is nearly isopotential for changes induced by an intracellularly applied current. The septal junctions of the muscle fibers are composed of collagenous fibers and their structure is similar to the muscle tendon. The low-frequency component of the electrotonic potential spreads into the neighboring compartments longitudinally with large attenuation, but a high-frequency component such as action potentials does not. An abdominal ganglion lies on each septum and innervates the caudally located segmental muscles. Application of a stimulus to the connectives of the ganglion causes a simultaneous contraction in the muscle fibers of this particular segment. The muscle contraction is therefore restricted within a segment. Intracellular recordings show that the muscle contraction is preceded by a large EPSP, which initiates an overshooting action potential. Stimulation of ganglia other than these near the recording site in the muscle segment are not very effective in producing a large junctional potential. Intracellular recordings or stimulating these ganglia reveal either one of the following responses: very small (less than 5 mV) depolarizing postsynaptic potential; very small hyperpolarizing junctional potential; or a composite of small de- and hyperpolarizing junctional potentials. The polarity and amplitude of these junctional potentials were not easily altered by the changes of the postsynaptic membrane potential. The hyperpolarizing junctional potential was not identical to the ordinary inhibitory synaptic potential. Stimulation of the segmental ganglion produced both large and small excitatory postsynaptic potentials in some fibers. Those muscle fibers appeared, therefore, to be innervated by at least two nerve fibers. Since each segmental muscle fiber is diffusely innervated by one or more nerve fibers and the length constant (λ) is longer than the length of the segment, the amplitude and the time course of EPSPs recorded from anywhere in a segmental fiber are almost identical. The following characteristics were obtained from large EPSPs and the discussion is confined to this response.

In the standard saline, 90% of muscle fibers examined produced all-or-none responses following a large EPSP evoked by external stimulation of the appropriate segmental ganglion. Therefore, in these preparations it was not possible to record a pure EPSP at the resting potential level, even though the muscle membrane potential was displaced by a large hyperpolarizing current (Cerf et al., 1959). Since the average resting potential of the muscle fibers was −40 mV and the firing level of the spike to direct stimulation was about −25 to −15 mV, EPSP amplitudes must be larger than 20 mV at the resting potential level. The inflection points on the rising phase of the neurogenic spikes ranged between 20 and 35 mV positive to the resting potential. Summation of EPSPs occurs with tetanic stimulation but facilitation is not observed for the large EPSP.

The height of the indirectly evoked action potential was greater than the height of the directly evoked spike. Sometimes the overshoot of the former response was twice the value of the latter. The difference of the maximum rate of rise between the neurogenic (18.6 V/sec) and myogenic action potential (9.35 V/sec) was especially significant. These differences are probably related to the fact that the area of muscle fiber which is excited by neural stimuli is larger than the area excited by direct stimulation. The finding is opposite to that of the frog end-plate spike and muscle spike but it is similar to that in the motor neuron in the cat spinal cord in which the orthodromic spike is larger than the antidromic (Coombs et al., 1955).

Several characteristics of the EPSP were estimated from preparations in which the spike electrogenesis did not occur in response to indirect stimulation. At the mean resting potential of -39 mV, the EPSP has a mean amplitude of 29 mV. The rise time was 6.4 msec at the maximum rate of rise of 10 V/sec. The maximum rate of fall was 1 V/sec and half-time of the decay was 17 msec. The depolarization during the EPSP was due to a conductance increase of as much as two fold of the resting value.

The EPSP Reversal Potential (E_{EPSP})

Since the muscle fibers are nearly isopotential, the EPSP reversal potential is assumed to be very close to the equilibrium potential of the ions involved in the postsynaptic electrogenesis. The E_{EPSP} was measured in two different ways: (a) by the changes in amplitude of the EPSP in relation to changes in membrane potential produced by applied current (Fig. 1, A1–2); (b) by the changes in membrane potential where an EPSP was superimposed on a directly evoked spike (B1–4) (Del Castillo and Katz, 1955). In many cases the first method could not be applied over an adequate range of membrane de- or hyperpolarization as already discussed and even an extrapolation technique could not be applied. The second method could not be applied with conditions where spikes were absent or the responses to direct stimulation were small. In some experiments the second method was applied after a prolonged TEA-spike was obtained by injecting TEA$^+$ into the muscle fiber (C1–4). Measurement of E_{EPSP} could then be carried out during the long-lasting plateau of the action potential. The E_{EPSP} before and after the TEA$^+$ injection did not show a significant difference. The reversal potential of the EPSP in the standard saline obtained from these techniques was almost zero membrane potential in 75% of 90 preparations and within ± 5 mV in the remainder.

The linear relationship between membrane potential and amplitude of EPSP broke down for hyperpolarizations which made the membrane more than 75 mV inside negative. This deviation results from a time-variant increase in membrane conductance analogous to that seen in the plateau stage of hyperpolarizing responses of lobster muscle fibers (Reuben et al., 1961). Linearity also broke down when the membrane was made inside-positive by more than about 20 to 25 mV. This is presumably due to an increased permeability of the inside positive membrane. The latency of the EPSP remained unaffected by the large changes in membrane potential. There was usually little or no change in the form of the EPSP except near the reversal potential, where the small responses sometimes appeared to be di- or triphasic. Such changes may be expected under the nonisopotential conditions in diffusely innervated muscle fibers (Bennett et al., 1966).

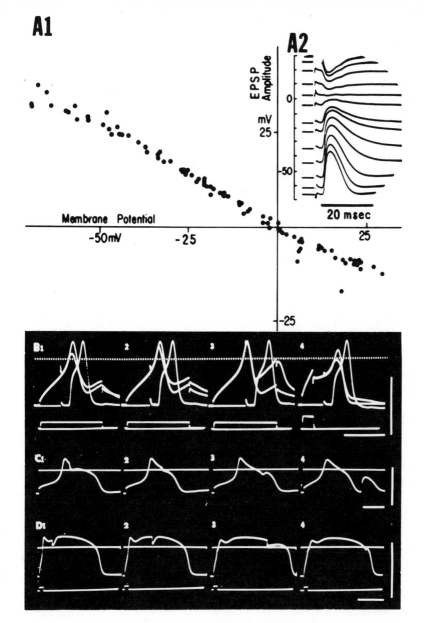

FIG. 1. Measurements of the reversal potential of EPSP. **A1–A2:** The reversal potential in the standard saline was measured by displacing the postsynaptic membrane potential by the application of sustained current. Graphical relationship between membrane potential and EPSP **(A1)**, and amplitude of EPSP and its time course at various membrane potential levels **(A2)** are shown. **B1–4:** The reversal potential in the standard saline was measured by the method of interaction between the directly evoked (myogenic) spike and a neurally evoked (neurogenic) spike. These superimposed responses in each set show a neurogenic spike, a myogenic spike, and a response produced by superimposing a neurally evoked spike on the various membrane potential levels of the myogenic spike. **C1–4:** The reversal potential in the standard saline was measured by the same method as **B1–4** but after intracellular injection of TEA$^+$ by a current of 1.5×10^{-7} A for 12 min. Since a large amount of intracellular TEA$^+$ was necessary to produce prolonged spikes in muscle fibers, the resting potential was decreased by more than 10 mV. Recovery of the resting potential was not seen. Only the responses produced by superimposing a neurally evoked spike on the various membrane potential levels of the TEA spike are shown. **D1–4:** The reversal potential in 20 mM TEA$^+$ in saline (equiosmolar glucose in standard saline was replaced) was determined by the same method used in **B1–4** and **C1–4**. Calibration: 50 mV, 20 msec **(B1–4)**, 40 msec **(C1–4)**, and 200 msec **(D1–4)**. Current calibration

Contributions of Various Ions

Effects of Na^+

The muscle fibers continue to produce spikes when directly stimulated in both Na^+-free glucose- or choline$^+$-substituted solutions. The neurally evoked responses however, are affected, the EPSP rising more slowly, becoming smaller, and eventually failing to elicit a spike in the muscle fiber (Woods, 1957). Similar behavior is seen in the frog end-plate (Fatt and Katz, 1952). Neuromuscular transmission was maintained in most of the fibers when Na^+ was reduced to half (35 mM) by substitution with choline$^+$. The reversal potential was determined by postsynaptic hyperpolarization using the extrapolation technique. The reversal potential shifted toward inside negative values with a decrease in $(Na^+)_0$. Changes in the E_{EPSP} of 0, -5, -13, and -18 mV were obtained from a particular preparation with Na^+ concentrations of 70, 35, 23 mM, and a few millimolar, which were substituted with appropriate amounts of sucrose. The average E_{EPSP} from seven neuromuscular junctions in choline substituted 35 mM Na^+ and in 17.5 mM Na^+ were -12.3 ± 3.6 mV ($\bar{X} \pm$ SD) and -20 ± 11.2 mV, respectively. The shift produced on increasing Na^+ up to 140 mM was not significant. Injection of Na^+ into the muscle fibers, as was done in the control experiment for the TEA$^+$ injection, also did not change the E_{EPSP} (Takeuchi and Takeuchi, 1960). Addition of 10 to 20 mM TEA Cl to the standard ionic medium did not shift E_{EPSP}, but the muscle fiber produced a typical prolonged TEA spike (Fig. 1, D-4).

When Li^+ replaced Na^+ in the standard saline the amplitude of the EPSP was markedly reduced and transmission was blocked. The rate of decrease of the EPSP in Li^+ saline was faster than in the Na^+-free glucose substituted medium, but a small depolarizing junctional potential remained for more than 30 min. This Li effect was reversible for a limited period. When Cs^+, Rb^+, $Tris^+$, or choline$^+$ replaced all the Na^+, the EPSP disappeared entirely. Muscle action potentials persist in these Na^+-free media. Presumably therefore, it is the nerve action potential that could not be maintained in these media.

Effects of K^+

The effects of changing K^+ within the range of 0 to 134 mM on neuromuscular transmission were examined. The K^+ level of the medium can be increased drastically without much affecting the resting potential of the muscle fibers (Belton and Grundfest, 1962). On increasing K^+ there was some indication that the reversal potential became positive but the neurally evoked activity was blocked rapidly in high-K^+ media. The difference in E_{EPSP} in 30 and 0 mM $(K^+)_0$ was compared in 2 mM Ca^{2+}-containing media.

Choline was substituted for K^+- and Mg^{2+}-substituted for Ca^{2+}. The average E_{EPSP} from eleven junctions was -4.2 ± 1.9 mV in 30 mM $(K^+)_0$ saline, which was within the range found in the standard saline. In the K^+-free saline the average E_{EPSP} was -10.4 ± 2.5 mV. Thus K^+ appears to be contributing in the generation of the EPSP. Experiments to test the relative effectiveness of $(Na^+)_0$ and $(K^+)_0$ on E_{EPSP} were unsuccessful.

Effects of Ca^{2+}

Removal of Ca^{2+} from the bathing solution caused blockage of transmission within 15 min. At this time muscle fibers continued to develop spikes in response to direct stimulation. When the Ca^{2+} concentration was varied between less than 1 and 18 mM the EPSP amplitude increased progressively, although the directly evoked muscle spikes decreased and became oscillatory graded responses. E_{EPSP} was not affected in low Ca^{2+} (5 to 1 mM) media. E_{EPSP} in high-Ca^{2+} media were estimated by both the extrapolation and interpolation techniques. In the presence of 16.3 mM Ca^{2+} the E_{EPSP} was about $+13$ mV. Measurements made by superimposing neurally evoked responses on TEA-induced prolonged muscle spikes also gave inside positive values for E_{EPSP} in high-Ca^{2+} media (Fig. 2). Both types of data

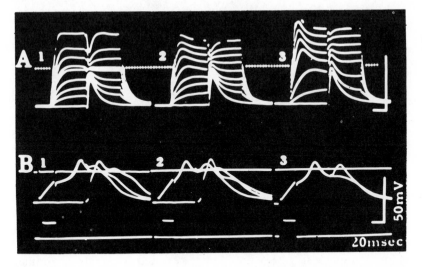

FIG. 2. Changes in reversal potential of EPSP in high-Ca^{2+} media. A1–3: E_{EPSP} was measured by the application of various amplitudes of postsynaptic depolarization. An electrically inexcitable muscle fiber was chosen. The dotted line shows zero reference potential. A1: in 5 mM Ca^{2+} (standard saline), the E_{EPSP} was obtained at the zero membrane potential level. A2: in 16.3 mM Ca^{2+}, E_{EPSP} was $+5.8$ mV. A3: in 38 mM Ca^{2+}, E_{EPSP} was 19.2 mV. When the preparation was transfered back to the standard saline (not shown), E_{EPSP} returned to the original level. B1–3: Reversal potential measurement in 16.3 mM Ca^{2+} medium by employing interaction method between myogenic and neurogenic response. TEA$^+$ was injected intracellularly as in Fig. 1.

therefore appear to indicate that the activated postsynaptic membrane is permeable to Ca^{2+}.

Neuromuscular transmission was blocked when 5 mM Ca^{2+} was substituted with an equal amount of Sr^{2+} or Ba^{2+}. Addition of these ions in the continued presence of 5 mM Ca^{2+} has little effect on the EPSP but the muscle action potential was greatly increased in amplitude and prolonged in duration. When the Ba^{2+} concentration was high (79 mM) neuromuscular transmission was irreversibly blocked (Werman et al., 1961).

Effects of Mg^{2+}

The EPSPs were reduced and eventually transmission was blocked on increasing Mg^{2+} from its normal level (10 mM), but reduction of Mg^{2+} to

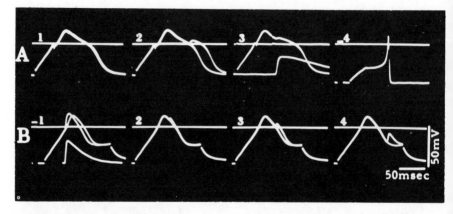

FIG. 3. Reversal potential measurements in high-Mg^{2+} media. TEA⁺ were previously injected into the muscle fiber as in Fig. 1. **A1–4:** in 56 mM Mg^{2+} medium. **A4** was taken before TEA⁺ injection. **B1–4:** in 84 mM Mg^{2+} medium. In **A3** and **B1** each EPSP at the resting potential level is shown.

less than 1 mM had little effect. When 5 mM Ca^{2+} was present, the addition of more than 100 mM Mg^{2+} was required to block the EPSP. This Mg^{2+} effect was reversible. In Mg^{2+}-free sucrose-substituted medium the E_{EPSP} was about -7 mV and appeared to shift to almost $+45$ mV (by extrapolation technique) in increasing Mg^{2+} to 84 mM. Reversal potentials determined by superimposing neurally evoked responses on TEA-induced spikes also gave a positive shift (Fig. 3). Even at the peak of the TEA spike, when the conductance of the muscle membrane is relatively high, the superimposed EPSP continued to be an additional positive-going change in the membrane potential. These data suggest that the postsynaptic membrane becomes permeable to Mg^{2+} during transmitter action.

Effects of Anion Substitution

Neuromuscular transmission was maintained more than an hour after replacement of Cl^- by other anions such as NO_3^-, acetate$^-$, propionate$^-$, and methylsulfate$^-$. Changes in E_{EPSP} were not observed in 100 mM methylsulfate medium in the presence of 30 mM Cl^-. The resting potentials increased by 10 to 30 mV on substituting acetate$^-$ for Cl^- in the standard saline. The E_{EPSP} appeared to shift in 83% of the preparations toward inside-negativity (range of E_{EPSP} -5 to -15 mV); in the other preparations no shift was observed.

DISCUSSION

The chemical nature of the transmitter substance at the mealworm neuromuscular junction is not known. The bath application of L-glutamate depolarizes the muscle fibers as has been observed in other insect preparations (Kerkut and Walker, 1966; Usherwood, 1969). However, we have neither succeeded to record a glutamate potential by its electrophoretic application onto the muscle surface nor did we observe the occurrence of spontaneous miniature EPSPs (Usherwood, 1961). Antagonistic actions of Ca^{2+} and Mg^{2+} on the transmission process were similar to those seen in many examples of excitatory synapses in a variety of preparations. The reversal potential of the EPSP at the mealworm neuromuscular junction was 0 mV, which is presumably the ionic equilibrium potential of the ions involved in generating the EPSP. The identical reversal potential has been observed in the locust jumping leg muscle (Del Castillo et al., 1953). The shift of the reversal potential in the negative direction in reduced $(Na^+)_0$ or $(K^+)_0$ media appears to indicate that both Na^+ and K^+ contribute in the generation of the EPSP. In the present study the permeability ratio of Na^+ and K^+ has not been determined. The postsynaptic membrane also appears to have undergone increases in permeability to Ca^{2+} and Mg^{2+}, since the E_{EPSP} shifted to the positive direction in increased $(Ca^{2+})_0$ or $(Mg^{2+})_0$ media. Although there are several examples of increased permeability of the postsynaptic membrane to Ca^{2+} during transmitter action the contribution of Ca^{2+} current to the EPSP in a normal saline is generally known to be very small (Del Castillo and Katz, 1955; Takeuchi, 1963; Katz and Miledi, 1969; Ruiz-Manresa and Grundfest, 1971; Kusano et al., 1974). Moreover, it has been observed in the amphibian preparations that an increase in $(Ca^{2+})_0$ shifts E_{EPSP} in a negative direction (Takeuchi, 1963; Koketsu, 1969). As explained by Takeuchi (1963) an increase in $(Ca^{2+})_0$ decreases the ratio of the Na^+ and K^+ conductance changes $(\Delta g_{Na}/\Delta g_K)$ at the endplate membrane during transmitter action specifically by reducing Δg_{Na}. The positive shift of E_{EPSP} in the mealworm neuromuscular junction in high-$(Ca^{2+})_0$

media is unique. Present data, however, do not specify whether a large Ca^{2+} current contributes directly to the EPSP or whether Ca^{2+} modifies the postsynaptic membrane permeability by altering other ionic conductances. Although it may not be applicable to the postsynaptic membrane, it has been observed that the Na^+ conductance of the electrically excitable muscle membrane of mealworm decreases in high-$(Ca^{2+})_0$ media, but the K^+ conductance increases (*unpublished*). In high-$(Mg^{2+})_0$ media the amplitude of the EPSP became smaller but the E_{EPSP} shifted in a positive direction. Mg^{2+} presumably reduced the transmitter output at the nerve terminal but like Ca^{2+} it appears to be permeant at the postsynaptic membrane, because of its effect on E_{EPSP}. This is perhaps significant in insects, which contain a high concentration of Mg^{2+} in their hemolymph. Results of anionic effects on E_{EPSP} are less concrete. As observed in other excitatory synapses the E_{EPSP} did not change when $(Cl^-)_0$ was substituted for by nonphysiological anions, such as methylsulfate. However, in some fibers, the E_{EPSP} shifted in the negative direction, for example, in the acetate-substituted saline. Since Ca^{2+} and Mg^{2+} concentrations were kept constant in these modified media, it is possible that the activities of these divalent cations might have been lowered, resulting in the observed negative shift of E_{EPSP}.

ACKNOWLEDGMENTS

This work was supported in part by grants from the Muscular Dystrophy Association of America, Inc., by Public Health Service Grants to Dr. Harry Grundfest, and by the National Institute of Neurological and Communicative Disorders and Stroke (NS 12275) to K. K.

REFERENCES

Belton, P., and Grundfest, H. (1962): Potassium activation and K-spikes in muscle fibers of the mealworm larva (*Tenebrio molitor*). *Am. J. Physiol.*, 203:588–594.

Bennett, M. V. L., Freeman, A. R., and Thaddeus, P. (1966): Reversal of post-synaptic potentials in non-isopotential system. *Abstr. Biophys. Soc.*, p. 122.

Buck, J. B. (1953): *Insect Physiology*, edited by K. D. Roeder, Chap. 6. John Wiley, New York.

Cerf, J. A., Grundfest, H., Hoyle, G., and McCann, F. V. (1959): The mechanism of dual responsiveness in muscle fibers of the grasshopper *Romalea microptera*. *J. Gen. Physiol.*, 43:377–395.

Coombs, J. S., Eccles, J. C., and Fatt, P. (1955): Excitatory synaptic action in motoneurons. *J. Physiol.*, 130:376–395.

Del Castillo, J., Hoyle, G., and Machne, X. (1953): Neuromuscular transmission in a locust. *J. Physiol.*, 121:539–547.

Del Castillo, J., and Katz, B. (1955): Local activity at a depolarized nerve-muscle junction. *J. Physiol.*, 128:396–411.

Fatt, P., and Katz, B. (1952): The effect of sodium ions on neuromuscular transmission. *J. Physiol.*, 118:73–87.

Katz, B., and Miledi, R. (1969): Spontaneous and evoked activity of motor nerve endings in calcium Ringer. *J. Physiol.*, 203:689–706.

Kerkut, G. A., and Walker, R. J. (1966): The effect of L-glutamate, acetylcholine and gamma-aminobutyric acid on the miniature end-plate potentials and contractures of the coxal muscle of the cockroach, *Periplaneta americana. Comp. Biochem. Physiol.,* 17:435–454.

Koketsu, K. (1969): *Calcium and excitable cell membrane.* In: *Neurosciences Research I,* edited by S. Ehrenpreis and O. C. Solnitzky, pp. 2–39. Academic Press, New York.

Kusano, K., and Grundfest, H. (1966): Ionic requirements for synaptic electrogenesis in neuromuscular transmission of mealworm larvae (*Tenebrio molitor*). *J. Gen Physiol.,* 50:1092.

Kusano, K., Miledi, R., and Stinnakre, J. (1974): Aequorin injections in the post-synaptic side of the squid giant synapse. XXVI. International Congress of Physiological Sciences (Abstract #458).

Reuben, J. P., Werman, R., and Grundfest, H. (1961): The ionic mechanism of hyperpolarizing responses in lobster muscle fibers. *J. Gen. Physiol.,* 45:243–265.

Ruiz-Manresa, F., and Grundfest, H. (1971): Synaptic electrogenesis in eel electroplaques. *J. Gen. Physiol.,* 57:71–92.

Takeuchi, N. (1963): Effects of calcium on the conductance change of the end-plate membrane during the action of transmitter. *J. Physiol.,* 45:243–265.

Takeuchi, A., and Takeuchi, N. (1960): On the permeability of end-plate membrane during the action of transmitter. *J. Physiol.,* 154:52–67.

Usherwood, P. N. R. (1961): Spontaneous miniature potentials from insect muscle fibers. *Nature,* 191:814–815.

Usherwood, P. N. R. (1969): *Electrochemistry of insect muscle. Advances in Insect Physiology,* edited by J. W. L. Beament, J. E. Treherne, and V. B. Wigglesworth, Vol. 6, pp. 205–271. Academic Press, New York.

Woods, D. W. (1957): The effect of ions upon neuromuscular transmission in a herbivorous insect. *J. Physiol.,* 138:119–139.

Werman, R., McCann, F. V., and Grundfest, H. (1961): Graded and all-or-none electrogenesis in arthropod muscle. I. The effects of alkali-earth cations on the neuromuscular system of *Romalea microptera. J. Gen. Physiol.,* 44:979–995.

Wyatt, G. R., and Kalf, G. F. (1957): The chemistry of insect hemolymph. II. Trehalose and other carbohydrates. *J. Gen. Physiol.,* 40:833–847.

Electrobiology of Nerve, Synapse, and Muscle,
edited by J. P. Reuben, D. P. Purpura, M. V. L. Bennett,
and E. R. Kandel. Raven Press, New York © 1976

Transmission at the Hatchetfish Giant Synapse

Michael V. L. Bennett, Stephen M. Highstein, and Pat G. Model

Department of Neuroscience, Albert Einstein College of Medicine, Yeshiva University, Bronx, New York 10461

The hatchetfish giant synapse was discovered in Harry Grundfest's Laboratory of Neurophysiology. In view of the celebratory nature of this volume, it may be appropriate to relate some of the unwritten synaptic history. Although the major experimental work was carried out in Harry's lab, the usual dilatory procedures delayed full publication until a number of us (including the first and third authors of this chapter) had left that island center of civilization and voyaged to the mainland for the greener pastures of the northeast Bronx.

The Grundfest environment of that period was most conducive to examination of a variety of preparations to establish the constellations of properties of excitable systems. At that time, one of us was looking in a number of preparations for electrotonic synapses. Electrical transmission had proved common in the highly synchronously responding nuclei controlling electric organs, but there was considerable resistance among physiologists to the idea that electrical synapses might be found more generally, even (perish the thought) in integrative centers of mammals (cf. Sloper, 1971). Thus, looking for electrical synapses in more conventional motor systems seemed to be a good approach for establishing a greater generality of electrical transmission, and, although at that time there were no obvious points of attack in the mammal, there were possibilities in lower vertebrates. A trip to the back country in Venezuela, in pursuit of electric fishes, produced the interesting rumor that hatchetfish flew, not by gliding as is obvious from the small size of their pectoral fins (Fig. 1), but by flapping like a bumblebee for which a similar large degree of wing loading has been often remarked. While daydreaming in a tropical fish store, an encounter with a tank full of hatchetfish elicited the notion that the controlling pectoral fin motoneurons would be electrically coupled to mediate the fast synchronous activity of flying. A few specimens were brought back to the lab, sent off to histology for silver staining, and casually examined. There were large motoneurons the location of which suggested that they were those innervating the pectoral fin depressor muscles, and preliminary physiological experiments so identified them and showed them to be coupled. Moreover, there were several re-

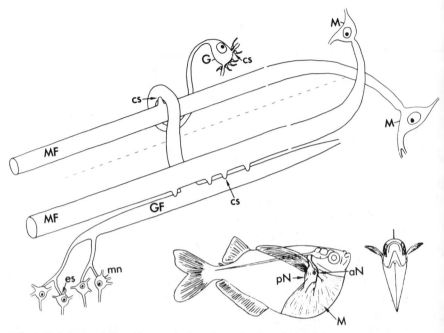

FIG. 1. Relations of Mauthner and giant fibers in the hatchetfish. In the large diagram, the course of a single giant fiber (GF) is shown with its relations to the two presynaptic Mauthner fibers (MF) and to the postsynaptic motoneurons (mn). Several giant fibers are found on each side. G, cell body of the giant fiber; M, cell body of the Mauthner fiber; es, electrical synapse; and cs, chemical synapse. The midline is indicated by the dashed line. **Inset:** Side and front views of the fish. The side view shows the brain and spinal cord, the muscles (M) that depress the pectoral fins, the anterior nerve (aN) to the depressor muscles, which is the principal nerve, and the smaller posterior nerve (pN). The anterior nerve arises from the base of the medulla. (From Model et al., 1975.)

markably large fibers in the medulla in addition to the Mauthner fibers. And, as destructive as paraffin embedding is, there were clear synapses between these giant fibers and the Mauthner fibers (Fig. 2). Each giant fiber synapsed with both Mauthner fibers (Figs. 1 and 2) and the flow of activity, subsequently verified, appeared to be that each Mauthner fiber excited giant fibers on both sides and that the giant fibers excited the pectoral fin motoneurons. Thus, a tail flip to either side mediated by a Mauthner fiber would be accompanied by pectoral fin depression on both sides. This connectivity requires that the Mauthner fiber–giant fiber synapses be unidirectional; otherwise, one Mauthner fiber would activate the other by way of the giant fibers, which would have the fish trying the impossible task of flipping its tail to both sides at the same time.

Another working hypothesis was that the giant synapses were electrotonic, to save on latency of the escape reflex. If they were electrotonic they would probably be rectifying in order to be unidirectional. However, when the hachetfish was proposed to Albert A. Auerbach as a subject for

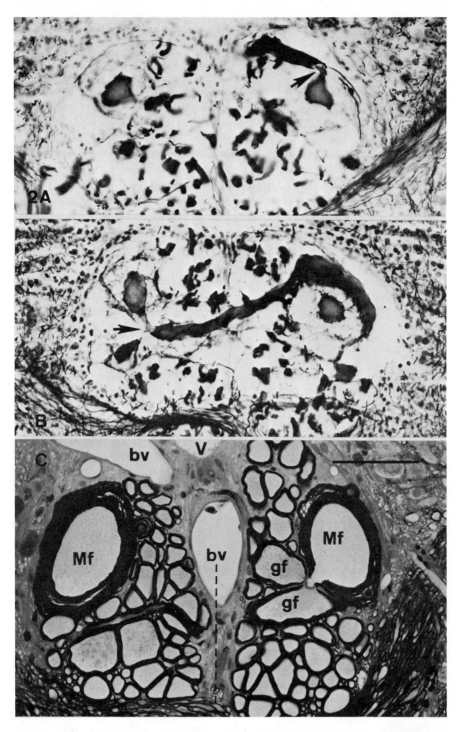

FIG. 2. Light micrographs of Mauthner fiber–giant fiber synapses. **A:** Silver-stained paraffin embedded cross section through the medulla showing a portion of a giant fiber proceeding from right to left after synapsing (*arrow*) with the near Mauthner fiber. **B:** Similar preparation showing a giant fiber proceeding from right to left across the midline to synapse (*arrow*) with the far Mauthner fiber. **C:** Epon-embedded 4-μm thick cross section stained with osmic acid and toluidine blue. On the right, a short myelinated process extends from the Mauthner fiber (Mf) to synapse with two postsynaptic giant fibers (gf). V, fourth ventricle; bv, blood vessel. The midline is indicated by the dashed line. ×380; scale, 50 μm. (**C** from Model et al., 1975.)

Ph.D. research, characterization of an axoaxonic synapse seemed a formidable problem to pose to a student. The motoneurons were thought to provide a more tractable subject for thesis work. As it turned out, he soon mastered the technical problems of working with the synapse (in what now is a rather simple preparation), and the betting concerning mode of transmission was proved wrong when he obtained convincing evidence that transmission at the synapse is chemical (Auerbach and Bennett, 1969a). That the preparation itself is more interesting than expected is some consolation for being wrong; little further consolation can be taken from the unexpected although reasonable finding that the giant fibers form rectifying electrotonic synapses on the motoneurons (Auerbach and Bennett, 1969b).

PROPERTIES OF THE SYNAPSE

The morphology and physiology of the hatchetfish giant synapse have been described in detail elsewhere (Auerbach and Bennett, 1969a; Model et al., 1975; Highstein and Bennett, 1975; Bennett et al., 1976; Highstein et al., 1976), and only a brief summary will be presented here. At the fine structural level, a synapse that has been stimulated little or not at all displays the typical characteristics associated with chemical transmission. The Mauthner fiber terminals contain numerous clear vesicles 400 to 600 Å in diameter (Fig. 3). There are dense projections into the Mauthner cytoplasm from the presynaptic membrane. Vesicles, which are clustered in the vicinity of the presynaptic membrane, closely approach the presynaptic membrane only in the immediate neighborhood of the dense projections. We presume that vesicles are released alongside the dense projections as is suggested by data from other central synapses (Pfenninger et al., 1969; Streit et al., 1972). We also presume that the vesicles close to the membrane comprise the "immediately available store" of transmitter that can be acted upon by action potentials in the presynaptic fiber. In the unstimulated synapse, there are a few tubular profiles of smooth membranes with occasional coated vesicles attached.

Tetanic stimulation drastically alters the morphological appearance. After 10 min at 10/sec (and several minutes rest during preparation for fixation by perfusion), the vesicles are largely depleted, and appear to be replaced by numerous irregular membranous compartments in the same region of the terminal (Fig. 4). Coated vesicles or pits are frequently attached to these compartments. Apparently the quantity of membrane in the ending is more or less preserved, but the membrane of the vesicles has been transferred to the irregular compartments. After an hour or two of rest, the irregular compartments disappear and the vesicles reappear, which suggests interconversion from one to the other.

The effects of cooling indicate that the vesicular membrane first becomes part of the external surface and then is reinternalized by coated vesicles.

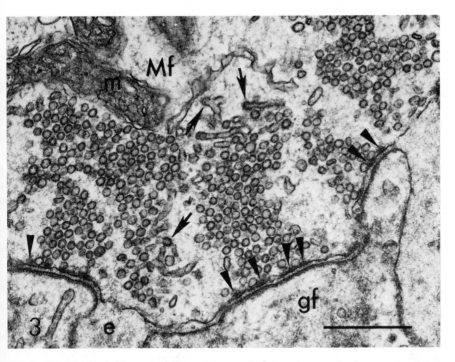

FIG. 3. The Mauthner fiber–giant fiber synapse, electron micrograph of an unstimulated control. The Mauthner terminal is in synaptic contact with a giant fiber. The numerous synaptic vesicles are of conventional morphology. Tubular smooth-surfaced endoplasmic reticulum extends into the synaptic region of the presynaptic terminal (Mf). Some coated vesicles are fused with the tubules (*arrows*). Dense cytoplasmic material is associated with both the pre- and postsynaptic membranes in the contact regions, and on the presynaptic membrane some of this material forms dense projections (*arrowheads*). Smooth vesicles closely approach the surface membrane only near these projections. Between the vesicles there is a fine filamentous meshwork. gf, postsynaptic giant fiber; m, mitochrondrion; e, extracellular channel. ×48,500; scale, 0.5 μm. (From Model et al., 1975.)

When a preparation is stimulated tetanically while cooling to 12 to 14°C, a picture is seen that is in dramatic contrast to that in Fig. 4. Vesicles are greatly depleted, but instead of irregular compartments there are great whorls of double membranes inside the Mauthner terminal (Fig. 5). The membranes prove to be still connected to the external surface, and they have attached to them large numbers of coated vesicles. Evidently, cooling to this level does not prevent the release of transmitter by exocytosis (Highstein et al., 1975) but does prevent reinternalization of membrane by coat material. Coated vesicles can still form but apparently are unable to break off from the surface.

Several possible reasons can be adduced for block of membrane reuptake by cooling, such as endothermic nature of the coat material reaction or stiffening of the lipids. It seems plausible that deforming planar membrane into a highly curved vesicular form would require energy, whereas

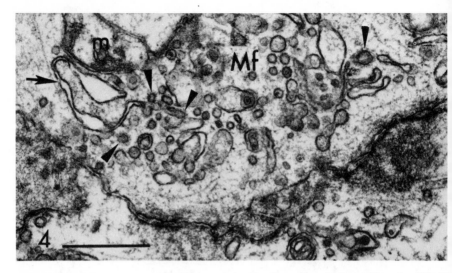

FIG. 4. A depleted synapse. Stimulation of the Mauthner fiber (Mf) at 10/sec for 10 min causes profound changes in the presynaptic element; synaptic vesicles are greatly reduced in number and there is a marked accumulation of irregular membranous compartments. Some of these compartments are in the form of flattened cysternae (*arrow*), but most are irregular in outline. Coated vesicles are fused with the membranes delimiting some of the irregular structures (*arrowheads*) and only an occasional apparently unattached coated vesicle is present. A few synaptic vesicles of normal appearance remain. The mitochondrion (m) is swollen. ×48,500; scale, 0.5 μm. (From Model et al., 1975.)

flattening of a vesicle into the rather planar external surface would not. The degree of cooling that we used would not be great for many cold-blooded forms, but it is much more severe than these tropical fish would normally see.

A similar effect is seen in the turtle retina in which cooling to 4°C appears to prevent membrane reuptake at photoreceptor synapses (Schaeffer and Raviola, 1975). However, no coated vesicles or pits are seen at this temperature, which may be too low even to allow them to form.

In the neuromuscular junction, it has been possible to trace membrane from external surface to internal compartment by peroxidase uptake (Heuser and Reese, 1973). The same techniques should be applicable to the hatchetfish synapse. The increase in external surface seen when the hatchetfish is cooled appears in some respects similar to the increase in surface that can be seen at the neuromuscular junction when fixation is applied during evoked release (Heuser and Reese, 1974); both fixation and cold block reuptake sooner than they block release and thus lead to an accumulation of membrane in the surface.

The giant synapse is a relay in that at low frequencies a single impulse in a Mauthner fiber produces a large postsynaptic potential (PSP) in each giant fiber that initiates one impulse. The synapse is chemically transmitting as indicated by the 0.3 to 0.4-msec irreducible delay between pre- and post-

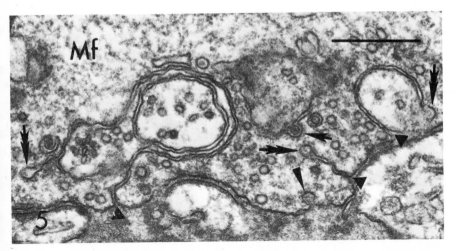

FIG. 5. A synapse stimulated during cooling to 12°C. Vesicles are depleted, but irregular compartments like those in Fig. 4 are absent. Instead, whorls of paired parallel membranes are present in the synaptic region. The parallel membranes are continuous with the plasma membrane of the terminal (*triangles*) and represent extensive invaginations of the presynaptic membrane. Many coated pits and vesicles are attached to the outer surface (*arrowhead*) and invaginating membranes (*arrow*), frequently at their innermost edges (*double arrows*). Mf, Mauthner fiber. ×48,500; scale, 0.5 μm. (From Model et al., 1975.)

synaptic responses (Fig. 6), and by inversion of the PSP when the inside is made sufficiently positive (Auerbach and Bennett, 1969a). A further indication is the absence of electrotonic coupling, a negative finding that is made reliable by the anatomical knowledge that the electrodes are very close to the synapse and that the synaptic projection of the Mauthner fiber is so short as to be isopotential.

It is easy to record miniature postsynaptic potentials (mPSPs) in the giant fiber. At least some of these arise from the Mauthner fibers, for when

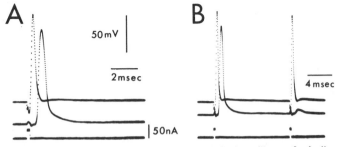

FIG. 6. Synaptic transmission between Mauthner and giant fibers. **A:** A directly evoked spike in a Mauthner fiber (*upper trace*, current on *lower trace*) is followed by a spike in a giant fiber (*middle trace*). **B:** Paired stimulation of the Mauthner fiber with a 12-msec interval between stimuli. The PSP is greatly reduced and fails to initiate an impulse in the giant fiber. (From Highstein and Bennett, 1975.)

directly depolarizing the Mauthner fiber, mPSPs can be evoked at a lower level than that at which an impulse is initiated (Auerbach and Bennett, 1969a; Auerbach, 1971). Almost as convincing as the effect of direct depolarization is the increase in frequency of mPSPs during tetanic stimulation, similar to that which is observed at the neuromuscular junction (Hurlbut et al., 1971). Moreover, curare which blocks the Mauthner fiber–giant fiber PSP also blocks the miniatures (Highstein and Bennett, 1975). Morphological study indicates that there are no other synapses on the giant fibers close to the Mauthner fiber synapses. However, in penicillin-treated preparations slow depolarizations are observed that may come from the giant fiber cell bodies or the postsynaptic motoneurons to which the giant fibers are electrotonically coupled (Model et al., 1972; Spira and Bennett, 1972). Unlike the mPSPs, these responses are not blocked by curare.

When the Mauthner fibers are stimulated at a gradually increasing frequency, the PSP in the giant fiber gets steadily smaller. The remarkable observation is that it can be run down essentially into the noise level, but it does not show failures under these conditions even though PSP amplitude becomes small compared to the size of a miniature (Auerbach and Bennett, 1969a; Fig. 7). (Some essentially normal sized mPSPs often persist during rundown. As discussed further below, we believe that these come from regions of the synapse not affected by the action potential and that they are irrelevant to the evoked PSPs.) The observation of very small PSPs without failures is not what one would expect from simple application of the quantal hypothesis (Katz, 1969). According to the theory, if mean PSP amplitude is in the neighborhood of the size of individual quanta, PSP amplitude becomes highly variable, and shows failures; that is, sometimes the PSP consists of one or two or more quanta and other times no quanta are released at all. Three simple explanations consistent with the quantal hypothesis can be adduced to explain our observations: (1) Quantal number is large to explain the absence of failures, but quantal size is reduced because vesicles are released before there is adequate time to fill them. This is the explanation we favor. (2) Quantal number is large, but quantal size is reduced through desensitization. (3) Only small numbers of quanta are released but with a high probability so that failures are not observed.

The last possibility is easiest to exclude because the PSP is smoothly graded in amplitude, even in the range of the size of a single quantum and below.

The desensitization hypothesis is made unlikely by the time courses of depression and recovery of PSP amplitude (Fig. 8). The PSP runs down fairly gradually during a long train of stimuli. If the train is interrupted briefly, for as little as a second, PSP amplitude recovers sufficiently so that the next PSP is adequate to initiate a spike. However, as the train is resumed, the PSP falls very rapidly again to its previous depressed level; the decline requires only a few stimuli and is much more rapid than the

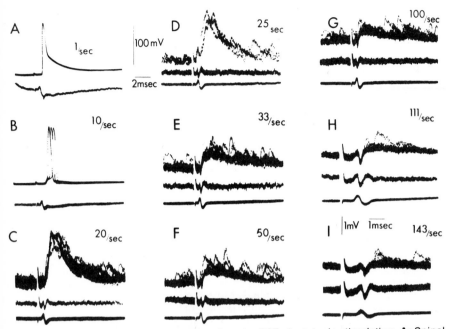

FIG. 7. Reduction of evoked PSPs to the size of mPSPs by tetanic stimulation. **A:** Spinal stimulation at a low rate (1/sec) showing the intracellularly recorded spike in the giant fiber (*upper trace*) and the field of the Mauthner and giant fibers recorded extracellularly on the lateral line lobe (*lower trace*). **B:** After some seconds of stimulation at 10/sec, the rate of rise of the PSP is reduced, but initiation of impulses in the giant fiber persists. Recorded as in **A. C:** At 20/sec stimulation, PSP amplitude is reduced below threshold. The upper trace is a high-gain intracellular recording. The middle trace is a just extracellular recording obtained subsequently at the same gain and stimulation frequency. The lower trace is a field recording as in **A. D–I:** Progressively increasing frequencies of stimulation (display as in **C,** faster sweep in **H** and **I**). The PSP becomes progressively and gradually smaller in amplitude until it is smaller than the mPSPs simultaneously recorded, which have changed little in amplitude. The evoked PSPs are longer in time course than the mPSPs. At the onset of stimulation, the frequency of mPSPs increases but then it decreases again, although not to zero. The mPSPs are generated at any time during the stimulation cycle, and show little preferential occurrence during the evoked PSPs. (From Highstein et al., 1975.)

initial rundown. This observation is unlike desensitization that has been observed at other synapses.

The partial filling hypothesis can explain the data provided vesicles are released before there is time to fill them completely. After prolonged stimulation that reduces PSPs to quantal size, the endings are largely depleted of vesicles; thus, the transmitter is likely to be released from newly formed vesicles that may not have had time to fill. One may then ask how long it takes to fill a vesicle. The rapid recovery of PSP amplitude following a tetanus suggests that vesicles can be filled in less than a second, which is remarkably fast. In this period, presumably only a few vesicles are filled since the subsequent rundown in PSP amplitude is so rapid. Furthermore,

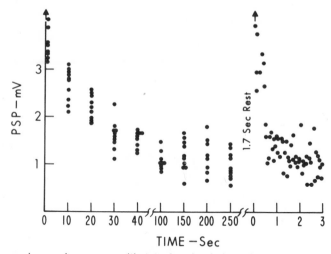

FIG. 8. Depression and recovery with tetanic stimulation. Successive PSP amplitudes are shown after the indicated periods of stimulation for up to 250 sec of stimulation, by which time a steady mean PSP level had been reached. At the onset of the tetanus the first 10 stimuli elicited spikes (*up-pointing arrow*), and PSP amplitudes are shown for immediately subsequent stimuli. The tetanus was stopped for 1.7 sec after 270 sec. During this rest, the PSP recovered sufficiently to initiate a spike but after 10 further stimuli, PSP amplitude had returned to its depleted value. This result suggests that PSP reduction is not due to desensitization.

after a prolonged rundown, as much as 45 min is required for recovery of amplitude of the last response to a brief train of three stimuli, which is consistent with the slow recovery of the vesicle population observed morphologically.

Further support for the rapidity of filling was obtained through analysis of amplitude variations of the recovering PSP. For this purpose, trains of 15 or more stimuli (20 to 25 msec apart) were given at various frequencies until a steady state of responding was reached. The first PSP thus had a known time for recovery with each presentation. From the assumption that PSP amplitude is Poisson distributed (that is, that individual quanta are released independently of each other), an estimate of quantal size and number could be calculated from the mean and coefficient of variation (Martin, 1966). In the experiment illustrated in Fig. 9, it was observed that with 750 msec between trains quantal size recovered completely, but with 500 msec between trains it was reduced below mPSP size observed prior to the onset of stimulation. Other experiments showed complete recovery of quantal size in as little as 200 msec. Although these times are surprisingly short, they are consistent with the rapid recovery of PSP amplitude shown in Fig. 8. Also, the rapid recovery of quantal size demonstrates that the recovery in Fig. 8 is not due simply to increase in quantum number.

Two assumptions were made in this calculation of recovery time, the ef-

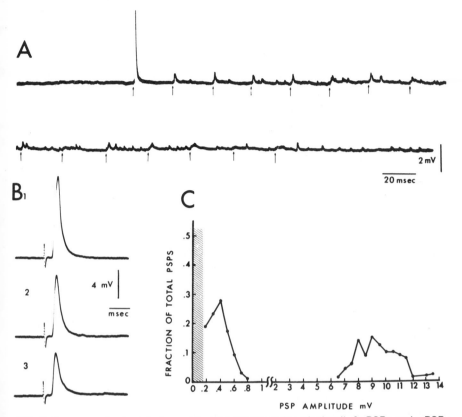

FIG. 9. Recovery of calculated quantal size between trains of stimuli. **A:** PSPs and mPSPs during a train of 15 stimuli at 25-msec intervals. The train had been repeated at 1/sec until a steady level of responding occurred. The amplitude of the last PSP in the train is comparable to the amplitude of the mPSPs. Continuous record from upper to lower trace. The mPSP frequency increased during the early part of the train. **B$_{1-3}$:** The first PSP in the train at faster sweep speed. **C:** Amplitude distributions of the first PSP and of miniature PSPs during repetition of the train at 1/sec. Mean mPSP amplitude is 0.38 mV and at this interval between trains (725 msec) quantal size calculated from variance is 0.32 mV. The noise level is indicated by cross-hatching along the ordinate. When 400 msec separated the trains, calculated quantal size was half the mPSP amplitude. (From Highstein et al., 1975.)

fects of which should be considered. First, variability of quantal size was neglected, which would at most slightly decrease the calculated recovery time over its actual value (Martin, 1966). Second, the distribution of PSP amplitudes might be a binomial instead of a Poisson distribution which would reduce variance for a given quantal size. The assumption of Poisson statistics would then tend to increase the calculated recovery time over its actual value. The probability of release is high as evaluated by the double-shock method; that is, the response to the second of a pair of stimuli separated by a short interval is greatly depressed suggesting that the first stimulus has released most of the immediately available store of vesicles. High probability of release would suggest that binomial statistics were more appropriate. However, if the number of vesicles in the immediately available store were Poisson distributed, the amplitude distribution would still be Poisson, even if probability of release were high. There appear to be many release sites (Fig. 3) and if the probability of occupation of one of these sites by a vesicle were low and independent of occupation of other sites, as is likely in the depleted synapse, then the number of vesicles in the store would be Poisson distributed.

The errors introduced by assumptions of uniform quantal size and Poisson distribution seem unlikely to be large and also should be in opposite directions. The rapidity of filling is remarkable and even a several-fold error would be unimportant at the present level of analysis.

To return to the main line of argument, recovery of PSP amplitude and of quantal size is very rapid. Furthermore, quantal size appears to decrease continually at shorter intervals between stimuli, and it follows that stimulated release can interrupt filling. From this conclusion it appears likely that filling takes place at or very close to the release sites. Certainly, the hypothesis that filling and release sites are the same would account for gradual recovery of quantal size following a tetanus. This hypothesis, although not immediately compelling, becomes more so if one considers alternatives. The rapidity of recovery strongly implies that vesicles are formed empty and filled rapidly. If vesicles were filled anywhere in the ending, it would be expected that they would arrive at the release sites after different delays and that some would be filled and some would be relatively empty. If one estimates a diffusion coefficient for synaptic vesicles of 10^{-7} cm^2/sec (A. Finkelstein, *personal communication*), the diffusion time for 1 μm is 0.1 sec. Since the distance between irregular compartments and release sites is about 1 μm, vesicles would occupy an appreciable fraction of a filling time in diffusing to the release sites. Although one might postulate (or even anticipate) active movement of vesicles via filaments, the times required would still appear to be rather long; yet, at high frequencies of stimulation few if any vesicles arrive full.

Another possibility might be that all the vesicles are filled anywhere in the ending and are in rapid equilibrium with each other through the cytoplasm. This suggestion seems unlikely because of the rapid re-rundown of quantal size following a brief interruption of a tetanus. A major change in total transmitter levels would have to occur very rapidly.

In the development of our analysis of transmission at this synapse, the properties of the mPSPs proved most confusing. An early concern was that if quantal size were reduced by tetanic stimulation, then one ought to see gradual recovery of spontaneous mPSPs following a tetanus. At most, small reductions in mean mPSP amplitudes were observed during and after tetani. The failure to observe small mPSPs is now completely understandable;

quantal size recovers so rapidly that we were sampling mPSPs after they had recovered fully in amplitude. Furthermore, the half time before a vesicle is released as a miniature is likely to be much longer than the time for filling. The mPSPs that persist during a tetanus led us down another false trail. We thought that the persistence of mPSPs at full size excluded desensitization. At first, it seemed that the persistent mPSPs could be vesicles from deep in the ending that were late in arriving at the release sites. However, since they are not released at all synchronously with evoked release (although they do show some tetanic increase in frequency), a different mechanism or site of release is indicated. If the site of release is different, then desensitization at the site of evoked release cannot be excluded.

The persistent mPSPs may after all be of some interest. In electron microscopy, stimulated endings often show a region where there are relatively large numbers of vesicles remaining and where the ending has an appearance not very different from the control. Perhaps these sites are responsible for the persistent mPSPs, but are insensitive to the action potential. If there is turnover of synaptic regions, these insensitive regions could represent new synaptic areas forming or old ones no longer mediating evoked release that will eventually be destroyed. A possible related form of nonfunctional synaptic area occurs at electrotonic synapses in which morphologically defined active zones for chemical transmission are frequently found without there being a demonstrable chemical component to the PSPs (Bennett, 1972).

FURTHER DISCUSSION

Given that a synaptic terminal synthesizes transmitter or takes it up from its environment and given that transmitter release involves exocytosis, membrane recycling in formation of new synaptic vesicles seems of obvious utility. Generality of the mechanism is made more likely by observations suggesting that recycling can occur in the absence of transmitter in the vesicles (Ceccarelli et al., 1973). However, for a neurosecretory cell secreting a peptide synthesized in the cell body, membrane recycling with local filling in the terminal probably does not occur. Nevertheless, membrane added to the surface by exocytosis of neurosecretory granules must be removed and apparently it is retrieved by endocytosis (Douglas et al., 1970). The retrieved membrane subsequently may be broken down in lysosomes as indicated for chromaffin cells of the adrenal medulla (Holtzman et al., 1973).

Even for a synapse locally packaging its transmitter the synthetic machinery must itself be synthesized in the cell body and transported down the axon, probably via the rapid axonal transport mechanism. The retrograde transport of extracellular proteins in membrane-bounded compartments, as revealed by peroxidase technique, provides another possible fate for membranes of a terminal (Teichberg et al., 1975). The relative levels of anterograde and retrograde transport and of membrane recycling are as yet incompletely determined for any cell and are certain to vary in different cell types and perhaps in different endings of the same cell.

A factor in local recycling and transport is likely to be the length of the axon. Although a given rate of transport can be equally well mediated by long and short axons, and rates shouldn't depend on axonal length, signaling to cause alterations of rates would require closer proximity of synthetic and secretory sites. A spectrum may be noted: at the neuro-muscular junction very little labeled material is transported in a retrograde fashion (Heuser and Reese, 1973). In tissue cultures of embryonic nerve and muscle, a large fraction of peroxidase taken up during activity is transported to the cell body (Teichberg et al., 1975).

It should be admitted that there is uncertainty as to how many vesicles comprise a quantum measured postsynaptically. At the neuromuscular junction, the observation of very small mPSPs and apparent multimodal distribution of quantal sizes has led to the suggestion that individual quanta may be due to multivesicular release (Kriebel and Gross, 1974). Further-more, when stimulating or recording in local areas, the number of quanta in the immediately available store corresponds more nearly to the number of morphologically described active zones than to the number of vesicles near them, which is consistent with simultaneous release of all the vesicles at an active zone (Wernig, 1975; Zucker, 1973). An alternative to the partial fill-ing hypothesis for the hatchetfish synapse might be that the quantum size is reduced because the number of vesicles contributing to the quantum is reduced. This explanation does not require the discharge of partially filled vesicles. It does however involve some mechanism of simultaneously activating release of a number of single vesicles. For miniatures this would require a short range interaction not mediated by membrane potential, and one would expect exocytotic figures to be clustered. No evidence for as-sociated release of closely neighboring vesicles has been found in freeze fracture preparations of the neuromuscular junction (Heuser et al., 1974). The case for multivesicular quanta is not convincing at this point and alternative explanations can be proposed. For example, if the cysternae from which the vesicles are formed contain a small amount of acetylcholine, small spontaneous miniatures could represent vesicles that had not visited a filling site and were discharged elsewhere.

A further uncertainty is present in the correspondence between vesicles and quanta. Although there is little doubt that the ultimate fate of a synaptic vesicle is exocytosis, a vesicle conceivably undergoes several transient contacts with the surface, each releasing transmitter, before it finally joins the external surface. A correspondence between mPSPs recorded and vesicle counts will not necessarily resolve this issue because the error introduced by multiquantal release could be opposite and canceling. It does seem more reasonable to us that once a vesicle opens to the exterior, surface tension forces it to fuse completely with the external membrane.

The demonstrability of vesicular depletion varies in different systems. The hatchetfish giant synapse, functioning as it does in an escape reflex, probably operates very phasically; that is, not at all most of the time and at high frequency for brief periods. With such a pattern of usage (and it would be pleasant to verify this with field observations) a high possible rate of release of vesicles with slow recovery is reasonable, and it would be interesting to know how the rates of muscle fatigue and adaptation in afferent pathways compare with the time course of depression at the synapse. In systems such as weakly electric organs that fire continuously at high frequencies (for example 300 to 600/sec in *Eigenmannia*), transmitter release and formation of vesicles are in a steady state. A normal complement of vesicles is present in active organs (Schwartz et al., 1975), and one would not expect that stimulation would produce vesicular depletion. An illustrative case is the crayfish neuromuscular junction in which 10/sec stimulation produces depletion only in 2,4-dinitrophenol (DNP)-treated preparations (Atwood et al., 1972). The poisoning apparently slows formation of new vesicles, and destroys the balance between release and formation in the untreated preparation.

Close proximity of filling and release sites not only best explains the responses in the hatchetfish; it is consistent with a number of other data in the literature. There is evidence from the sympathetic ganglion and from the cerebral cortex that transmitter released by stimulation is enriched in recently synthesized material as compared to the total transmitter pool (Barker et al., 1972; Birks and Fitch, 1974; Chakrin et al., 1972; Collier, 1969). This could arise if filling of newly formed vesicles occurred at the release sites. Of course, the time scale of the tracer experiments is much longer than that of our physiological observations. Preferential release of newly synthesized transmitter could occur if transmitter were loaded into the vesicles as it was synthesized, but presumably free cytoplasmic transmitter is also available for loading into vesicles and release. There are physiological data from the neuromuscular junction that are consistent with filling at release sites. In hemicholinium-poisoned muscle that has been stimulated to the point where quantal size is greatly reduced, a rest of several minutes allows a marked recovery that is quite rapidly reversed as stimulation is resumed (Elmqvist and Quastel, 1965). Elmqvist and Quastel suggest that one explanation of their findings is that "the most readily releasable [quanta], perhaps those closest to the presynaptic membrane, are those most rapidly filled as new synthesis takes place."

We suppose that in the rested synapse, vesicles away from the presynaptic membrane are for the most part filled with transmitter. If filling occurs only at release sites, it would be expected to be delayed with respect to formation of new vesicles. Thus, vesicles of stimulated endings that lack what are presumably Ca granules may represent newly formed vesicles that have not yet visited a filling site (Boyne et al., 1974; Politoff et al., 1974; Pappas and Rose, 1976). Observations on the hatchetfish do not yet exclude slow filling of vesicles away from the release sites, but following a depleting tetanus, comparison of the vesicle population and responsiveness to trains of stimuli might shed light on this question.

The hypothesis that filling and release sites are the same or very close together is subject to further experimental test. Part of the recovery of PSP amplitude is due to increase in quantum size, part is due to increase in quantum number. During the initial recovery period from a tetanus that depresses quantal size, it is likely that new empty vesicles are continuing to arrive at the filling and release sites. We plan to give subthreshold pulses to the Mauthner fiber during this period to evoke asynchronous release of quanta. Thus, we should be able to directly observe the spectrum of quantal sizes rather than infer a mean quantal size from variance and mean amplitude. We also plan to directly test for desensitization by iontophoretic application of the transmitter, which appears to be acetylcholine (Spira et al., 1970).

The diagram of Fig. 10 summarizes our conclusions. The outline of membrane recycling is similar to that proposed for the neuromuscular junction, but in this case it is based on observations of depletion, recovery, and block of reuptake of surface membranes by cold. In addition, it may be supposed that formation of new smooth vesicles from irregular compartments involves coat material just as does reinternalization of membrane in the external surface. The electrophysiological observations provide an important

PRESYNAPTIC ELEMENT

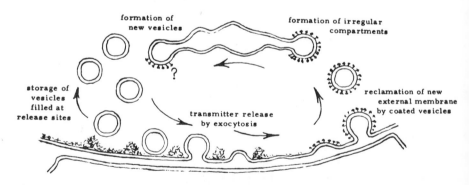

POSTSYNAPTIC ELEMENT

FIG. 10. Diagram of membrane recycling. Coat material may participate in the formation of new vesicles from the irregular compartments, a possibility suggested here by the coat material with a question mark along side. Filling is suggested to occur at or near the release sites. Newly formed vesicles are empty but may be filled at the release sites and then returned to the center of the ending to comprise a mobilizable store. (From Bennett et al., 1975.)

extension of the morphological data in suggesting that the filling of vesicles occurs at or near the sites of release.

ACKNOWLEDGMENTS

This work was supported in part by grants from the National Institutes of Health (NS-11431, NS-07512, and HD-04248) and the Alfred P. Sloan Foundation.

Dr. Highstein was supported by New York City Health Research Council Career Scientist Award I-781 and a National Institutes of Health Research Career Development Award.

REFERENCES

Atwood, H. L., Lang, F., and Morin, W. A. (1972): Synaptic vesicles: Selective depletion in crayfish excitatory and inhibitory axons. *Science*, 176:1353–1355.

Auerbach, A. A. (1971): Spontaneous and evoked quantal transmitter release at a vertebrate central synapse. *Nature*, 234:181–183.

Auerbach, A. A., and Bennett, M. V. L. (1969a): Chemically mediated transmission at a giant fiber synapse in the central nervous system of a vertebrate. *J. Gen. Physiol.*, 53:183–210.

Auerbach, A. A., and Bennett, M. V. L. (1969b): A rectifying synapse in the central nervous system of a vertebrate. *J. Gen. Physiol.*, 53:211–237.

Barker, L. A., Dowdall, M. J., and Whittaker, V. P. (1972): Choline metabolism in the cerebral cortex of guinea pigs. *Biochem. J.*, 130:1063–1080.

Bennett, M. V. L. (1972): A comparison of electrically and chemically mediated transmission. In: *Structure and Function of Synapses*, edited by G. D. Pappas and D. P. Purpura, pp. 221–256. Raven Press, New York.

Bennett, M. V. L., Model, P. G., and Highstein, S. M. (1976): Stimulation induced depletion of vesicles, fatigue of transmission and recovery processes at a vertebrate central synapse. *Cold Spring Harbor Symp. Quant. Biol.*, Vol. 40 (*in press*).

Birks, R. I., and Fitch, S. J. G. (1974): Storage and release of acetylcholine in a sympathetic ganglion. *J. Physiol.*, 240:125–134.

Boyne, A. F., Bohan, T. P., and Williams, T. H. (1974): Effects of calcium-containing fixation solutions on cholinergic synaptic vesicles. *J. Cell Biol.*, 63:780–795.

Ceccarelli, B., Hurlbut, W. P., and Mauro, A. (1973): Turnover of transmitter and synaptic vesicles at the frog neuromuscular junction. *J. Cell Biol.*, 57:499–524.

Chakrin, L. W., Marchbanks, R. M., Mitchell, J. F., and Whittaker, V. P. (1972): The origin of the acetylcholine released from the surface of the cortex. *J. Neurochem.*, 19:2727–2736.

Collier, B. (1969): The preferential release of newly synthesized transmitter by a sympathetic ganglion. *J. Physiol.*, 205:341–352.

Douglas, N. W., Nagasawa, J., and Schultz, R. (1970): Electron microscope studies on the mechanism of secretion of posterior pituitary hormones and the significance of microvesicles (synaptic vesicles): Evidence of secretion by exocytosis and formation of microvesicles as a by-product of this process. *Mem. Soc. Endocrinol.*, 19:353–377.

Elmqvist, D., and Quastel, D. M. J. (1965): Presynaptic action of hemicholinium at the neuromuscular junction. *J. Physiol.*, 177:463–482.

Heuser, J. E., and Reese, T. S. (1973): Evidence for recycling of synaptic vesicle membrane during transmitter release at the frog neuromuscular junction. *J. Cell Biol.*, 57:315–344.

Heuser, J. E., and Reese, T. S. (1974): Morphology of synaptic vesicle discharge and reformation at the frog neuromuscular junction. In: *Synaptic Transmission and Neuronal Interaction*, edited by M. V. L. Bennett, pp. 59–77. Raven Press, New York.

Heuser, J. E., Reese, T. S., and Landis, D. M. D. (1974): Functional changes in frog neuromuscular junctions studied with freeze-fracture. *J. Neurocytol.*, 3:109–131.

Highstein, S. M., and Bennett, M. V. L. (1975): Fatigue and recovery of transmission at the Mauthner fiber–giant fiber synapse of the hatchetfish. *Brain Res.,* 98:229–242.

Highstein, S. M., Model, P. G., and Bennett, M. V. L. (1975): Effects of cooling on the Mauthner fiber–giant fiber synapse of the hatchetfish. *Neurosci. Abs.,* 1:646.

Highstein, S. M., Model, P. G., and Bennett, M. V. L. (1976): Repetitive stimulation, fatigue and recovery of the Mauthner fiber–giant fiber synapse of hatchetfish. In: *Mechanisms in Transmission of Signals for Conscious Behavior,* edited by T. Desiraju. Elsevier, Amsterdam (*in press*).

Holtzman, E., Teichberg, S., Abrahams, S. J., Citkowitz, E., Crain, S. M., Kawai, N., and Peterson, E. R. (1973): Notes on synaptic vesicles and related structures, endoplasmic reticulum, lysosomes, and peroxisomes in nervous tissue and the adrenal medulla. *J. Histochem. Cytochem.,* 21:349–385.

Hurlbut, W. P., Longenecker, H. B., Jr., and Mauro, A. (1971): Effects of calcium and magnesium on the frequency of miniature end-plate potentials during prolonged tetanization. *J. Physiol.,* 219:17–38.

Katz, B. (1969): *The Release of Neural Transmitter Substances.* The Sherrington Lectures. X. Liverpool Univ. 60 pp.

Kriebel, M. E., and Gross, C. (1974): Multimodal distribution of frog miniature and end plate potentials in adult, denervated, and tadpole leg muscles. *J. Gen. Physiol.,* 64:85–104.

Martin, A. R. (1966): Quantal nature of synaptic transmission. *Physiol. Rev.,* 46:51–66.

Model, P. G., Highstein, S. M., and Bennett, M. V. L. (1975): Morphological correlates of fatigue and recovery of transmission at the Mauthner fiber–giant fiber synapse of the hatchetfish. *Brain Res.,* 98:209–228.

Model, P. G., Spira, M. E., and Bennett, M. V. L. (1972): Synaptic inputs to the cell bodies of the giant fibers of the hatchetfish. *Brain Res.,* 45:288–295.

Pappas, G. D., and Rose, S. (1976): Localization of calcium deposits in the frog neuromuscular junction at rest and following stimulation. *Brain Res.,* 103:362–365.

Pfenninger, K., Sandri, C., Akert, K., and Eugster, C. H. (1969): Contribution to the problem of structural organization of the presynaptic area. *Brain Res.,* 12:10–18.

Politoff, A. L., Rose, S., and Pappas, G. D. (1974): The calcium binding sites of synaptic vesicles of the frog sartorius neuromuscular junction. *J. Cell Biol.,* 61:818–823.

Pysh, J. J., and Wiley, R. G. (1974): Synaptic vesicle depletion and recovery in cat sympathetic ganglia electrically stimulated *in vivo. J. Cell Biol.,* 60:365–374.

Schaeffer, S. M., and Raviola, E. (1976): Ultrastructural analysis of functional changes in the synaptic endings of turtle photoreceptor cells. *Cold Spring Harbor Symp. Quant. Biol.,* Vol. 40 (*in press*).

Schwartz, I. R., Pappas, G. D., and Bennett, M. V. L. (1975): The fine structure of electrocytes in weakly electric teleosts. *J. Neurocytol.,* 4:87–114.

Sloper, J. J. (1971): Dendro-dendritic synapses in the primate motor cortex. *Brain Res.,* 34:186–192.

Spira, M. E., and Bennett, M. V. L. (1972): Penicillin induced seizure activity in the hatchetfish. *Brain Res.,* 43:235–241.

Spira, M. E., Model, P. G., and Bennett, M. V. L. (1970): Cholinergic transmission at a central synapse. *J. Cell Biol.,* 47:199a–200a.

Streit, P., Akert, K., Sandri, C., Livingston, R. B., and Moor, H. (1972): Dynamic ultrastructure of presynaptic membranes at nerve terminals in the spinal cord of rats. Anesthetized and unanesthetized preparations compared. *Brain Res.,* 48:11–26.

Teichberg, T., Holtzman, E., Crain, S. M., and Peterson, E. R. (1975): Circulation and turnover of synaptic vesicle membrane in cultured fetal mammalian spinal cord neurons. *J. Cell Biol.,* 67:215–230.

Wernig, A. (1975): Estimates of statistical release parameters from crayfish and frog neuromuscular junctions. *J. Physiol.,* 244:207–221.

Zucker, R. S. (1973): Changes in the statistics of transmitter release during facilitation. *J. Physiol.,* 229:787–810.

Electrobiology of Nerve, Synapse, and Muscle,
edited by J. P. Reuben, D. P. Purpura, M. V. L. Bennett,
and E. R. Kandel. Raven Press, New York © 1976

On the Physiological Role of Slow Inhibitory Postsynaptic Potential in the Neurons of Sympathetic Ganglia

Vladimir I. Skok

Bogomoletz Institute of Physiology, Kiev, U.S.S.R.

Since the first evidence was obtained that stimulation of preganglionic fibers evokes primary hyperpolarization in the neurons of sympathetic ganglia (Lorento de Nó and Laporte, 1949), several studies have tried to clarify the neuronal pathways involved in generation of this hyperpolarization and the underlying ionic mechanisms. It has been suggested that this hyperpolarization, called the slow inhibitory postsynaptic potential (slow IPSP) is mediated by muscarinic cholinergic transmission from preganglionic fibers into small intensely fluorescent cells (SIF cells) which exert a hyperpolarizing action upon the neurons of the ganglion through the release of catecholamines (Eccles and Libet, 1961; Libet and Owman, 1974).

Evidence has been obtained that the slow IPSP is produced by the activity of an electrogenic sodium pump (Nishi and Koketsu, 1968). Other authors consider slow IPSPs to be the result of a decrease in the passive ion flux through the membrane (Engberg and Marshall, 1971). It has been commonly accepted that electrogenesis of slow IPSP differs essentially from that of the fast IPSP observed in other neurons. The slow IPSP is not followed by an increase in ionic permeability of the membrane (Nishi and Koketsu, 1968; Kobayashi and Libet, 1968; Libet, 1970; Dun and Nishi, 1974); it is small and can be observed only if high-frequency preganglionic stimulation is used to produce a summation of single slow IPSPs (Libet, 1970).

Little or no evidence has been obtained to explain the functional role of the slow IPSP, although it has been accepted that it modulates synaptic transmission through the ganglion causing inhibition (Libet et al., 1968). No direct inhibition was found in normal (uncurarized) amphibian (Libet et al., 1968) and mammalian (Skok, 1973) sympathetic ganglia. Since the slow IPSP is not associated with decrease in membrane resistance and its amplitude is rather small, the question arises as to whether this potential inhibits transmission at the ganglion. In the case of the IPSPs that operate through an increase in conductance of the postsynaptic membrane, the inhibitory effect is independent of the sign of the potential (Grundfest and Reuben, 1961) and is due to the "clamping" of the EPSP generator toward the inside-negative electromotive force of the IPSP generator. Hyperpolarization, if present, plays a secondary role (see Eccles, 1964). Recent studies have suggested that dopamine acting at the site that generates slow IPSPs in the neurons of a sympathetic ganglion augments rather than depresses the amplitude of fast EPSP (Dun and Nishi, 1974), which might facilitate rather than inhibit transmission through the ganglion.

Thus there is considerable uncertainty about the inhibitory role of slow IPSP in sympathetic ganglia. This makes it important to know whether the slow IPSP occurs in the natural electrical activity of the neurons in sympathetic ganglia, especially during the inhibitory sympathetic reflex. The data presented below have been obtained with this purpose.

Figure 1 illustrates the spontaneous activity recorded intracellularly from the neurons of the superior cervical (A:2) and lumbar sympathetic ganglia of the rabbit (A:3), and ciliary ganglion of the cat (B:2). A recording was made from the ganglia with the intact blood supply in experiments under slight urethane–cloralose anesthesia; the ganglia were left connected to the spinal cord via preganglionic fibers (disconnection from the spinal cord immediately stops spontaneous activity in all neurons of the ganglion).

In the superior cervical and lumbar sympathetic ganglia neurons stimulation of preganglionic fibers evokes slow IPSPs (as well as fast EPSPs and slow EPSPs), which are illustrated by Fig. 1(A:1). A recording with sucrose-gap technique from curarized ganglion (curarization is used to prevent spike generation in the neurons of the ganglion) reveals a large positive potential (P-potential) which occurs after the negative potential (N-potential). The P-potential corresponds to intracellularly recorded slow IPSP, and the N-potential corresponds to intracellularly recorded fast EPSP. Atropine abolishes the P-potential, whereas the N-potential is not affected [Fig. 1(A:1)], which corresponds to data obtained previously in numerous experiments (Eccles and Libet, 1961; Nishi and Koketsu, 1968; Libet et al., 1968). No P-potential occurs in the ciliary ganglion [Fig. 1(B:1)].

Figure 1 indicates that there are only EPSPs and spikes but no IPSPs in the spontaneous activity of ganglion neurons recorded intracellularly, regardless of whether slow IPSP can be evoked by stimulation of preganglionic fibers. In this way, the ganglion neurons differ from central neurons where fast spontaneous IPSPs are observed (Creutzfeldt and Ito, 1968).

It seemed important to test whether slow IPSPs can be evoked in the neurons of sympathetic ganglia by stimuli which cause strong inhibition of spontaneous sympathetic activity in normal ganglia. Such inhibition may be evoked by stimulation of depressor nerves. Although the main inhibitory locus is in the central nervous system (Pitts and Bronk, 1942; Iggo and Vogt, 1960), some authors suggest the inhibition may also occur in sympathetic ganglia (Beck et al., 1966).

Figure 2 illustrates effects produced in two neurons of superior cervical ganglia by stimulation of depressor nerves. Most neurons (77%) respond with a decrease or stop in their spontaneous activity; the rest (23%) do not

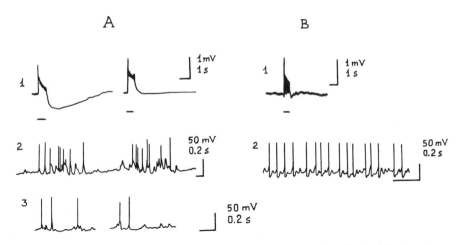

FIG. 1. Slow potentials evoked in curarized isolated autonomic ganglia by orthodromic stimulation, and spontaneous electrical activity recorded from the neurons of noncurarized ganglia *in situ.*

A:1—N-potential and P-potential recorded from isolated curarized (*d*-turbocurarine 5×10^{-5} M) cervical sympathetic ganglion of the cat with sucrose-gap technique in response to a train of repetitive stimuli (30/sec) applied to preganglionic fibers. The time of stimulation is indicated by the horizontal bar. Before (*left record*) and after (*right record*) treatment of the ganglion with atropine (0.5×10^{-6} M). Note that atropine abolishes P-potential (A. J. Ivanov, *unpublished data*). **2,3**—Spontaneous activity recorded intracellularly from superior cervical ganglion of the rabbit and from fifth lumbar sympathetic ganglion of the cat, respectively. The recording was performed from the ganglion *in situ;* preganglionic fibers were left intact (Skok, 1974).

B:1—N-potential recorded from isolated curarized ciliary ganglion of the cat with sucrose-gap technique similarly to **A:1**. Note that P-potential does not appear (Ivanov and Melnichenko, 1971). **2**—Spontaneous activity recorded intracellularly from ciliary ganglion of the cat similarly to **A:2,3** (Skok, 1974).

respond to this stimulation. In both types of neurons, no fast or slow IPSPs were observed during stimulation of the depressor nerves.

Although according to Libet (1970) slow IPSP can be evoked by stimulation of preganglionic fibers in most neurons of superior cervical ganglia, one cannot exclude the possibility that stimulation of the depressor nerve evokes IPSPs only in a small group of neurons which have escaped penetration by intracellular electrode. To test this possibility the sucrose-gap technique was used, which allows the recording of the average electrical response simultaneously from almost all neurons of the ganglion. The results obtained are shown in Fig. 3. In these experiments the ganglion was isolated from the body except for the connection through the cervical sympathetic nerve which contains preganglionic fibers connecting the ganglion to the spinal cord.

As Fig. 3:1 shows, stimulation of the depressor nerve evokes a large positivity of the ganglion neurons. But unlike the P-potential shown in Fig. 1(A:1), the P-potential evoked by stimulation of the depressor nerve is not affected by atropine [Fig. 3(A:2)]. A positivity of the same or higher

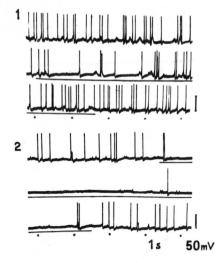

1

2

1 s   50mV

FIG. 2. The effect of stimulation of depressor nerves on the spontaneous activity recorded intracellularly from two neurons (**1** and **2**) of superior cervical ganglia of the rabbit (V. N. Mirgorodskii, *unpublished data*). Time of stimulation is indicated by the horizontal bar.

amplitude than produced by stimulation of depressor nerves may be produced by blocking the conduction of impulses in preganglionic fibers or by section of the nerve containing preganglionic fibers. The effect of blocking of conduction in preganglionic fibers produced by constant current is shown in Fig. 3(B:2), and the effect of sectioning of preganglionic fibers is shown in Fig. 3(C:2); no response to stimulation of depressor nerves occurs after preganglionic fibers are cut.

It thus seems likely that spontaneous preganglionic activity makes the ganglion negative in relation to preganglionic fibers, and this negativity disappears when preganglionic spontaneous activity stops. Sustained negativity recorded from the whole ganglion is probably produced by summation of numerous discrete processes (EPSPs and spikes) occurring in each neuron, for no sustained depolarization produced by presynaptic influence is recorded intracellularly. The same results were obtained from another sympathetic ganglion, the lumbar sympathetic ganglion of the rabbit (Skok et al., 1974). It thus follows that stimulation of depressor nerves does not evoke slow IPSPs in the neurons of sympathetic ganglia.

The results obtained indicate that stimulation of depressor nerves inhibits the spontaneous activity of preganglionic neurons or other neurons in the central nervous system and does not produce a direct inhibition in sympathetic ganglia. Another possibility is that stimulation of depressor nerves triggers in the ganglion the inhibitory mechanisms described above (activation of SIF cells), whereby catecholamines released in the ganglion act upon presynaptic nerve terminals rather than upon the neurons of the ganglion. The depressant action of catecholamines upon the presynaptic nerve terminals has been shown by Christ and Nishi (1971) and by Dun and Nishi (1974). This action may explain the well-known inhibitory effect of catecholamines on the transmission through sympathetic ganglia (Marrazzi,

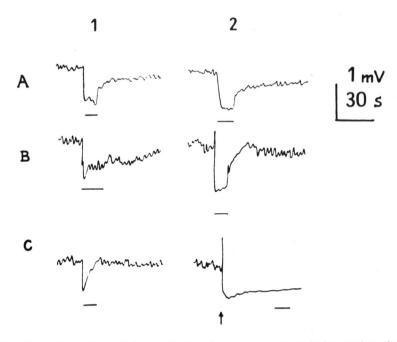

FIG. 3. The effects of stimulation applied to depressor nerves and of cessation of spontaneous preganglionic activity on the spontaneous activity recorded from superior cervical ganglia of the rabbit with sucrose-gap technique (Skok et al., 1974).
A: Effects of stimulation of depressor nerves before **(1)** and after **(2)** the treatment of the ganglion with atropine $(1 \times 10^{-6}$ M). **B:** Effect of stimulation of depressor nerves **(1)** and effect of blocking of impulse conduction in preganglionic fibers produced by constant electric current **(2)**. **C:** Effect of stimulation of depressor nerves **(1)** and effect of section of preganglionic fibers **(2)**. The moment of section is indicated by the arrow.
The records were obtained from three preparations **(A, B,** and **C)**. Horizontal bar indicates the time of stimulation of depressor nerves **(A, B:1, C)** or the time of passing the current blocking impulse conduction in preganglionic fibers **(B:2)**.

1939) or through parasympathetic ganglia (De Groat and Saum, 1972) without the assumption that this inhibitory effect is due to slow IPSPs.

It may be concluded that there is no evidence supporting the suggestion that the slow IPSP exerts an inhibitory action similar to the inhibitory action of the fast IPSP. The slow potential may play no inhibitory role but may be related to other functions, e.g., to extrusion of the excess of sodium from the neuron (cf. Nishi and Koketsu, 1968).

REFERENCES

Beck, L., Du Charme, D. W., Gebberg, L., Levin, J. A., and Pollard, A. A. (1966): Inhibition of adrenergic activity at a locus peripheral to the brain and spinal cord. *Circ. Res., Suppl. 1,* 18:55–59.
Christ, D. D., and Nishi, S. (1971). Site of adrenaline blockade in the superior cervical ganglion of the rabbit. *J. Physiol. (Lond.),* 213:107–117.
Creutzfeldt, O., and Ito, M. (1968): Functional synaptic organization of primary visual cortex neurones in the cat. *Exp. Brain Res.,* 6:324–352.

De Groat, W., and Saum, W. R. (1972): Sympathetic inhibition of the urinary bladder and of pelvic ganglionic transmission in the cat. *J. Physiol. (Lond.)*, 220:297–314.

Dun, N., and Nishi, S. (1974): Effects of dopamine on the superior cervical ganglion of the rabbit. *J. Physiol.*, 239:155–164.

Eccles, J. C. (1964): *The Physiology of Synapses.* Springer-Verlag, Berlin-Göttingen-Heidelberg.

Eccles, R. M., and Libet, B. (1961): Origin and blockade of the synaptic responses of curarized sympathetic ganglia. *J. Physiol. (Lond.)*, 157:484–503.

Engberg, I., and Marshall, K. C. (1971): Mechanism of noradrenaline hyperpolarization in spinal cord motoneurones of the cat. *Acta. Physiol. Scand.*, 83:142–144.

Grundfest, H., and Reuben, J. P. (1961): Neuromuscular synaptic activity in lobster. In: *Nervous Inhibition*, pp. 92–104. E. Florey, Ed., Pergamon Press. London, England.

Iggo, A., and Vogt, M. (1960): Preganglionic sympathetic activity in normal and in reserpine-treated cats. *J. Physiol. (Lond.)*, 150:114–133.

Ivanov, A. J., and Melnichenko, L. V. (1971): Effect of *d*-tubocurarine upon the synaptic transmission in cat ciliary ganglion. *Fiziol. Zh.*, 17:94–95 (in Ukrainian).

Kobayashi, H., and Libet, B. (1968): Generation of slow postsynaptic potentials without increases in ionic conductance. *Proc. Natl. Acad. Sci. USA*, 60:1304–1311.

Libet, B. (1970): Generation of slow inhibitory and excitatory postsynaptic potentials. *Fed. Proc.*, 29:1945–1956.

Libet, B., Chichibu, S., and Tosaka, T. (1968): Slow synaptic responses and excitability in sympathetic ganglia of the bullfrog. *J. Neurophysiol.*, 31:383–395.

Libet, B., and Owman, Ch. (1974): Concomitant changes in formaldehyde-induced fluorescence of dopamine interneurones and in slow inhibitory postsynaptic potentials of the rabbit superior cervical ganglion, induced by stimulation of the preganglionic nerve or by a muscarinic agent. *J. Physiol. (Lond.)*, 237:635–662.

Lorente de Nó, R., and Laporte, Y. (1949): Synaptic transmission in a sympathetic ganglion. *Arch. Sci. Physiol.*, 3:465–466.

Marrazzi, A. S. (1939): Adrenergic inhibition at sympathetic synapses. *Am. J. Physiol.*, 127:738–744.

Nishi, S., and Koketsu, K. (1968): Analysis of slow inhibitory postsynaptic potential of bullfrog sympathetic ganglion. *J. Neurophysiol.*, 31:717–728.

Pitts, R. F., and Bronk, D. W. (1942): Excitability cycle of the hypothalamic-sympathetic neurone system. *Am. J. Physiol.*, 135:504–521.

Skok, V. I. (1973): *Physiology of Autonomic Ganglia.* Igaku Shoin Ltd., Tokyo.

Skok, V. I. (1974): Convergence of preganglionic fibres in autonomic ganglia. In: *Mechanisms of Neuronal Integration in Nervous Center*, edited by P. G. Kostyuk, pp. 27–33. Nauka, Leningrad (in Russian).

Skok, V. I., Bogomoletz, V. I., Ivanov, A. J., and Mirgorodskii, V. N. (1974). Electrical activity of sympathetic ganglia during depressor reflex. *Neirofiziologiia*, 2:216–224 (in Russian).

Electrobiology of Nerve, Synapse, and Muscle,
edited by J. P. Reuben, D. P. Purpura, M. V. L. Bennett,
and E. R. Kandel. Raven Press, New York © 1976

Mechanism of Electroreception in Ampullae of Lorenzini of the Marine Catfish *Plotosus*

S. Obara

Department of Physiology, Teikyo University, School of Medicine, Itabashi-ku, Tokyo 173, Japan

An increasing number of both behavioral and electrophysiological evidence has established the electroreceptive function of ampullae of Lorenzini of elasmobranchs (for review, see Bennett, 1971*b*). Because of their unique structure, they provide an excellent preparation for the detailed analysis of receptor operation (see Obara and Bennett, 1972; Steinbach, 1974). Among teleosts, organs similar to the elasmobranch ampullae have been known so far only in a marine catfish, *Plotosus* (Friedrich-Freska, 1930; Lekander, 1949). Their function, however, appears to be unexplored until recently.

The *Plotosus* ampullae are highly sensitive tonic electroreceptors, similar to those of elasmobranchs. However, they also differ in several respects from the latter. This chapter presents a summary of the operation of the *Plotosus* ampullae, with particular reference to an active contribution of receptor cell activity in the tonic mode of operation of the system. Short communications dealing with several aspects of this operation have appeared elsewhere (Obara and Oomura, 1973; Akutsu and Obara, 1974; Obara, 1974; Obara et al., 1974; Umekita et al., 1975).

MATERIALS

Plotosus anguillaris (*Lacépède*) is one of a few marine species among nonelectric silurid fish. They are widely distributed in the tropical and subtropical seas of southeast Asia, and commonly found in large schools along the Pacific coast of Japan. They are usually considered as pests rather than of any commercial value, because of their venomous stinging dorsal and pectoral fins. The fish were collected by net, and transported to the laboratory in plastic bags containing sea water and filled with oxygen. They were fed on frozen shrimp, and survived well for up to several months in a laboratory aquarium with circulating sea water at 18° to 20°C.

MORPHOLOGY

A number of young and adult specimens, both fresh and preserved in 10% formalin, were examined. The general organization of ampullae of

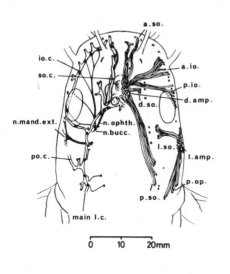

FIG. 1. Lateralis receptors in the head of *Plotosus*. Dorsal view. *Left side,* canal system with canal organs indicated as dark spots. Infraorbital (io.c.), supraorbital (so.c.), postorbital (po.c.), and main lateralis (main l.c.) canals are shown. *Right side,* ampullae of Lorenzini with long ducts. Dorsal ampullae (d.amp.) send their ducts to anterior, dorsal and posterior supraorbital fields (a.so., d.so. and p.so.) and to anterior and posterior infraorbital fields (a.io. and p.io.). Lateral ampullae (l.amp.) are shown only with the ducts to lateral supraorbital (l.so.) and preopercular fields (p.op.). Innervation (VII) is also shown in left side. Superficial ophthalmic nerve (n.ophth.) supplies the dorsal ampullae and also the so.c. organs. Buccalis nerve (n.bucc.) supplies exclusively the io.c. organs. External mandibular nerve (n. mand. ext.) supplies the lateral ampullae (modified from Lekander, 1949).

Lorenzini of *Plotosus* was similar to that described first by Friedrich-Freska (1930), except that, as for the groupings of ampullae, the revision proposed by Lekander (1949) was confirmed. The schematic illustration summarizing these reports is given in Fig. 1; further description will be limited to the dorsal group of ampullae, from which most of the physiological data has been obtained because of the technical feasibility.

Ampullae of Lorenzini of *Plotosus* are similar in structure to those of elasmobranchs (Murray, 1965). The sensory epithelium consists of a single layer of receptor cells, and forms a nearly spherical ampulla. A large number of ampullae occurs in a cluster, slightly anterior to and between the eyes. From each ampulla a jelly-filled transparent duct runs out in subcutaneous tissue to reach a distant site in the skin and to open to the outside. This radiating array of long ducts is one of the characteristics of the ampullae both of *Plotosus* and elasmobranch, in sharp contrast to the ampullary receptors of fresh water species which are scattered over much of the body surface, and embedded in the skin with only short ducts (see Bennett, 1971*b*).

The second characteristic appears to be the presence of numerous receptor cells aligned parallel to the wall of each individual ampulla, which is innervated only by six to eight afferent nerve fibers. Histological estimate indicates a probable convergence of 250 to 750 receptor cells onto a single afferent fiber, even without considering the most likely innervation overlap (Obara, 1974), whereas in fresh water species much smaller innervation ratios have been reported (Lissman and Mullinger, 1968; Wachtel and Szamier, 1969). The afferent innervation comes from the anterior lateralis nerve (Friedrich-Freska, 1930), as the superficial ophthalmic nerve, VII

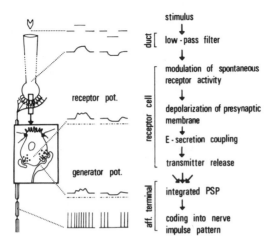

FIG. 2. The mode of operation of ampullae of Lorenzini of *Plotosus. Left,* anatomical diagram of a single ampulla. Convergence of many receptor cells onto a single afferent nerve fiber is depicted. In the thick square is shown a single receptor cell with apical microvilli and with afferent synapses on the basal surface. *Center,* Schematic illustration of potential changes at different places of the ampullary system shown to left. Note that the receptor potential must be superimposed on the electrotonic potential, and the generator potential has the afferent spikes riding on it, but that the different components are shown separately for the purpose of schematic presentation. Positivity is shown as upward deflections. The broken lines under receptor and generator potentials indicate their fully suppressed levels. At rest, both potentials are shifted to more depolarized levels, because of the spontaneous receptor activity. *Right,* causal sequence of intermediate steps in electroreception (from Obara, 1974).

(Herrick, 1901). After splitting several times, the final branch of six to eight myelinated fibers of approximately 10 μm in diameter first comes into close apposition with the duct, and proceeds along it toward the ampulla, finally making synaptic contact with the receptor cells.

Fine structure (see Fig. 2) was studied by Nishihara and Yamamoto (1971). The receptor cells are nonciliated, but bear microvilli on the apical surface (also see Lissmann et al., 1968). Synapses are only of the afferent type and occur at several places on the basal and lateral surface of the receptor cells. Synaptic projections of the receptor cells contain characteristic synaptic rods surrounded by an accumulation of vesicles. Tight junctions are found between the supporting cell and the receptor cell near their lumenal border.

PHYSIOLOGY

Methods

Several procedures have been devised according to various experimental requirements, details of which are found in earlier papers. The ampullae and the afferent terminal branches can be visualized in a curarized fish under the dissecting microscope (as is shown in Fig. 1) by simply removing the overlying skin and the ampullary capsule, since the whole system lies in loose subcutaneous tissue and is connected to the skin only at the pores.

Most of the experiments described in this paper were carried out *in situ* by recording with glass microelectrodes from inside the ampulla, and also by recording either intracellularly or externally from the afferent terminal branch. Electrical stimulation was given either to the pore through a low resistance electrode, or by penetrating the duct with another microelectrode. Antidromic stimulation was given to the trunk of the superficial ophthalmic nerve, which involved only the afferent fibers since efferent innervation is reportedly absent.

Results

General Properties and Mode of Operation

The electrosensitivity of the ampullary system could be readily demonstrated on a single unit activity which was obtained from the nerve trunk at its exit from the cranium. With this approach, no dissection in the ampullary field was required, and the ampullae remained completely undisturbed. The single fiber usually carried fairly regular afferent discharges of 30 to 50 per sec in the absence of stimuli. Positive current pulses given to the pore gradually increased the frequency of afferent discharges, and negative ones reduced it, as in other teleost receptors (Bennett, 1965, 1971a; Roth, 1968, 1969), but opposite that of the skate ampullae (Murray, 1965; Obara and Bennett, 1972). Termination of the stimuli was followed by reversed aftereffects. Although these responses were of tonic nature, adaptation did occur to stimuli of both polarities. A discernible change in the frequency could be produced by a few microvolt potential variations at the pore. The "overstimulation" phenomenon described for the skate ampullae (Murray, 1965; Obara and Bennett, 1972), however, was not observed even with extremely strong stimuli of more than 1,000 times above the threshold.

Mechanical sensitivity is small; a firm pressure over the ducts or the ampullary field induced only a transient facilitation. In contrast, the afferent units from the canal organs of the same fish showed a vigorous response to minute disturbances in the water, but were quite insensitive to electrical pulses at the intensities employed to stimulate the ampullae. The difference in their electrical sensitivity, however, may reflect in part the difference in the accessory structures of the respective receptor systems. The long duct, the most conspicuous accessory structure in the ampullae, showed an extremely long space constant *in situ,* so that potential variations at the pore were transmitted to the ampulla without noticeable attenuation. This exactly duplicates the situation in the skate ampulla, although their electrical properties appear to be somewhat different (see Waltman, 1966).

Before proceeding further with presentation of experimental data, the overall operation of *Plotosus* ampullae may be summarized (Obara, 1974) in order to outline the main issues under consideration (Fig. 2). In this working hypothesis the receptor cells are assumed to be already gradually activated in the absence of stimuli—"spontaneous receptor activity." The receptor activity thus induced (receptor potential) is due to a Ca-dependent depolarization at the basal or presynaptic membrane of the cell, causing a steady release of an excitatory transmitter. Because of the extensive convergence at this receptor–afferent synapse, the induced excitatory postsynaptic potentials (EPSPs) in an afferent terminal are smoothed to result in a small maintained depolarization (generator potential), which in turn sets up a regular "resting or spontaneous" afferent discharge. The incoming sensory input at the pore, namely the extrinsic electrical field variation, will modulate the spontaneous receptor activity gradually and linearly within a certain range, hence modulating the afferent impulse frequency, through the successive intermediate steps of transmitter release and action.

Within the framework of the present hypothesis, the *receptor potential* may be defined as an intermediate process in the receptor cell, which serves as a presynaptic potential as well as a stimulus-dependent response. Similarly the *generator potential* in the afferent terminal are PSPs which serve as a coding mechanism in forming the afferent impulse pattern.

Transmission at the Receptor–Afferent Synapses

The tonic mode of operation was defined from the input–output characteristics between afferent impulse frequency and applied electric stimulus. A greater amount of information can be gained by an intracellular recording from the afferent terminal (Furukawa and Ishii, 1967a; Obara et al., 1974). Intracellular recording in the afferent nerve was often found feasible near the final bifurcation of the nerve bundle close to the ampulla. This part is still composed of myelinated nerves and the nearest synaptic terminations may be as far as 100 μm away from the recording site. In view of the following data, however, the recording will be considered as that of the afferent terminal for the sake of simplicity.

On successful penetration signaled by a sudden negative DC shift, the afferent terminal showed a regular afferent spike discharge. Stimulation of the ampulla now induced graded slow potential changes of either polarity on which the afferent spikes were superimposed. Since the slow potential in depolarizing direction is associated with facilitation of the spikes (Fig. 3A–C), and the hyperpolarization with suppression (D–E), they will be called the depolarizing and hyperpolarizing *generator potentials* (GP), respectively (see Davis, 1965).

Termination of stimuli was followed by similar slow potentials but of reversed polarity, as would be expected by the response patterns of the afferent discharge. Also a temporal summation could be observed for the

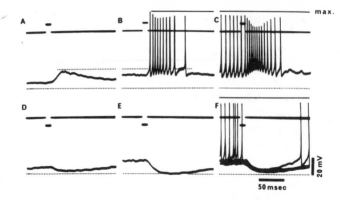

FIG. 3. Intracellular recordings from the afferent terminal. Repetitive short current pulses given to the ampulla induced a gradual membrane fluctuation, as well as the depolarizing GP, either appearing alone **(A)** or with facilitation of the afferent discharge (**B** and **C**). Note the time course of the subthreshold slow potential and also of the spike peak and the afterpotentials. The line marked by *max*. indicates the maximum height of the spike. The upper dotted line shows the firing level, while the lower one the most negative membrane potential. **D** to **F:** the hyperpolarizing GP with concomitant afferent suppression. Several sweeps are superimposed in F. Note the distinct inflection at the onset of GPs of both polarities (*unpublished data*).

GP of either polarity. Taking advantage of these features, a gradual fluctuation of the membrane potential may be induced in the afferent terminal by adjusting the repetition rate of the stimuli. When the membrane potential was shifted to a more hyperpolarized level in this way, the GP could be observed with no contamination of the afferent spikes (Fig. 3 A,D, and E). The graded GP thus revealed had a long and gradual time course, far outlasting the stimulus. Small slow ripples might be superimposed, but no discrete component suggestive of either quanta or unitary postsynaptic potentials was ever observed. The onset of the GP of both polarities could be quite distinct, although their latency was usually over several milliseconds.

The depolarizing GP clearly represents EPSPs. Presumably a given single afferent fiber is receiving synaptic inputs from numerous receptor cells (see Morphology section), and integrating them over space and time. The conductance increase associated with a PSP of this type might be expected to last throughout the slow potential changes. Presence of such a conductance increase was suggested by the decreased spike height and also by the raised levels of the afterhyperpolarization of the spikes (Fig. 3B and C) (Eccles, 1964; Katz, 1969; Obara and Bennett, 1972). The time course of these measures follows approximately that of the subthreshold depolarizing GP. Simultaneous recording of the ampullary potential further indicated that the depolarizing GP in a single afferent terminal was closely correlated though not directly with the ampullary potential, but with an active response in the ampulla that was superimposed on the electrotonic potential (Obara et al., 1973). This will be discussed in connection to the ampullary response

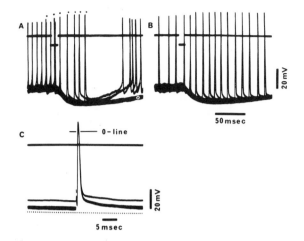

FIG. 4. The hyperpolarizing GP as indicative of disfacilitation. **A** and **B:** superimposed sweeps showing nearly constant hyperpolarizing GP. Antidromic stimuli were given to the nerve trunk once in each sweep at varying times. **A:** Antidromic spikes were not blocked (marked by dots near the peak), while orthodromic spikes were suppressed during the hyperpolarizing GP. **B:** at a more hyperpolarized level with no orthodromic spikes. All the spikes were antidromically evoked. Note the increase of spike size during the GP. **C:** antidromic spikes superimposed over the hyperpolarizing GP shown on expanded sweeps (*unpublished data*).

in a later section. Antidromic spikes superimposed on the depolarizing GP showed similar reduction of size (Obara et al., 1973). A direct conductance measurement of the afferent terminal by the bridge method also indicated the conductance increase, although less explicitly.

On the other hand, the hyperpolarizing GP shown in Fig. 3D to F cannot be considered as an inhibitory PSP. The antidromic spike invading the afferent terminal was never blocked during the hyperpolarizing GP. Instead, the spike size was even increased (Fig. 4), suggesting a conductance decrease rather than increase (Obara et al., 1973). The increased spike height might in part be due to a removal of the inactivation process in spike initiation which depends on the membrane potential (Hodgkin and Huxley, 1952). The bridge measurements did reveal that there was at least no conductance increase. The hyperpolarizing GP, therefore, must be regarded as a repolarization, or disfacilitation, from a previous level of maintained depolarization.

The implications here will be clear enough that there is a maintained effect of an excitatory transmitter even prior to stimulus application. Furthermore, since this effect can be turned off quite rapidly as is shown by the distinct onset of the hyperpolarizing GP (Fig. 3D,E, and F; Fig. 4), the maintained effect must be due to a continuous release of transmitter, but not due to its accumulation in the synaptic gap (Obara et al., 1973). Thus, this single piece of evidence clearly indicates that the receptor cells in the ampulla must be continuously releasing an excitatory, though still unidentified, transmitter in the absence of extrinsic stimuli.

Input–Output Relation Across the Sensory Synapse

Transmission at the synapse can be characterized more quantitatively by observing the extracellular potential from the afferent terminal in the presence of tetrodotoxin (TTX) (Steinbach, 1974; Umekita et al., 1975). By recording from the afferent nerve branch close to ampulla with a pair of Pt wire electrodes, a massive resting afferent discharge was observed. On stimulation to the ampulla, slow potential changes of either polarity were recorded from the nerve in addition to the expected changes in afferent discharges. Simultaneous intraaxonal recording indicated that these extracellular slow potentials closely resembled the GPs shown in Fig. 3. In the following experiments, a long conditioning pulse was first given to the ampulla to induce a maximal hyperpolarizing GP in the nerve. A shorter test pulse was then superimposed to produce a positive deflection in the ampulla and a clearly definable depolarizing GP in the nerve (Fig. 5B).

The presynaptic *control or reference level* may be defined as the ampullary potential prior to stimulation that is associated with the steady "resting" rate of afferent impulses. Preliminary tests revealed that the size of the hyperpolarizing GPs on maximal conditioning could serve as a good measure in assessing recovery of the ampullary potential to the reference level follow-

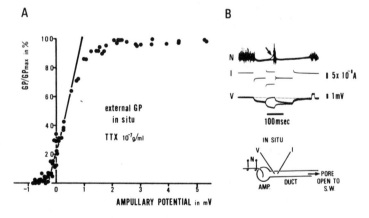

FIG. 5. Input–output relation across the receptor-afferent synapse. **A:** abscissa; ampullary potential with respect to the reference level prior to stimulation, and ordinate; relative amplitude of the initial peak of the depolarizing GP in response to test pulse. **B:** sample records from a different preparation without TTX. N, external recording from the afferent terminal. I, test pulses of both polarities are superimposed on a conditioning hyperpolarizing pulse. V, ampullary potential with a dotted line indicating the reference level. Arrow in N trace indicates the depolarizing GP in response to the lumen positive ampullary potential, but no further hyperpolarizing GP on additional negativity in the ampulla. **Lower diagram:** electrode arrangement (modified from Umekita et al., 1975).

ing any perturbation, even when the afferent spikes were eliminated by TTX.

The external depolarizing GPs in response to varying test pulses in the combined stimulation were recorded in the presence of TTX. Relative amplitude of the initial GP peaks was plotted against the presynaptic receptor response which was taken as the deviation of the corresponding ampullary potential from the reference level (Fig. 5A). The input-output relation thus obtained was found to follow an approximately S-shaped curve, similar to that reported for the squid giant synapse (Katz and Miledi, 1967; Kusano, 1970). Significant differences from the latter, however, may be pointed out. First, the linear portion around the reference level is very steep, showing at least a 10-fold increase for 1 to 2 mV change in the ampulla, while in the squid synapse a corresponding increase in the PSP requires a 12 mV increment in the presynaptic membrane (Kusano, 1970). The slope may be even steeper, since the ampullary potential is recorded extracellularly, and the effective depolarization across the presynaptic membrane may be still smaller. Secondly, the input–output relation is clearly shifted along the presynaptic voltage axis toward the negative region. The reference level with the ampulla unstimulated corresponds to about 20% of the maximum output, indicating the maintained effect of a depolarizing transmitter at the reference level. Both of these characteristics support the conclusions derived in the previous sections.

Responses of the Ampulla In Situ

The responses observed in the ampullary lumen can be taken as a mass response of the sensory epithelium, recorded extracellularly (see Morphology section). Serious technical difficulties in measuring the ampullary potential may be immediately recognized in view of the extraordinary sensitivity and also of the tonic nature of responses of the receptor system. However, since it was found that a reference level of the ampullary potential could be assessed by observing the hyperpolarizing GP extracellularly, the ampullary responses could be evaluated more quantitatively.

The ampullary responses to positive and negative pulses are shown superimposed in the lowermost traces in Fig. 6, with simultaneous external GP in the uppermost traces. The ampullary responses to stimulation of both polarities were graded and almost symmetrical up to $\pm 200 \mu V$, with little tendency to oscillate (Fig. 6A and B). The off-responses observed in the afferent nerve corresponded to the oscillatory rebounds in the ampulla. When the intensity of the pulses was increased gradually, the responses started to become nonlinear, particularly in the depolarizing direction. A damped oscillation began to appear at the onset (Fig. 6C and D), and finally a regenerative response was evoked, both associated with marked facilitation in the nerve (D). On the other hand, the responses in the hyper-

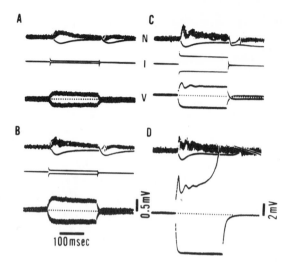

FIG. 6. Responses of the *in situ* ampulla. *Uppermost trace* (N), external recording from the afferent terminal showing both GPs and afferent discharges. *Middle trace* (I), stimuli given to the ampulla, which is omitted in record D. *Lowermost trace* (V), ampullary potential with positivity upward. Negative ampullary potentials are associated with the hyperpolarizing GP and afferent suppression, and positive ones with the depolarizing GP and afferent facilitation. In each record are superimposed responses to successive stimuli of opposite sign (negative first). The responses to smaller stimuli are symmetrical with rebounds of opposite polarities **(A)**. A complete afferent suppression required ampullary hyperpolarization of less than 80 μV in this case. The ampulla shows oscillatory **(B–D)** and regenerative responses **(D)** to depolarizing stimuli (*unpublished data*).

polarizing direction were much simpler, and soon became flattened (Fig. 6C and D). On withdrawal of the microelectrode only a small DC potential was registered.

The polarity of the nonlinear responses is consistent with the supposition that they are derived from a depolarizing activity generated at the innervated or basal surface of the receptor cells, just as was proposed in the phasic electroreceptors of fresh water teleosts (Bennett, 1965). The proposed site of electrogenesis in the receptor cell means that positivity in the ampullary potential is associated with depolarization of the innervated surface of receptor cell, and the ampullary negativity is associated with hyperpolarization. Histological considerations also suggest that the transition from graded to regenerative responses represents an increasing synchronization of activity of many receptor cells in the sensory epithelium. These hypotheses will be further substantiated in later sections.

The Receptor Cell Activity and the Ampullary Potential

The sequence from the ampullary potential to the afferent output was already shown in terms of the input–output relation across the sensory synapse (Fig. 5). A finer evaluation is required because of the presence of non-

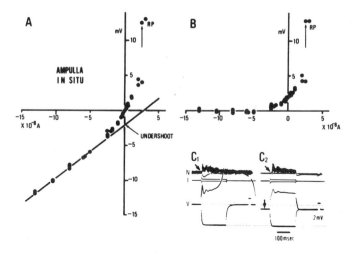

FIG. 7. Nonlinearity in the *in situ* ampulla and estimation of the active component. **A:** *I-V* relation around the reference level as the origin. The straight line is extrapolated from the linear portion of the curve below about −6 which intersects the voltage axis at a level corresponding to the undershoot after the regenerative ampullary response (RP). **B:** active component estimated from **A** by extrapolation and subtraction of the linear region. **C:** sample records from a different preparation. **C₁:** responses at the reference level, same as in Fig. 6D. **C₂:** responses during the undershoot (*arrow* in V trace) immediately after the regenerative response in **C₁**. Note the absence of spontaneous afferent discharge and of a hyperpolarizing GP (*arrow* in N trace) (*unpublished data*).

linearities in the ampullary response. Careful plotting of the *I-V* relation of a given ampulla revealed a marked graded nonlinearity around the reference level (Fig. 7). As shown in the plot, however, the responses became quite linear when the ampulla was hyperpolarized. The straight line was obtained from the linear parts below −10 to −30 mV, and it was seen to intersect the V-axis at about 2 mV negative to the reference level. A deviation from this straight line began to appear at about −6 mV and kept on increasing, finally to give rise to the regenerative response, marked by RP in the plot. The intersecting level ranged from −1 to −3 mV among ampullae, and was found approximately to correspond to the level of undershoot after the regenerative ampullary response. During the undershoot, the transmitter release appeared to be completely turned off, because there was no afferent discharge, and also because even a strong cathodal pulse given to the ampulla evoked no hyperpolarizing GP during this period (Fig. 7C). As the ampullary potential gradually returned to the reference level, the afferent discharge as well as the hyperpolarizing GP on stimulation reappeared.

Since the graded depolarizing potential in the ampulla has been correlated with the afferent facilitation (Fig. 6), the graded nonlinearity around the reference level may also be considered as an active process which is continuous to the regenerative ampullary response. Presumably, the straight line in the plot in Fig. 7A represents a passive *I-R* drop, over which the ampulla is giving an active and graded contribution (Fig. 7B) that may be termed a *receptor potential* (RP). The intersection negative to the reference level, then, implies that even without extrinsic stimuli the ampulla is actively depolarized by about 2 mV, causing the continuous transmitter release which has been proposed previously (Fig. 4).

Finally it may be pointed out that the nonlinearity or the excitability of the ampulla should be still compatible with the linear operation of the system as a whole. The ampullary response around the reference level may be regarded as quite linear within the linear working range of the system which spans less than 1 mV (Fig. 5).

Regenerative Responses of the Ampulla Under Electrical Isolation

When the ampulla was electrically isolated, the ampullary response could be converted into a fully regenerative activity with a response having a sharp threshold. Ionic requirements for this regenerative response (RR) were studied by perfusing the medium surrounding the ampulla isolated in this way. The results explicitly indicate that the regenerative RP is due to a Ca-dependent depolarizing activity originating at the basal face of the receptor cells (Akutsu et al., 1974). This particular series of experiments was performed with the ampulla which was *physically* isolated from the fish, together with a length of its duct. However, the procedure of the *electrical isolation* can be similarly applied to the ampulla remaining in its original position, as will be shown in a later section.

The ampulla electrically isolated shows several characteristics (Fig. 8B) which are quite different from those of the ampulla *in situ* described in the previous section. First, there was a larger DC standing potential of 16 to 20 mV negative inside the ampulla. Secondly, the responses to electrical stimuli were much larger in both polarities. With anodal stimulation, a de-polarizing and almost fully regenerative response could be triggered which long outlasted the stimulus duration. This regenerative response was apparently only very slowly inactivated, and then was followed by little under-shoot. Usually an additional strong cathodal pulse was given to the ampulla in order to abolish the sustained response, and to minimize refractoriness. The voltage threshold was near the zero potential level. No oscillatory response was observed below this threshold level. The subthreshold responses and those in the hyperpolarizing direction which gave a nearly exponential rise and fall were quite linear down to over -100 mV.

The afferent discharge was absent, or much sparser in the isolated ampulla, and furthermore, it was never suppressed even by a large hyper-polarization in the ampulla (Fig. 8B). No hyperpolarizing GP was observed either. After the strong afferent facilitation associated with the regenerative ampullary response (Akutsu et al., 1974), however, this persisting resting discharge was seen to disappear for some period. The large amount of transmitter released following the regenerative ampullary response may have fatigued the afferent fiber or induced a desensitization of the postsynaptic membrane in the afferent terminal (see Katz and Thesleff, 1957).

Comparison of the Ampullary Responses, In Situ and Isolated

The alteration in the response characteristics of the ampulla and of the afferent output pattern under electrical isolation from those of the intact organ raised an intriguing possibility, that the ampulla became fully suppressed under electrical isolation, so that it ceased to release the transmitter, and that the ampulla *in situ* was activated somehow through being communicated to outside sea water by its own duct, and hence induced to release certain amount of transmitter in the absence of stimuli.

The response characteristics of a given ampulla under these two conditions are compared in this section (Obara, 1974). The I-V relation of the ampulla was first determined for a wider range around the reference level which was continually monitored by observing the afferent output. The same ampulla was subsequently isolated in its original position. The response patterns characteristic for both conditions have been already described, and sample records for each are shown in Fig. 8A and B. Two sets of I-V relations of the same ampulla under different conditions are plotted in Fig. 9B.

On the basis of morphological considerations and also of the electrical properties of the ampullary duct, a simple equivalent circuit may be given in order to simulate the linear parts of the curves both in de- and hyperpolarizing quadrants (Fig. 9C). The switch, S_1, introduces an active EMF (E_a) in the ampulla. The ampullary duct is represented by a single longitudinal element (R_d), since there is little leakage along the duct resulting in the extremely long length constant. The resistance (R_e) looking outside from the pore should be small, and may be lumped together with R_d. The junction potential at the pore between the jelly in the duct and the sea water is represented by E_e, which may include potential differences at the gill and so forth along the current path. The two conditions shown in Fig. 8 are switched by S_2.

The values of each component in the equivalent circuit can be estimated for the linear parts of the plots. Only a summary description based upon these estimates will be given. The short-circuiting load ($R_d + R_e$) has nearly the same value as that of the fully activated ampulla ($R_r//R_a$) under isolated condition. The *in situ* ampulla is apparently heavily loaded and depolarized in the face of this much short-circuit. The ampullary potential may be assumed to be nearly clamped to E_e which is close to zero, or near the threshold level of the isolated ampulla. The conductance of the *in situ* ampulla reaches only to about 21% of that of the isolated ampulla even when fully activated, suggesting an inactivation process (hence the variable R_a).

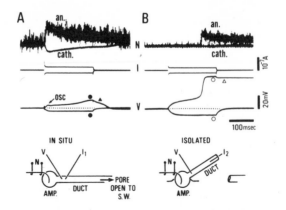

FIG. 8. Sample records taken from a single ampulla under two conditions. **A:** *in situ.* **B:** electrically isolated, which are schematically illustrated by diagrams under each record. *Uppermost trace* (N), external recording from the afferent terminal. *Middle trace* (I), current pulses given to the ampulla. *Lowermost trace* (V), ampullary responses with depolarization upward. Successive responses first to lumen negative cathodal (cath.) and then to anodal (an.) stimuli are superimposed as marked for N traces. OSC, oscillatory depolarizing response in *in situ* ampulla, similar to those in Fig. 6. The ampullary oscillation and also a hyperpolarizing GP are absent in the isolated ampulla **(B).** Symbols attached to V traces correspond to those in Fig. 9A and B (modified from Obara, 1974).

If the steady depolarization of about 2 mV from the level projected from the linear region in the hyperpolarizing quadrant is assumed to result from graded activation as already suggested (Fig. 7), the active conductance at this level would be about 17% of the maximum for the *in situ* ampulla.

To summarize, it appears that the electrically excitable, Ca-dependent process in the ampulla proper is under *in situ* conditions, being electrically short-circuited through its own duct opening to outside sea water, and held biased near the original threshold level. An excitable element thus biased will be expected to develop both the activation and inactivation processes and to exhibit graded and oscillatory responses. A classical example of the response of this type is the subthreshold "local response" in the axon (Hodgkin and Rushton, 1946). The inactivation is evident by the conductance measurement in the present system. The nonlinear responses observed in the *in situ* ampulla also imply a development of the activation process concomitant with the inactivation. Presumably, the nonlinearity with a small steady depolarization around the reference level represents a dynamic balance of these processes, resulting in a graded and/or partial activation of the excitable elements in the *in situ* ampulla. Considering the histological data of the sensory epithelium, this may suggest the *presence of a certain population of activated receptor cells* in the absence of any extrinsic stimuli. Furthermore, the causal sequences described in the preceding sections suggest that this state of ampulla is the initial process leading to the "resting" afferent discharge.

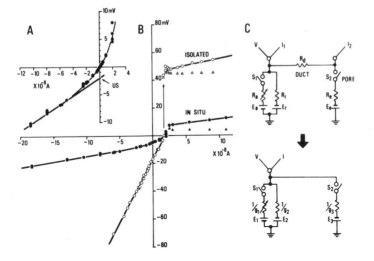

FIG. 9. *I-V* relations of a single ampulla under two conditions. A different preparation, but from records similar to those shown in Fig. 8. *Circles,* ampullary responses to 200 msec current pulses. *Triangles,* sustained levels of the regenerative response after the pulse. Filled symbols for the *in situ* ampulla, and open ones for the isolated ampulla, as in Fig. 8. **A:** nonlinearity around the reference level of *in situ* ampulla. shown at higher voltage gain. US, undershoot level after the regenerative response. **B:** *I-V* relations for a wider range are superimposed together with DC standing potentials under two conditions. **C:** equivalent circuit. Capacitative components are omitted for simplicity. *Upper diagram,* original circuit representing the two experimental situations. R_r and E_r, resistance and emf of the resting or fully suppressed ampulla. R_a and E_a, those of the active channel during the depolarizing ampullary response, which is introduced by S_1. R_d, longitudinal resistance of the ampullary duct. R_e and E_e, resistance and EMF looking outside from the pore. The *in situ* conditions are represented by closure of switch S_2. I_1 and I_2, stimuli applied as in diagrams in Fig. 8. *Lower diagram,* R_d and R_e in the upper diagram are lumped for the convenience of calculation (modified from Obara, 1974).

CONCLUSIONS AND COMMENTS

The summary of operation of the *Plotosus* ampullae has been already given (Fig. 2), and little further comment will be required. In both general morphology and tonic mode of operation, the *Plotosus* ampullae closely resemble those of marine elasmobranchs. Most probably an adaptation to the highly conductive medium of sea water common to both cases has led to such a remarkable convergent evolution (see Waltman, 1966; Bennett, 1971*b*). The teleost traits of *Plotosus* ampullae are apparent in the effective stimulus polarity and in the site of Ca activity which are similar to those of the phasic receptors of fresh water teleosts (Bennett, 1967; Zipser and Bennett, 1971). The spontaneous receptor cell activity described in the present system may deserve further consideration.

The extraordinary sensitivity of electroreceptors (see Lissmann, 1958; Dijkgraaf and Kalmijn, 1963; Bennett, 1971*b*) as well as of sensory receptors of other modalities in general remains as a challenging problem. In the case of *Plotosus* ampullae, it is tempting to ascribe the high sensitivity to the electrical excitability of receptor cells (Bennett, 1965, 1967; Obara and Bennett, 1972). Signal amplification through electrical excitability per se, however, appears to be insignificant, because the ampulla is heavily loaded to give only graded responses within the system's working range. An estimate of the amplification factor may be obtained by comparing slopes of the *I-V* relation of *in situ* ampulla and of the passive component in Fig. 7, which amounts to only about twofold. In this respect two mechanisms may be depicted from the causal sequence shown in Fig. 2.

The *modulation mechanism* primarily operating at the receptor cell level (Fig. 2) presumably gives the first step responsible for the remarkable sensitivity, since such a system should show essentially no threshold, given sufficient time for analysis (Bennett, 1971b), the only limitation being posed by the stability of carrier signal—namely of the spontaneous activity of receptor cells. The second mechanism of functional significance appears to be the *extensive convergence* at the receptor-afferent synapse. The experimental data indicate chemical transmission at this sensory synapse (Obara et al., 1973; Akutsu and Obara, 1974; Umekita et al., 1975). Apart from the chemical amplification inherent in the synaptic transmission (see Katz, 1969; Eccles, 1964), the integrating mechanism through the extensive convergence at this sensory synapse presumably operates as a sort of signal averaging process which contributes to improve the signal-to-noise ratio. This will result in an increase in effective sensitivity, but at the expense of loss of time resolution. The frequency characteristics of the present system have not been determined accurately, but the tonic responsiveness of the ampulla and the filtering characteristics of the ampullary duct both suggest that the ampullae of Lorenzini are low-frequency receptors.

Having deduced these mechanisms, however, it is perhaps salutary to note that they are not completely unique to the ampullae of Lorenzini, but appear to be common among higher-order sensory receptors. Both in the acoustico-lateralis system and vertebrate retina the *convergence* from receptor cells to afferent nerves has been established histologically. In the retina there are two distinct systems, one with fewer or no convergence which serves for more discriminative reception, and another with extensive convergence which shows a greater sensitivity.

The *modulation* of receptor activity through the sensory input also has been repeatedly suggested for sensory receptors of various modalities, although mechanisms proposed in each case may vary diversely. In fact, so-called transducer action in sensory receptors involves complex mechanisms. Certainly, it is rarely a simple energy conversion process even in engineering terms, and never in biological systems. Direct experimental evidence against the energy conversion is provided in cochlear microphonics (Békésy, 1960). Thus, in biological systems the sensory inputs always work, either releasing a potential energy of the membrane potential or modulating a steady energy flow across the receptive membrane (see Davis, 1965). A directly comparable example has been reported in the vertebrate retina. The photoreceptor is held depolarized in darkness, releasing a depolarizing transmitter to subsequent cells. Illumination acts to modulate the ongoing receptor activity gradedly. The hyperpolarizing receptor potential in photoreceptors is associated with a conductance decrease (Toyoda et al., 1969), and with a reduced transmitter release (Dowling and Ripps, 1972). Perhaps the mechanisms found in the ampullae of Lorenzini, a specialized lateralis receptor, are more widely applicable to other sensory receptors, which may not be too surprising in view of the phylogenetic origin of the ampullae from the acoustico-lateralis system (see Lissmann and Mullinger, 1968).

What is unique in the present system, however, is the demonstration of a mechanism by which an electrically excitable element, hence essentially nonlinear, is adapted to contribute to a linearly graded signal transmission. Similar modulation of electrically excitable membrane has been proposed in the skate ampullae, but at the apical surface of the receptor cells, in which both the effective stimulus and the ampullary response are of opposite polarity from the teleost receptor (Obara and Bennett, 1968, 1972; Waltman, 1968). The spontaneous receptor activity of skate ampullae, however, was tentatively assumed to be oscillatory (Obara and Bennett, 1972). Whether the activity of a single receptor cell is oscillatory or a gradedly continuous DC shift will have to be determined by intracellular recording.

The demonstration of electrically excitable response in two tonic receptors of skate and *Plotosus* suggests a contribution of similar mechanism in other tonic electroreceptors, as well as in acousticolateralis mechanoreceptors. Electrical nonlinearity has not been shown in tonic electroreceptors of fresh water teleosts, presumably because the conductance increase due to Ca-dependent activity is too small (Bennett, 1967, 1971b). Microphonics of canal organ (Flock, 1965) and of fish macula (Furukawa and Ishii, 1967b) exhibit marked nonlinearity, but whether it is due purely to mechanical coupling, or also to electrical nonlinearity is not known.

ACKNOWLEDGMENTS

The author is particularly grateful to staffs of Mito Aquarium, Numazu-city, Shizuoka and of Kanazawa Aquarium, Kanazawa-city, Ishikawa for the generous supply and maintenance of the fish. The initial part of this project was done in the Department of Physiology, Kanazawa University. Professor Y. Oomura, the chairman of the institution at the time who is now in the Department of Physiology, Kyushu University, is acknowledged for his support. The work was supported in part by grants from the Ministry of Education of Japan, 7004, 90958, 96050, and 99054, and from NIH,

NS-07201-03 to Professor Y. Oomura. The work in Teikyo University was also supported in part by grants from the Ministry of Education of Japan, 837005 and 811009.

REFERENCES

Akutsu, Y., and Obara, S. (1974): Ca-dependent receptor potential of the electroreceptor of marine catfish. *Proc. Jap. Acad.,* 50:247–251.

Békésy, G. von (1960): *Experiments in Hearing.* McGraw-Hill, New York.

Bennett, M. V. L. (1965): Electroreceptors in Mormyrids. *Cold Spring Harbor Symp. Quant. Biol.,* 30:245–262.

Bennett, M. V. L. (1967): Mechanism of electroreception. In: *Lateral Line Detectors,* edited by P. Cahn, pp. 313–393. Indiana University Press, Bloomington, Indiana.

Bennett, M. V. L. (1971a): Electrolocation in fish. *Ann. NY Acad. Sci.,* 188:242–269.

Bennett, M. V. L. (1971b): Electroreception. In: *Fish Physiology,* edited by W. S. Hoar and D. J. Randall, Vol. V, pp. 493–574. Academic Press, New York.

Davis, H. (1965): A model for transducer action in the cochlea. *Cold Spring Harbor Symp. Quant. Biol.,* 30:181–190.

Dijkgraaf, S., and Kalmijn, A. J. (1963): Untersuchungen über die Funktion der Lorenzinischen Ampullen an Haifischen. *Z. Vergleich. Physiol.,* 47:438–456.

Dowling, J. E., and Ripps, H. (1972): Effects of Mg^{2+} on skate horizontal cells: evidence for release of transmitter from receptors in darkness. *Biol. Bull.,* 143:458–459.

Eccles, J. C. (1964): *The Physiology of Synapses.* Springer-Verlag, Berlin.

Flock, Å. (1965): Electron microscopic and electrophysiological studies on the lateral-line canal organ. *Acta Oto-Laryngol.,* Suppl. 199:1–90.

Furukawa, T., and Ishii, Y. (1967a): Neurophysiological studies on hearing in goldfish. *J. Neurophysiol.,* 30:1377–1403.

Furukawa, T., and Ishii, Y. (1967b): Effects of static bending of sensory hairs on sound reception in the goldfish. *Jap. J. Physiol.,* 17:572–588.

Friedrich-Freska, H. (1930): Lorenzinische Ampullen bei dem Siluroiden, *Plotosus anquillaris* Bloch. *Zool. Anz.,* 87:49–66.

Herrick, C. J. (1901): The cranial nerves and cutaneous sense organs of the North American siluroid fishes. *J. Comp. Neurol.,* 11:177–249.

Hodgkin, A. L., and Huxley, A. F. (1952): A quantitative description of membrane current and its application to conduction and excitation and nerve. *J. Physiol. (Lond.),* 117:500–544.

Hodgkin, A. L., and Rushton, W. A. H. (1946): The electrical constants of a crustacean nerve fibre. *Proc. Roy. Soc. B.,* 133:444–479.

Katz, B. (1969): *The Release of Neural Transmitter Substances. Sherrington Lectures X.,* Liverpool University Press, Liverpool.

Katz, B., and Miledi, R. (1967): A study of synaptic transmission in the absence of nerve impulses. *J. Physiol. (Lond.),* 192:407–436.

Katz, B., and Thesleff, S. (1957): A study of the "desensitization" produced by acetylcholine at the motor end-plate. *J. Physiol. (Lond.),* 138:63–80.

Kusano, K. (1970): Influence of ionic environment on the relationship between pre- and post-synaptic potentials. *J. Neurobiol.,* 1:435–457.

Lekander, B. (1949): The sensory line system and the canal bones in the head of some ostariophysi. *Acta Zool. Stockh.,* 30:1–131.

Lissmann, H. W. (1958): On the function and evolution of electric organs in fish. *J. Exp. Biol.,* 35:156–191.

Lissmann, H. W., and Mullinger, A. M. (1968): Organization of ampullary electric receptors in Gymnotidae (Pisces). *Proc. Roy. Soc. B.,* 169:345–378.

Murray, R. W. (1965): Electroreceptor mechanisms: The relation of impulse frequency to stimulus strength and responses to pulsed stimuli in the ampullae of Lorenzini of elasmobranchs. *J. Physiol. (Lond.),* 180:592–606.

Nishihara, H., and Yamamoto, T. (1971): Fine structure of the ampullary organs of Lorenzini in marine catfish, *Plotosus anguillaris. J. Electron Microscop.,* 20:231.

Obara, S. (1974): Receptor cell activity at 'rest' with respect to the tonic operation of a specialized lateralis receptor. *Proc. Jap. Acad.,* 50:386–391.

Obara, S., Akutsu, Y., and Oomura, Y. (1974): Receptor mechanism in a tonic electroreceptor of marine catfish, *Plotosus anguillaris. Proc. Internat. Union Physiol. Sci.* XI, New Delhi.

Obara, S., and Bennett, M. V. L. (1968): Receptor and generator potentials of ampullae of Lorenzini in the skate, *Raja. Biol. Bull.,* 135:430.

Obara, S., and Bennett, M. V. L. (1972): Mode of operation of ampullae of Lorenzini of the skate, *Raja. J. Gen. Physiol.,* 60:534–557.

Obara, S., and Oomura, Y. (1973): Disfacilitation as the basis for the sensory suppression in a specialized lateralis receptor of the marine catfish. *Proc. Jap. Acad.,* 49:213–217.

Roth, A. (1968): Electroreception in the catfish, *Amiurus nebulosus. Z. Vergleich. Physiol.,* 61:196–202.

Roth, A. (1969): Elektrische Sinnesorgane beim Zwergwels, *Ictalurus nebulosus* (Amiurus nebulosus). *Z. Vergleich. Physiol.,* 65:368–388.

Steinbach, A. B. (1974): Transmission from receptor cells to afferent nerve fibers. In: *Synaptic Transmission and Neuronal Interaction,* edited by M. V. L. Bennett, pp. 105–140. Raven Press, New York.

Toyoda, J., Nosaki, H., and Tomita, T. (1969): Light-induced resistance changes in single photoreceptors of *Necturus* and *Gekko. Vis. Res.,* 9:453–463.

Umekita, S., Sugawara, Y., and Obara, S. (1975): Input-output relation across the receptor–afferent synapses in a tonic electroreceptor of marine catfish. *Proc. Jap. Acad.,* 51:485–490.

Wachtel, A. W., and Szamier, R. B. (1969): Special cutaneous receptor organs of fish: IV. Ampullary organs of the non-electric catfish, *Kryptopterus. J. Morphol.,* 128:291–308.

Waltman, B. (1966): Electrical properties and fine structure of the ampullary canals of Lorenzini. *Acta Physiol. Scand.,* Suppl. 264:1–60.

Waltman, B. (1968): Electrical excitability of the ampullae of Lorenzini in the ray. *Acta Physiol. Scand.,* 74:29A-30A.

Zipser, B., and Bennett, M. V. L. (1973): Tetrodotoxin resistant electrically excitable responses of receptor cells. *Brain Res.,* 62:253–259.

Electrobiology of Nerve, Synapse, and Muscle,
edited by J. P. Reuben, D. P. Purpura, M. V. L. Bennett,
and E. R. Kandel. Raven Press, New York © 1976

The Taste Response Modification by Salt in the Single Gustatory Cell of Rats

Masahiro Ozeki

Department of Biology, Faculty of Education, Yamanashi University, Kofu 400, Japan

Ozeki and Sato demonstrated in 1972 in the rat tongue that the gustatory responses to each of the four taste stimuli were modified by the addition of NaCl to the substance being tested. However, they did not examine the relationship between the magnitude of the receptor potential in response to the gustatory stimuli and the concentration of NaCl added to the test solutions.

The present study reports on the effects caused by adding saline to each of the four taste solutions on the magnitude of receptor potentials recorded intracellularly from the gustatory cells.

MATERIALS AND METHODS

Adult, female Sprague-Dawley rats were used. Each rat, anesthetized with an intravenous injection of sodium amobarbital (50 mg/kg body weight) into the tail, was fixed on a stereotactic table with a head-holder, and the trachea was cannulated. To stop small muscular movements of the tongue, the hypoglossal nerves on both sides were cut under the jaw. The tongue was pulled out and pinned at the tip onto a plastic plate. The tongue was usually soaked in saline solution containing 0.0414 M NaCl, which is the same as the average sodium concentration in the saliva (Hiji, 1969). Procedures of inserting a microelectrode filled with 3 M KCl into a gustatory cell in the rat fungiform papilla and methods of intracellular recording receptor potentials have been fully described elsewhere (Ozeki and Sato, 1972).

As the standard test gustatory stimuli, 0.5 M NaCl, 0.5 M sucrose, 0.01 N HCl, and 0.02 M quinine hydrochloride were used. Taste solutions were applied slowly to the tongue at a rate of about 1 ml/50 sec with an injection syringe. After stimulation, the tongue was rinsed with saline.

RESULTS AND DISCUSSION

Effects of Addition of NaCl to Each of the Four Basic Gustatory Solutions on the Magnitude of Receptor Potential

After the microelectrode penetrated into a gustatory cell in a fungiform papilla of the rat tongue, the receptor potential of the cell in response to various chemical stimulating substances could be recorded (Ozeki and Sato, 1972). Magnitudes of the receptor potentials in response to sucrose, quinine, and HCl were modified by addition of 0.0414 M NaCl to the test solutions (Fig. 1). This concentration of NaCl is the same as in rat saliva.

Response profiles of 14 cells examined in experiments in which the cells were stimulated by four basic stimuli and by the stimuli with the addition of saline are shown in Fig. 2. The magnitude of response to each basic stimulus was influenced characteristically by the addition of saline. Comparing the left section in which the cells stimulated by four basic stimuli only with

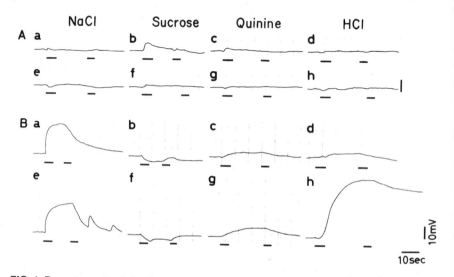

FIG. 1. Receptor potentials of two gustatory cells **(A, B)** produced by 0.5 M NaCl (a); 0.5 M sucrose (b); 0.02 M quinine (c); 0.01 N HCl (d); 0.5414 M NaCl (e); 0.5 M sucrose with 0.0414 M NaCl (f); 0.02 M quinine with 0.0414 M NaCl (g); and 0.01 N HCl with 0.0414 M NaCl (h). The left horizontal bar underneath each record indicates the time of application of stimuli; the right bar indicates rinsing of the papilla with saline solution. (Reproduced from Ozeki and Sato, 1972, by permission of *Comp. Biochem. Physiol.*)

the right section in which the stimuli included saline, by the addition of saline the magnitude of response to NaCl was little enhanced (as would be expected), the magnitude of response to HCl was often markedly enhanced, whereas that to sucrose was depressed. After the addition of saline to the test solutions, the mean magnitude of response to NaCl increased slightly from 12.6 ± 8.2 mV (mean ± SD of 12 cells) to 13.4 ± 8.4 mV; that to sucrose decreased from 4.3 ± 4.0 mV (mean ± SD of six cells) to 1.5 ± 0.5 mV; that to quinine showed a slight increase from 2.9 ± 1.9 mV (mean ± SD of eight cells) to 3.9 ± 4.3 mV; and that to HCl increased from 13.3 ± 13.5 mV (mean ± SD of 10 cells) to 30.4 ± 18.7 mV. The changes in mean values of the response to NaCl, sucrose, and quinine were not significant, that for HCl showed a significant increase ($p = 0.05$).

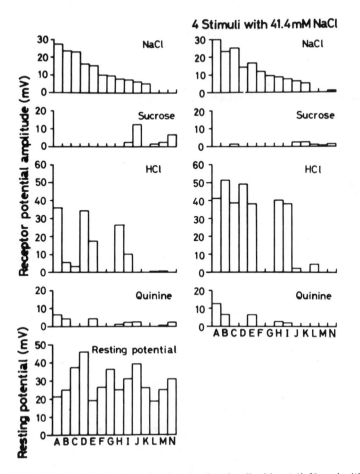

FIG. 2. Response profiles of 14 cells for four basic stimuli without (*left*) and with (*right*) saline and resting potentials of each cell (*bottom left*). The cells are arranged in order of decreasing response amplitude to 0.5 M NaCl. From the top, stimuli are: 0.5 M NaCl, 0.5 M sucrose, 0.01 N HCl, and 0.02 M quinine. Response magnitudes for all four stimuli in each cell and magnitudes of resting potentials of each cell are demonstrated by the blocks at the same point on the x axis.

Relationship between Magnitude of Receptor Potential
and the Concentration of Four Basic Gustatory Stimuli with NaCl

Figure 3 shows the effect of the addition of NaCl to HCl on the magnitude of receptor potentials recorded from two gustatory cells. When a cell was stimulated by 0.001 N HCl, a small depolarization was observed (A). The magnitude of response to 0.001 N HCl was increased by the addition of saline (B), but the amplitude of the response to 0.001 N HCl with 0.5 M NaCl was smaller than that to 0.5 M NaCl only (compare C and D). On the other hand, in another cell the magnitude of response to 0.01 N HCl was

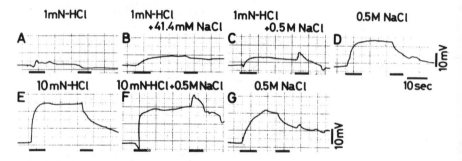

FIG. 3. Receptor potentials of two gustatory cells produced by HCl, NaCl, or mixture of them. **A–D** are recorded from one cell that did not respond to sucrose but did respond to NaCl, quinine, and HCl in that order of magnitude of response. **E–G** are recorded from another cell that responded to HCl, NaCl, and sucrose in that order of magnitude of response (this cell was not tested with quinine). Test stimuli employed were: 0.001 N HCl **(A)**; 0.001 N HCl with 0.0414 M NaCl **(B)**; 0.001 N HCl with 0.5 M NaCl **(C)**; 0.5 M NaCl **(D, G)**; 0.01 N HCl **(E)**; and 0.01 N HCl with 0.0414 M NaCl **(F)**. In C and F, saline rinses were followed by off-responses. The left horizontal bar underneath each record indicates the time of application of stimuli; the right bar indicates rinsing of the papilla with saline solution.

decreased by the addition of saline (compare F and E). However, in this cell the magnitude of the response to 0.01 N HCl with saline was larger than that to 0.5 M NaCl only (compare F and G).

In 9 of 10 cells examined, the magnitude of receptor potentials in response to HCl was increased by the addition of saline, and in one cell the magnitude was decreased. The enhancement of the response to 0.001 and 0.01 N HCl by the addition of saline is shown in Fig. 4C. When the concentration of NaCl added was as high as 0.5 M, the magnitude of response to HCl was slightly depressed. It is not clear from this experiment if the HCl receptor site in the microvilli of the cell was actually modified by the addition of NaCl. These results indicate that the magnitude of response to HCl is augmented or depressed by the addition of low and high concentrations of NaCl, respectively. The reversal point of the receptor potential produced by 0.5 M NaCl is not the same as that produced by 0.01 N HCl (Ozeki, 1973), since when the cell is stimulated by HCl with high concentration of NaCl, the magnitude of receptor potential is decided by the lower potential level of reversal point in each stimulus.

When a cell was stimulated with sucrose, the magnitude of receptor potential in response to sucrose with saline was frequently smaller than that to sucrose only (Fig. 1). This decreasing phenomenon was observed in four of six cells examined. The relationships between magnitude of receptor potential and concentration of sucrose only or sucrose with saline were divided into two classes by the following results as shown in Fig. 4A and B. The ratios between the magnitude of receptor potential in response to 0.5 M sucrose (S) and to 0.5 M NaCl (Na) in Fig. 4A and B were 1.4 and 0.01,

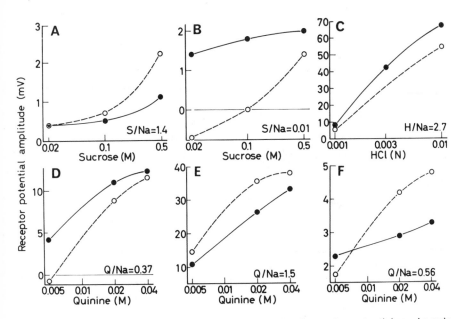

FIG. 4. Relationships between the maximum magnitude of receptor potentials and a pair of stimulus concentrations of sucrose **(A, B)**, HCl **(C)**, and quinine **(D–F)** without (open circles) and with (filled circles) saline solution.

respectively. When the cell had a relatively high sensitivity to sucrose in comparison with that to NaCl, the magnitude of receptor potential in response to a low concentration of sucrose was not modified, while that to a high concentration of sucrose was depressed by the addition of saline (class A; five cells). When the cell has very low sensitivity to sucrose in comparison with that to NaCl, the magnitude of receptor potential in response to a low concentration of sucrose was markedly increased and that to a high concentration of sucrose was not as increased by the addition of saline (class B; one cell).

The effect of the addition of NaCl to quinine solution at 0.005, 0.02, and 0.04 M on the magnitude of receptor potential was also examined. The relationships between the magnitude of receptor potentials and the concentration of quinine with or without saline are plotted. The cells were grouped into three classes according to the ratio of the magnitude of receptor potential in response to 0.02 M quinine (Q) and to 0.5 M NaCl (Na). When the cell showed as small a ratio of Q/Na as 0.37 (Fig. 4D), the magnitude of response to quinine with saline was larger than that to quinine only within the range of these concentrations (class D). When the cell showed as large a ratio of Q/Na as 1.5 (Fig. 4E), the magnitude of response to quinine plus saline was smaller than that to quinine only (class E). When the cell showed an intermediate ratio of Q/Na such as 0.56 (Fig. 4F), the magnitude of responses to quinine at low concentration with saline was larger than that to quinine only but the magnitude for quinine at high concentration with saline was smaller (class F). Of the eight cells examined, four were in class D, two in class E, and two in class F.

When the cell responded to both quinine and NaCl, the direction of modification of the magnitude of receptor potential by the addition of saline might be determined by whether the cell has a higher sensitivity to quinine than to NaCl. In general, NaCl has a slight depressive effect on the response to quinine because the magnitude of receptor potential in response to a mixture of quinine and NaCl was smaller than that of the sum of responses to individual solutions.

When one compares each modification of the magnitude of receptor potential in response to NaCl, sucrose, quinine, and HCl by the addition of saline, the gustatory cell showed a remarkable potentiation of the response to HCl and a depression to sucrose. Hidaka (1972) has also showed that the magnitude of response to HCl at relatively weak concentration in the paletal chemoreceptors of the carp was potentiated by the addition of NaCl.

SUMMARY

The gustatory response to the four taste qualities was recorded intracellularly from the single cell of the rat. The taste responses to sucrose, quinine, and HCl were modified by the addition of saline (0.0414 M NaCl). The response to sucrose decreased in five cells and increased in one. The response to quinine decreased in four cells, increased in three, and did not change in one. The response to HCl increased in nine cells and decreased slightly in one. The magnitude of receptor potential in response to HCl was significantly increased by the addition of saline ($p = 0.05$).

ACKNOWLEDGMENTS

I gratefully acknowledge the helpful suggestions and criticisms provided by Professor M. Sato, in whose laboratory part of this work was done.

REFERENCES

Hidaka, I. (1972): Stimulation of the paletal chemoreceptors of the carp by mixed solutions of acid and salt. *Jap. J. Physiol.*, 22:39–51.

Hiji, Y. (1969): Gustatory response and preference behavior in alloxian diabetic rats. *Kumamoto Med. J.*, 22:109–118.

Ozeki, M., and Sato, M. (1972): Responses of gustatory cells in the tongue of rat to stimuli representing four taste qualities. *Comp. Biochem. Physiol.*, 41A:391–407.

Ozeki, M. (1973): Electrical activities of gustatory cells in the tongue of rat to stimuli representing four taste qualities. *Mem. Fac. Lib. Art Educ. Yamanashi Univ.*, No. 23:74–78.

Electrobiology of Nerve, Synapse, and Muscle,
edited by J. P. Reuben, D. P. Purpura, M. V. L. Bennett,
and E. R. Kandel. Raven Press, New York © 1976

Proteins in the Squid Giant Axon

Harold Gainer and Vivian S. Gainer*

*Behavioral Biology Branch, National Institute of Child Health and Human Development,
National Institutes of Health, Bethesda, Maryland 20014; and *Marine Biological Laboratory, Woods Hole, Massachusetts 02543*

The squid giant axon has been extremely valuable as a model system for
fundamental studies in electrobiology (Adelman, 1971; Cole, 1968; Hodgkin, 1964; Tasaki, 1968). However, comparatively little biochemical work
has been done on this model [see Lasek (1974) for a brief review of this
subject]. Our interest in this experimental preparation was stimulated by
the fact that it was possible to obtain relatively uncontaminated axoplasm
for biochemical analysis (Bear, et al., 1937).

In this paper, we present recent studies on the composition and synthesis
of proteins in the squid giant axon. These studies bear on two neurobiological issues: (1) the characterization of the major protein subunits found in
axoplasm and an evaluation of their possible relationship to the various subcellular structures that are present in axoplasm; and (2) whether the axon is
capable of *de novo* protein synthesis, as has been proposed for other systems (Koenig, 1965; Alvarez and Chen, 1972). In using the squid giant axon
as a model preparation to deal with these issues, one must always keep in
mind the problem of biological diversity. However, in view of the successful
generalizations that have been derived from comparative electrobiology
(Grundfest, 1966), it is hoped that equivalent biochemical generalizations
will also emerge.

ANALYSIS OF THE MAJOR PROTEIN SUBUNITS
IN SQUID AXOPLASM

The resolving power of disc electrophoresis, first described by Ornstein
and Davis (Ornstein, 1964), allows for excellent fractionation and characterization of various macromolecules (Maurer, 1971). In addition to being
the method of choice for the separation of proteins, it can also be used
analytically. Proteins may be separated on the basis of their size only [by
electrophoresis in sodium dodecyl sulfate (SDS)], or by exploiting their
intrinsic electrical properties (i.e., isoelectric focusing). In some cases it is
desirable to separate proteins on polyacrylamide gels using a combination
of their electrical and molecular size properties, and an analytical theory

exists for this approach (Ferguson, 1964; Rodbard and Chrambach, 1971).

In this paper, we use an acid-urea gel system (Davis et al., 1972) to analyze the major proteins of squid axoplasm. Separation of the axoplasmic proteins by polyacrylamide electrophoresis in SDS was also done, using methods described elsewhere (Gainer, 1971). The advantage of the acid-urea over the SDS gel system is primarily due to the preservation of the electrical charge characteristics of the proteins in the acid-urea method. In both methods all the proteins are unidirectionally charged. In the case of acid-urea gel which runs at pH 2.7 the proteins are positively charged, whereas in SDS they are negatively charged. However, the SDS gel separates complex mixtures of proteins into molecular weight classes, whereas the acid-urea gel has a higher resolution, since in this system a difference of one positively charged residue on the protein would provide a detectable 3% change in electrophoretic mobility (Panyim and Chalkley, 1969).

Figure 1 illustrates the acid-urea gel separations of proteins extracted from various types of axons in the squid. In each case the isolated axons were cleanly dissected (axoplasm from the giant axon was extruded by conventional methods) and then homogenized in the appropriate buffers for each gel system (Davis et al., 1972; Gainer, 1971). A reducing agent,

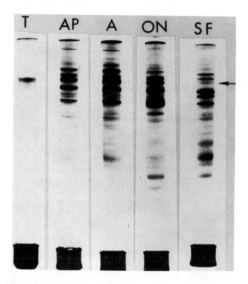

FIG. 1. Polyacrylamide gel electrophoresis of proteins extracted from various types of axons in the squid. Electrophoresis was done using an acid-urea system (see text) that separates proteins on the basis of their size and charge. The top of the gel is the origin, and electrophoresis was toward the cathode (*bottom*). The proteins on the gel were stained with Coomassie Blue. For comparison, isolated chick-brain tubulin (T) is shown on the left, and the mobility of T is depicted on the right side by an arrow. AP, A, ON, and SF represent proteins extracted from extruded axoplasm (of squid giant axon), intact squid giant axon (but cleaned free of surrounding small fibers), optic nerve, and small fibers surrounding the giant axon, respectively.

β-mercaptoethanol, was included in all the buffers, and the extract was centrifuged at $10,000 \times g_{max}$ for 1 hr before application of the supernatant to the gels. The mobility of isolated chick-brain microtubule protein (or tubulin, designated T), obtained from Dr. Lionel Rebhun (University of Virginia), is also shown for comparison (Fig. 1). The tubulin consists of two protein subunits that are separated only slightly by the acid-urea gel system. Extruded axoplasm from the squid giant axon (AP), when electrophoresed on this gel system, revealed five major protein subunits and a number of minor bands. One of these major bands appears to correspond to the tubulin (in electrophoretic mobility). Electrophoresis of proteins extracted from the entire giant axon, which included the axoplasm, plasma membrane, and sheath (i.e., Schwann cells, basal lamina, etc.), provided a similar protein distribution, except that a number of more mobile, minor protein bands were also detected. Since the axoplasm in the giant axon contains about 10-fold the amount of protein found in the plasma membrane plus sheath, it was to be expected that the bands in A would be dominated by the bands seen in AP. The smaller axons of the optic nerve (ON) and small fibers surrounding the giant axon (SF), which contain a greater proportion of nonaxoplasmic proteins from their sheaths, were also extracted and electrophoresed (Fig. 1). The five major bands observed from AP were also represented in varying amounts on the ON and SF gels. In addition to these five major axoplasmic protein subunits, both the ON and SF gels also contained prominent bands with considerably higher mobilities. Whether these rapidly moving bands are unique to the optic nerve and small fiber axons, or represent a greater contribution of their contaminating sheath tissues (e.g., glia, etc.) remains to be determined. One unexpected finding was the relatively low content of microtubule protein (see arrow in Fig. 1) in the SF axons. The main point of these data is that five major and distinct protein subunits were detectable in axoplasm from the giant axon, and that these subunits also appeared in the electrophoretic profile of the optic nerve and small fiber axons.

This distribution of the major proteins of axons depicted in Fig. 1 appears to be axon specific. Comparison of the electrophoretic patterns of proteins extracted from the stellate ganglion, and various nonneuronal tissues to that of axoplasm (AP) is presented in Fig. 2. The differences are apparent. The proteins of mantle muscle (M) provided seven major bands, only two of which corresponded in electrophoretic mobility to the bands in AP. The proteins extracted from the stellate ganglion (G), gill (GL), and gastrointestinal tract (GI) of the squid were by comparison very complex and exhibited a wide range of electrophoretic mobilities.

Further analysis of the five major proteins in axoplasm was made by application of the Ferguson equation (Ferguson, 1964; Chrambach and Rodbard, 1971; Rodbard and Chrambach, 1971). The axoplasmic proteins were electrophoresed on acid-urea gels at three different monomer concentra-

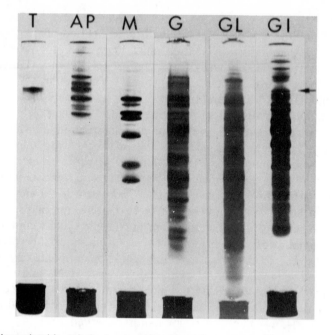

FIG. 2. Polyacrylamide gel electrophoresis of proteins extracted from various nonneural tissues of the squid. (See Fig. 1 for description of electrophoresis system.) T, AP, M, G, GL, and GI represent isolated chick-brain tubulin, extruded axoplasm, muscle from mantle, stellate ganglion, gill, and gastrointestinal tract, respectively.

tions. The mobilities of the five major bands relative to methyl green (R_f) were plotted against the percent gel concentration (%T). The relationship between these parameters is given by:

$$\log R_f = -K_R T + \log Y_0$$

where R_f is the relative mobility of a protein at gel concentration T, Y_0 is the apparent, free relative mobility (i.e., the R_f when $T = 0$), and K_R is the retardation coefficient that is a function of molecular radius. From the "Ferguson plot," described above, it is possible to calculate the K_R and Y_0 values of the various protein subunits from the slopes and intercepts (at $T = 0$). Since the $\sqrt{K_R}$ is linearly related to the geometric mean molecular radius of globular proteins (Chrambach and Rodbard, 1971; Rodbard and Chrambach, 1971), the sizes (radii) of the major axoplasmic proteins could be determined from a standard curve generated from the electrophoresis of marker proteins on acid-urea gels (see Fig. 3, right).

The "Ferguson plot" of the major axoplasmic proteins is illustrated in Fig. 3 (left). Since the slopes of the lines (A–E in Fig. 3) were very close to each other, it was apparent that the separation between these proteins on the acid-urea gel was primarily on the basis of their different charge properties

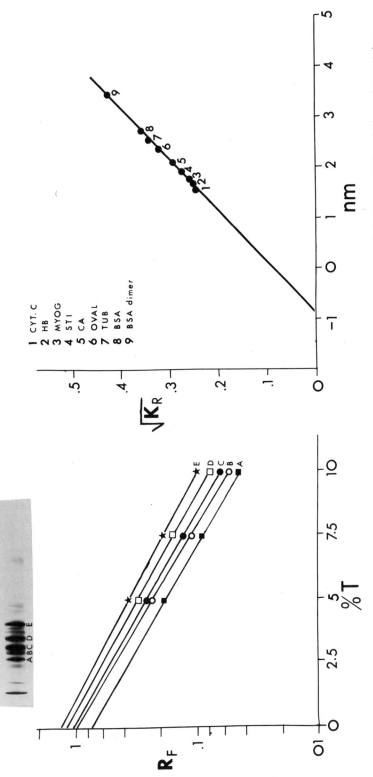

FIG. 3. Ferguson plot analysis of the major protein subunits in the axoplasm of the giant axon. **Left:** The mobility of the major proteins (A–E) relative to methyl green (R_F) are plotted against the acrylamide concentration (%T) of the gel. Inset shows 10% acid-urea gel with proteins from axoplasm. **Right:** Plot of retardation coefficient (K_R) against mean geometric radius (nm) for various standard proteins: (1) cytochrome c; (2) hemoglobin; (3) myoglobin; (4) soybean trypsin inhibitor; (5) carbonic anhydrase; (6) ovalbumin; (7) chick-brain tubulin; (8) bovine serum albumin monomer; (9) dimer.

at pH 2.7. Using the above equation, the free mobilities (Y_0) and mean geometric radii of these five proteins were calculated. These results are presented in Table 1. Whereas the radii of these proteins ranged from 2.4 to 2.75 nm, their Y_0 values were more diverse (i.e., ranging from 0.74 to 1.35). When chick-brain tubulin was subjected to the same treatment and analysis, a Y_0 equal to 1.05- and 2.6-nm radius was obtained, thereby strengthening the suggestion that band C represents microtubule protein. Although it is not possible to easily convert the mean geometric radii of proteins to molecular weight values (Rodbard and Chrambach, 1971), it is probably fair to conclude (from the relationship of the radii of the standard proteins shown in Fig. 3 to their known molecular weights) that the five major axoplasmic proteins ranged in molecular weights from about 40,000 to 71,000 daltons.

An alternative method of determining the sizes of the major axoplasmic proteins is by polyacrylamide gel electrophoresis in SDS. Figure 4 depicts a densitometric scan at 560 nm of an SDS gel containing separated axoplasmic proteins stained by Coomassie Blue. Since the electrophoretic mobility of proteins on this gel system is a direct function of their size and the molecular sieving properties of the gel, it is possible to obtain a direct estimate of the molecular weights of proteins by comparison with the mobilities of standard proteins of known molecular weights (see upper abscissa in Fig. 4). Five major protein classes were detected on the SDS gel — at approximately 71,000, 57,000, 54,000, 46,000 and 43,000 daltons (arrows, Fig. 4). The mobility of the 57,000-dalton class corresponded to the mobility of chick-brain tubulin on the same system. (The tubulin actually ran as two bands close together in this position of the gel.) The 57,000-dalton protein shown in Fig. 4 is represented by a broad band that appears to be composed of two bands, which are clearly resolved when less protein is loaded onto the gel. Thus, five major axoplasmic protein subunits were detected in squid axoplasm by two separate methods (the C band in the acid-

TABLE 1. *"Ferguson-plot" analysis of major protein subunits in squid axoplasm (acid-urea gel electrophoresis)*[a]

Protein band	Y_0	Mean geometric radius ($\overline{nm}$)
A	0.74	2.4
B	0.98	2.75
C	1.05	2.60
D	1.20	2.60
E	1.35	2.55

[a] The proteins (A–E) correspond to those shown on the gel in Fig. 3 (inset). Y_0 represents the free mobility of the protein. Values were calculated from data in Fig. 3 using Ferguson equation (see text). The Y_0 and $\overline{nm}$ values for chick-brain tubulin equal 1.05 and 2.6, respectively.

MW/1000

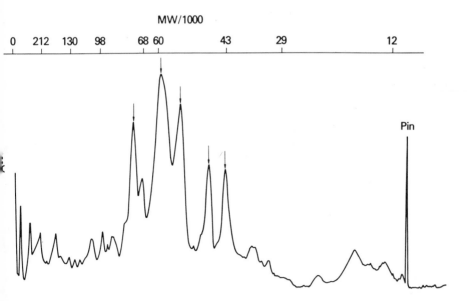

FIG. 4. Molecular weight distribution of proteins isolated from pure axoplasm extruded from the squid giant axon. The proteins were separated in SDS on an 11% polyacrylamide gel and stained with Coomassie Blue. The destained gel was scanned at 560 nm to provide the densitometric trace shown. The deflection, marked Pin, represents the bromphenol blue marker position. *Upper abscissa,* positions on the gel of various marker proteins of known molecular weights (which were coelectrophoresed on a separate gel). 0, origin of the gel. *Arrows,* five major protein peaks.

urea gel, and the 57,000-dalton band in the SDS gel, are each probably composed of the two subunits of tubulin). Because of the relatively large quantities of these proteins in axoplasm, it is likely that they are representative of structural proteins.

RELATIONSHIP OF THE MAJOR PROTEIN SUBUNITS TO STRUCTURAL COMPONENTS IN AXOPLASM

Electron microscopic studies have revealed at least six distinct structures in nervous tissue; microtubules, neurofilaments, microfilaments, astrocyte filaments, smooth endoplasmic reticulum, and mitochondria (Peters et al., 1970; Schmitt, 1968; Wuerker and Kirkpatrick, 1972). With the exception of astrocyte filaments, all of these are amply found in invertebrate and vertebrate axons.

Probably the best known of all the fibrous structures are the 20- to 26-nm microtubules, which have been shown to be composed of a 120,000-dalton protein (dimer) and can be reduced to two subunits: 54,000 to 57,000 daltons (Weisenberg et al., 1968). The microtubule protein (tubulin) from a variety of experimental preparations appears to be similar. The protein composition of the 10-nm neurofilament, however, is still unresolved. In the mammalian nervous system, the major neurofilament protein has been variously reported as 60,000 daltons (Shelanski et al., 1971), 85,000 daltons (Wuerker and Kirkpatrick, 1972), and 50,000 daltons (Davison and Winslow, 1974). The astrocyte filament, approximately 5 to 7 nm, contains protein dimers that coelectrophorese with tubulin (about 57,000 daltons), but do not resemble tubulin when peptide mapping studies are done (Johnson and Sinex, 1974). The 5-nm microfilaments appear to contain an actin-like protein, around 45,000 daltons (Fine and Bray, 1971), that binds heavy meromyosin (Chang and Goldman, 1973). Compelling evidence for the presence of an actomyosin-like protein in mammalian brain has been reported (Berl et al., 1973). Recent studies have demonstrated that the slowly transported component in mammalian nerves contains primarily proteins that coelectrophorese with tubulin, actin, and a triplet of proteins (68,000, 160,000, and 212,000 daltons) suggested as possibly being associated with neurofilaments (Hoffman and Lasek, 1975).

Similar attempts to associate specific proteins with fibrous structures have been made on the squid giant axon. Electron microscopic studies have demonstrated the usual fibrous and membrane structures (Villegas, 1969; Metuzals, 1969; Schmitt, 1959). The colchicine binding protein in squid axoplasm (Borisy and Taylor, 1967) has been identified as the microtubule protein (Davison and Huneeus, 1970). In their studies on isolated 10-nm neurofilaments from the squid giant axon, Huneeus and Davison (1970) reported obtaining a protein ranging in molecular weight from 74,000 to 80,000 daltons (depending on the methods used), which they termed filarin. Similar estimates of 68,000 to 75,000 daltons for squid axon filarin have been obtained by other workers (Maxfield, 1953; Lasek, 1974; Metuzals, *personal communication*).

From the above brief review of the literature, it would appear that the 57,000-dalton protein (Fig. 4, SDS gel) and band C (Table 1, acid-urea gel), which we have detected in squid axoplasm, represents tubulin, and that our 71,000-dalton protein (band B, Table 1) probably corresponds to the protein termed filarin. By analogy, the 46,000-dalton protein found in squid axoplasm (band E, Table 1) probably corresponds to the 45,000-dalton protein isolated from microfilaments (Fine and Bray, 1971). However, this leaves two *major* protein subunits in squid axoplasm for which we cannot account—the 54,000-dalton protein (band D, Table 1) and the 43,000-dalton protein (band A, Table 1). These two distinct proteins, found in large quantity in axoplasm, may be loosely bound to the fibrous (intraaxonal) structures, and therefore, are lost when these structures are isolated for analysis. Another possibility is that they are associated with another structure entirely (e.g., the agranular reticulum). The above correlations are, of course, quite speculative, and further work utilizing subcellular fractionation and peptide mapping procedures in combination with electrophoresis is necessary before any definite conclusions can be drawn. In any case, the axoplasm of the squid giant axon contains a number of identifiable major proteins (and minor proteins as well) which are potential candidates for structural proteins in axoplasm.

THE ORIGIN OF AXOPLASMIC PROTEINS

It has been well established that axonal proteins are derived largely from the intraaxonal transport of proteins from the neuron soma (Weiss and Hiscoe, 1948; Droz and Leblond, 1963; Grafstein, 1969; Lasek, 1970; Ochs, 1972. However, various studies indicate that some axonal proteins may be derived from local synthesis mechanisms, either within the axon itself (Koenig, 1965), or by the synthesis of proteins in satellite cells (e.g., glia) which are subsequently transported into the axon (Singer, 1967, 1968). The former mechanism seems unlikely since ribosomes are rarely found, if at all, in axons (Zelena, 1972). Indeed, Lasek et al. (1973) have analyzed the RNA in squid axoplasm and found virtually no ribosomal RNA. However, these authors did find a substantial amount of 4S RNA, which may be transfer RNA. The sheath surrounding the axon does contain 28, 18, and 4S RNA (presumably mostly in the Schwann cells). Thus, the axon *itself* would appear incapable of *de novo* protein synthesis. However, when Giuditta et al. (1968) incubated the giant axon (isolated from its cell bodies) in ³H-amino acids, labeled proteins appeared in the axoplasm.

In view of the above results, one of us (H. G.)—in collaboration with R. J. Lasek, R. J. Pryzblyski, J. L. Barker, and I. Tasaki—set out to study the origin of these labeled proteins. A preliminary report of some of this work has been published (Lasek et al., 1974). Incubation of isolated giant axons in media containing ³H-leucine confirmed the findings of Giuditta et al. (1968), and showed that the synthesis of the labeled proteins was inhibited by puromycin and cyclohexamide, but not by chloramphenicol. This indicated that the labeled proteins were synthesized by conventional ribosomal mechanisms. Autoradiographs of squid giant axons, after various incubation times in ³H-leucine, showed that most of the labeled proteins were in the regions of the sheath that corresponded to the Schwann cells, but a considerable number of grains were found in the axoplasm. The ratio of grains in axoplasm to sheath was comparable to the trichloroacetic acid precipitable radioactivity ratios found when the axoplasm was isolated from the sheath by extrusion, thus discounting the possibility that the labeled proteins found in the extruded axoplasm were due to damage of the sheath during the extrusion procedure. About 40% of the total radioactivity of the preparation was found in the axoplasm after 2 hr of incubation. The newly synthesized proteins from the extruded axoplasm and sheath were subjected to isoelectric focusing and SDS gel electrophoresis, and a correspondence in labeled protein patterns was found (Lasek et al., 1974). The labeled proteins found in the axoplasm coelectrophoresed with some but not all of the major proteins in squid axoplasm (Fig. 5). The data in Fig. 5 compare the densitometric trace of a 7.5% SDS–polyacrylamide gel containing axoplasmic proteins (axoplasm was not centrifuged before application to gel), with the radioactive profile of an identical gel containing labeled axoplasmic proteins. Incubation of extruded axoplasm with ^{3}H-amino acids did not generate labeled proteins, and thus, it was concluded that these data were consistent with the interpretation that proteins were synthesized *de novo* in the Schwann cells and then transferred to the axon (Lasek et al., 1974). The sizes of the labeled proteins ranged from about 12,000 to greater than 200,000 daltons (the bulk being between 40,000 and 80,000 daltons, Fig. 5; also see Fig. 2 in Lasek et al., 1974), thus precluding the possibility that these proteins were passively moving through channels in the electrotonic junctions (Villegas, 1972).

Given the above hypothesis of the transfer of newly synthesized proteins from Schwann cells to axon, we attempted to demonstrate that synthesis could be uncoupled from transport. Removal of calcium ions from the incubation media had no effect on synthesis, but decreased the radioactivity in the axoplasm to less than half (Lasek et al., *in preparation*). Thus, the

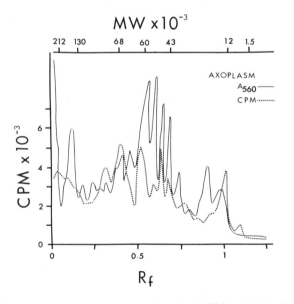

FIG. 5. Molecular weight distribution of proteins on 7.5% SDS gel isolated from axoplasm extruded from the squid giant axon. The solid line shows the densitometric profile of the major axoplasmic proteins, and the dotted line shows the profile of labeled proteins found in the axoplasm after 2 hr of incubation in ^{3}H-leucine (the cpm data calculated from Lasek et al., 1974). *Lower abscissa,* mobility relative to cytochrome c (= 1.0). *Upper abscissa,* gel positions of standard proteins of known molecular weight.

transport mechanism appeared to be dependent on extracellular calcium. Kinetic analysis of the rates of appearance of labeled proteins in axoplasm versus sheath tended to confirm the notion that the Schwann cells were the source of labeled proteins. There was a 30- to 60-min lag period between the presence of labeled proteins in the sheath and axoplasm. This lag period was more clearly demonstrated in giant axons that were intracellularly perfused by the method of Lehrman et al. (1969), while incubating in media containing ^{3}H-leucine. In these perfusion studies, the axons conducted propagated spikes throughout the incubation, and labeled proteins appeared in the perfusate only after 30 to 60 min of incubation. After this initial lag period, the rate of appearance of labeled proteins in the perfusate was linear for 8 hr (Gainer et al., *in preparation*). Inclusion of RNAase (50 mg/ml) in the perfusion fluid did not influence the rate or extent of appearance of labeled proteins in the perfusate, whereas the extracellular application of puromycin prevented it completely.

One possible mechanism for the transfer of these large proteins is an exocytosis by the Schwann cells coupled to endocytosis (i.e., pinocytosis) in the giant axon. Evidence for pinocytosis in the giant axon comes from the work of Giuditta et al. (1971) who showed that labeled bovine serum albumin (BSA) is actively taken up by squid axoplasm (confirmed by Lasek et al., *in preparation*). However, the kinetics of uptake of the labeled BSA differed greatly from the transfer kinetics seen with endogenously synthesized proteins from the Schwann cells (*in preparation*). This difference was found in both extrusion and perfusion experiments, and the inclusion of large amounts of BSA in the medium did not effect the transfer rate of endogenous proteins. The evidence for exocytosis from the Schwann cells is less direct. Electron microscopic studies show that the Schwann cells contain golgi bodies (Villegas and Villegas, 1960; Villegas, 1969) presumably for packaging secretory material. The dependence of the transfer process on extracellular calcium ions is also consistent with an exocytotic process (Douglas, 1966). No morphological evidence that shows pinocytotic vesicles in the squid giant axon exists at present.

Although the data now available strongly support the hypothesis that large quantities of newly synthesized, Schwann cell proteins are transferred to squid axoplasm, the functional roles of these proteins are unclear. Some possibilities are: (1) because of the large size of the giant axon, the proteins transported from the neuron soma are inadequate, and, therefore, must be supplemented by this mechanism (for nutritional purposes, and structural or membrane replacement); and (2) these proteins represent "information (trophic) macromolecules" for the axon. Probably similar processes, to varying extents, occur in other axons. There may be a continuum ranging from axons that are highly dependent on local synthesis mechanisms (e.g., in the crustacea, where motoneurons isolated from their cell bodies can remain functional for as long as 1 year; see Hoy et al., 1967; Bittner, 1973), to axons in which the proteins are primarily derived from the neuron cell body (Singer, 1967, 1968; Joseph, 1973). The fact that the squid axon can degenerate (Sereni and Young, 1932) places it somewhere between these two extremes.

POSSIBLE SIGNIFICANCE OF INTERCELLULAR TRANSPORT OF MACROMOLECULES

The observation that large macromolecules are transferred from Schwann cells to the giant axon of the squid may reflect a general biological phenomenon. The literature is replete with examples of molecular exchanges and metabolic cooperation between adjacent cells (Loewenstein, 1973; Bennett, 1973; Kolodny, 1971, 1972; Subak-Sharpe et al., 1969; Martz and Steinberg, 1971; Stoker, 1967; Cox et al., 1970). In this manner, transport of macromolecules could be involved in the regulation of intracellular metabolism by the immediate environment (i.e., an adjacent cell). The exquisite regulatory controls in differentiation (Hamburgh, 1971) may make use of such a mechanism.

REFERENCES

Adelman, W. J., Jr., editor (1971): *Biophysics and Physiology of Excitable Membranes*. Van Nostrand Reinhold Corp., New York.

Alvarez, J., and Chen, W. Y. (1972): Infection of leucine into a myelinated axon: Incorporation in the axoplasm and transfer to associated cells. *Acta Physiol. Lat. Am.*, 22:266–269.

Bear, R. S., Schmitt, F. O., and Young, J. Z. (1937): Investigations on the protein constituents of nerve axoplasm. *Proc. R. Soc. Lond. [Biol.]*, 123:520–529.

Bennett, M. V. L. (1973): Function of electrotonic junctions in embryonic and adult tissues. *Fed. Proc.*, 32:65–75.

Berl, S., Puzkin, S., and Nicklas, W. J. (1973): Actomyosin-like protein in brain. *Science*, 179:441–446.

Bittner, G. D. (1973): Degeneration and regeneration in crustacean neuromuscular systems. *Am. Zool.*, 13:379–408.

Borisy, F. G., and Taylor, E. W. (1967): The mechanical action of colchicine. *J. Cell Biol.*, 34:525–533.

Chang, C., and Goldman, R. D. (1973): The localization of actin-like fibers in cultured neuroblastoma cells as revealed by heavy meromyosin binding. *J. Cell Biol.*, 57:867–874.

Chrambach, A., and Rodbard, D. (1971): Polyacrylamide gel electrophoresis. *Science*, 172: 440–451.

Cole, K. S. (1968): *Membranes, Ions and Impulses*. Univ. of California Press, Berkeley.

Cox, R. P., Krauss, M. R., Balis, M. E., and Dancis, J. (1970): Evidence for transfer of enzyme product as the basis of metabolic cooperation between tissue culture fibroblasts of Lesch–Nyhan disease and normal cells. *Proc. Natl. Acad. Sci. USA*, 67:1573–1579.

Davis, R. H., Copenhaver, J. H., and Carver, M. J. (1972): Characterization of acidic proteins in cell nuclei from rat brain by high-resolution acrylamide gel electrophoresis. *J. Neurochem.*, 19:473–477.

Davison, P. F., and Huneeus, F. C. (1970): Fibrillar proteins from squid axons. II. Microtubule protein. *J. Mol. Biol.*, 52:429–439.

Davison, P. F., and Winslow, B. (1974): The protein subunit of calf brain neurofilament. *J. Neurobiol.*, 5:119–133.

Douglas, W. W. (1966): Calcium-dependent links in stimulus-secretion coupling in the adrenal medulla and neurohypophysis. In: *Mechanisms of Release of Biogenic Amines*. Proc. Wenner-Gren Symposium, pp. 267–290. Pergamon Press, Oxford.

Droz, B., and Leblond, C. P. (1963): Axonal migration of proteins in the central nervous system and peripheral nerves as shown by radioautography. *J. Comp. Neurol.,* 121:325–346.

Ferguson, K. A. (1964): Starch gel electrophoresis–Application to the classification of pituitary proteins and polypeptides. *Metabolism,* 13:985–1002.

Fine, R. E., and Bray, D. (1971): Actin in growing nerve cells. *Nature [New Biol.],* 234:115–118.

Gainer, H. (1971): Micro-disc electrophoresis in sodium dodecyl sulfate: An application to the study of protein synthesis in individual, identified neurons. *Anal. Biochem.,* 44:589–605.

Giuditta, A., Dettbarn, W. D., and Brzin, M. (1968): Protein synthesis in the isolated giant axon of the squid. *Proc. Natl. Acad. Sci., USA,* 59:1284–1287.

Giuditta, A., Udine, B. D., and Pepe, M. (1971): Uptake of protein by the giant axon of the squid. *Nature [New Biol.],* 229:29–30.

Grafstein, B. (1969): Axonal transport: Communication between soma and synapses. In: *Advances in Biochemical Pharmacology,* edited by E. Costa and P. Greengard, pp. 11–25. Raven Press, New York.

Grundfest, H. (1966): Comparative electrobiology of excitable membranes. In: *Advances in Comparative Physiology and Biochemistry,* edited by O. E. Loewenstein, pp. 1–116. Academic Press, New York.

Hamburgh, M. (1971): *Theories of Differentiation.* American Elsevier Publishing Co., New York.

Hoffman, P. N. and Lasek, R. J. (1975): The slow component of axonal transport. Identification of major structural polypeptides of the axon and their generality among mammalian neurons. *J. Cell. Biol.,* 66:351–366.

Hodgkin, A. L. (1964): *The Conduction of the Nervous Impulse.* Charles C Thomas Co., Springfield, Ill.

Hoy, R. R., Bittner, G. D., and Kennedy, D. (1967): Regeneration in crustacean motoneurons: Evidence for axonal refusion. *Science,* 156:251–252.

Huneeus, F. C., and Davison, P. F. (1970): Fibrillar proteins from squid axons. I. Neurofilament protein. *J. Mol. Biol.,* 52:415–428.

Johnson, L. S., and Sinex, F. M. (1974): On the relationship of brain filaments to microtubules. *J. Neurochem.,* 22:321–326.

Joseph, B. S. (1973): Somatofugal events in wallerian degeneration: A conceptual overview. *Brain Res.,* 59:1–18.

Koenig, E. (1965): Synthetic mechanisms in the axon–I. Local axonal synthesis of acetylcholinesterase. *J. Neurochem.,* 12:343–355.

Kolodny, G. M. (1971): Evidence for transfer of macromolecular RNA between mammalian cells in culture. *Exp. Cell Res.,* 65:313–324.

Kolodny, G. M. (1972): Cell to cell transfer of RNA into transformed cells. *J. Cell. Physiol.,* 79:147–150.

Lasek, R. J. (1970): Protein transport in neurons. *Int. Rev. Neurobiol.,* 13:289–324.

Lasek, R. J. (1974): Biochemistry of the squid giant axon. In: *A Guide to Laboratory Use of the Squid, Loligo peali,* edited by J. M. Arnold, pp. 69–74. Marine Biological Laboratory, Woods Hole, Mass.

Lasek, R. J., Dabrowski, C., and Nordlander, R. (1973): Analysis of axoplasmic RNA from invertebrate giant axons. *Nature,* 244:162–165.

Lasek, R. J., Gainer, H., and Pryzbylski, R. J. (1974): Transfer of newly synthesized proteins from Schwann cells to the squid giant axon. *Proc. Natl. Acad. Sci. USA,* 71:1188–1192.

Lehrman, L., Watanabe, A., and Tasaki, I. (1969): Intracellular perfusion of squid giant axons: Recent findings and interpretations. *Neurosci. Res.,* 2:71–105.

Loewenstein, W. R. (1973): Membrane junctions in growth and differentiation. *Fed. Proc.,* 32:60–64.

Martz, E., and Steinberg, M. S. (1971): The role of cell–cell contact in "contact" inhibition of cell division: A review and new evidence. *J. Cell. Physiol.,* 79:189–210.

Maurer, H. R. (1971): *Disc Electrophoresis.* Walter de Gruyter, Berlin.

Maxfield, M. (1953): Axoplasmic proteins of the squid giant nerve fiber with particular reference to the fibrous protein. *J. Gen. Physiol.,* 37:201–216.

Metuzals, J., and Izzard, C. S. (1969): Spatial patterns of thread-like elements in the axoplasm of the squid. *J. Cell Biol.,* 43:456–479.

Ochs, S. (1972): Rate of fast transport in mammalian nerve fibers. *J. Physiol. (Lond.),* 277:627–645.

Ornstein, L. (1964): Disc electrophoresis—I. Background and theory. *Ann. NY Acad. Sci.,* 121:321–349.

Panyim, S., and Chalkley, R. (1969): High resolution acrylamide gel electrophoresis of Histones. *Arch. Biochem. Biophys.,* 130:337–346.

Peters, A., Palay, S. L., and Webster, H. DeF., (1970): *The Fine Structure of the Nervous System: The Cells and their Processes.* Harper and Row, New York.

Rodbard, D., and Chrambach, A. (1971): Estimation of molecular radius, free mobility, and valence using polyacrylamide gel electrophoresis. *Anal. Biochem.,* 40:95–134.

Schmitt, F. O. (1959): The structure of the axon filaments of the giant nerve fibers of *Loligo* and *Myxicola. J. Exp. Zool.,* 113:499–516.

Schmitt, F. O. (1968): Fibrous proteins—neuronal organelles. *Proc. Natl. Acad. Sci. USA,* 60:1092–1101.

Sereni, E., and Young, J. Z. (1932): Nervous degeneration and regeneration in cephalopods. *Pubb. Staz. Zool. Napoli,* 12:173–208.

Singer, M. (1967): Transport of materials into the axon from nonperikaryal sites. *Neurosci. Res. Program Bull.,* 5:351–355.

Singer, M. (1968): Penetration of labeled amino acids into the peripheral nerve fibers from surrounding body fluids. In: *Ciba Foundation Symposium on Growth of the Nervous System,* edited by G. E. W. Wolstenholme and M. O'Conner, pp. 200–215, J. A. Churchill, London.

Shelanski, M. L., Albert, S., DeVries, G. H., and Norton, W. T. (1971): Isolation of filaments from brain. *Science,* 174:1242–1245.

Stoker, M. G. P. (1967): Transfer of growth inhibition between normal and virus-transformed cells. *J. Cell Sci.,* 2:293–304.

Subak-Sharpe, H., Burk, R. R., and Pitts, J. D. (1969): Metabolic cooperation between biochemically marked mammalian cells in tissue culture. *J. Cell Sci.,* 4:353–367.

Tasaki, I. (1968): *Nerve Excitation. A Macromolecular Approach,* Charles C Thomas, Springfield, Ill.

Villegas, G. M., and Villegas, R. (1960): The ultrastructure of the giant nerve fiber of the squid: Axon–Schwann cell relationship. *J. Ultrastruct. Res.,* 3:362–373.

Villegas, G. M. (1969): Electron microscopic study of the giant nerve fiber of the giant squid *Dosidicus gigas. J. Ultrastruct. Res.,* 26:501–514.

Villegas, J. (1972): Axon-Schwann cell interaction in the squid nerve fiber. *J. Physiol. (Lond.),* 225:275–296.

Weisenberg, R. C., Borisy, G. G., and Taylor, E. W. (1968): The colchicine binding protein of mammalian brain and its relation to microtubules. *Biochemistry,* 7:4466–4479.

Weiss, P., and Hiscoe, H. B. (1948): Experiments on the mechanism of nerve growth. *J. Exp. Zool.,* 107:315–396.

Wuerker, R. B., and Kirkpatrick, J. B. (1972): Neuronal microtubules, neurofilaments, and microfilaments. *Int. Rev. Cytol.,* 33:45–75.

Zelena, J. (1972): Ribosomes in myelinated axons of dorsal root ganglia. *Z. Zellforsch.,* 124:217–229.

Electrobiology of Nerve, Synapse, and Muscle,
edited by J. P. Reuben, D. P. Purpura, M. V. L. Bennett,
and E. R. Kandel. Raven Press, New York © 1976

Development of Denervatory Action Potentials in Slow Muscle Fibers of the Toad and Its Trophic Dependence

René Epstein and Arturo Jorge Bekerman

Instituto de Biologia Celular, Facultad de Medicina, Universidad de Buenos Aires, Paraguay 2155, 2°, Buenos Aires, Argentina

It has been demonstrated that the membrane electrophysiological properties of the extrafusal skeletal muscle fibers develop defined denervatory changes such as: (1) an increase in the membrane resistance due to the reduction in potassium permeability (Nicholls, 1956); (2) fibrillatory potentials and slow oscillations of the membrane potentials (Li et al., 1957; Belmar and Eyzaguirre, 1966; Muchnik et al., 1972); (3) a decrease in the sensitivity to tetrodotoxin (TTX) of the action potential in rat skeletal muscle (Redfern and Thesleff, 1971); (4) the appearance of action potentials in the slow muscle fibers (SMF) of the frog, demonstrated by Miledi et al. (1971). These authors described the fully developed state of this denervatory action potential, that appears in muscle fibers which normally do not generate an all-or-none response (Kuffler and Vaughan Williams, 1953; Burke and Ginsborg, 1956).

Our interest was in studying the evolution of this last denervatory phenomenon, first, to get a more precise idea on the membrane mechanisms involved, since it has been shown that the development of the denervatory action potential can be prevented by the timely administration of an RNA-synthesis blocker (Schmidt and Tong, 1973). Secondly, we wanted to see if the lack of action potentials in the SMF depended on a trophic regulation of presynaptic origin. Stefani and Schmidt (1972b) have reported that the reinnervated SMF lose the action potential before neuromuscular transmission is restored.

We have found that the denervatory action potential develops progressively, starting from an initial stage as a very small depolarizing response to end up as an overshooting spike, that this development takes several days, and that already the initial response is sensitive to TTX. We were also able to show that the onset of the phenomenon depends on the length of the axon stump left distal to the site of transection. This observation points to the intervention of a presynaptic trophic factor. In the course of these experiments we had to characterize partially the toad slow muscle fibers, since it was more convenient for us to use a toad muscle preparation.

METHODS

We used the SMF of the *m. pyriformis* of the toad *Bufo arenarum* H. Two to seven fibers could be recognized in the region of the medial border of each muscle. To minimize displacement due to contraction the muscles were wrapped around and pinned onto a Lucite rod covered with polyethylene tubing (Stefani and Schmidt, 1972a), and then mounted in a Lucite chamber placed on Pelltier batteries to control the temperature. The preparation between was bathed in a high-Ca^{2+} saline for better differentiation between the SMF and the fast muscle fibers (Stefani and Steinbach, 1969), of the following composition: 115 mM NaCl, 2.5 mM KCl, 8 mM $CaCl_2$, and 2 mM Tris buffer. The temperature was kept at 18° to 22°C.

The electrical activity was studied with the usual intracellular microelectrode technique. The recording electrode, filled with 3 M KCl solution, was connected to a NFl Bioelectric Instruments amplifier in series with a plug-in amplifier 3A72 on a Tektronix oscilloscope. In some cases dV/dT records were performed simultaneously by parallel recording on the second beam of the oscilloscope through a plug-in 3A8 differential amplifier. The current injection electrode was filled with saturated potassium citrate solution, and connected to an isolation unit activated by a pulse generator in series with a DC source which could supply steady polarizing currents.

The denervations were performed by sectioning the sciatic nerves at the hip under ether anesthesia. This left a distal axon stump 1 to 1.5 cm long.

RESULTS

The Development of the Action Potential in the Denervated SMF

The SMF were already recognized on penetration with the recording microelectrode, since their resting potential (E_{RP}) after an initial instantaneous value of -70 to -80 mV fell to -45 to -65 mV. To confirm this initial identification the fibers were hyperpolarized to -100 mV (this steady hyperpolarization was maintained throughout the study of each fiber), and the membrane time constant was determined by the application of a pulse of inward current. Values of more than 1 sec were regularly found (see Fig. 2) and served as conclusive criteria for considering the fiber a SMF (Miledi et al., 1971). Not denervated or recently denervated SMF presented a delayed rectification with a threshold at approximately -40 mV.

The other fibers which were found, the fast muscle fibers, presented an E_{RP} of -80 to -100 mV, a short time constant (less than 100 msec) and generated fast action potentials (5 to 10 msec time to peak) with 20 mV overshoot. All the electrophysiological elements of the slow and fast muscle fibers in the toad were coincident with those described for the frog (see Stefani and Steinbach, 1969).

The capacity of the SMF to generate an overshooting action potential (AP) appeared progressively after denervation. We computed five stages in this process: (1) a minimum initial response, which was detected as an upward inflection in the depolarization of exponential time course due to a rectangular current pulse; (2) a clear-cut small AP (of less than 20 mV voltage for the depolarizing phase); (3) an AP with a rapid rising phase which did not reach the 0 mV membrane potential (E_m) at its peak; (4) an AP reaching an $E_m = 0$ mV at the peak; (5) an overshooting AP (Fig. 1; also see Fig. 2). In many cases stage 1 was confirmed after visual detection by a simultaneous dV/dT record, to verify clearly the point of inflexion. We called stage 0 the response of those recently denervated SMF which only showed the usual delayed rectification.

In an experimental series conducted during the months of January to April (summer and early autumn) in which 17 muscles were studied successfully (Fig. 2), the AP started to develop 5 to 6 days after denervation (stages 1 and 2), increased its amplitude reaching an E_m of 0 mV at the peak at 7 to 8 days (stages 3 and 4) and a maximum of 10 mV overshoot at 9 to 11 days (stage 5). There was a great homogeneity in the stage of development of the AP in the different SMF of each denervated muscle: In 77% of the muscles all the fibers of one muscle showed the same stage of development of the denervatory AP, whereas the remaining 23% had the responses of its fibers distributed in no more than two stages of development.

The timing of development of the denervatory AP was quite different in other periods of the year. In experiments conducted through the winter we observed muscles with up to 18 days of denervation without any response

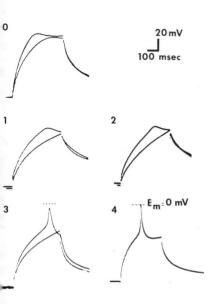

FIG. 1. Different stages in the development of the denervatory AP. Stage **0** corresponds to a nondenervated SMF. The delayed rectification can be seen. Stages **1** to **4** have been recorded in different SMF at various times after denervation (for explanation of the stages, see text). E_m of the different fibers: stages **0** to **3** = −120 mV; stage **4** = −100 mV.

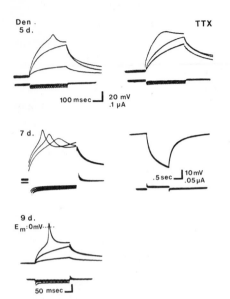

FIG. 2. Timing of the denervatory AP development (January to April series), sensitivity to TTX of the denervatory AP, and time constant of the SMF. *Left column:* denervatory APs at 5, 7, and 9 days after denervation, as indicated (E_m = −105, −115, and −90 mV, respectively). *TTX:* the same fiber as in 5d (E_m = −110 mV) after 10 min in saline with tetrodotoxin (10^{-7} g/liter). *Lower right record:* time constant of the same fiber as in **7d** (E_m = −110 mV). *Calibration:* for the time constant record, as indicated; for the other records: 20 mV, 0.1 μA, and 100 msec, except the time base of the **9d** record (50 msec).

to depolarization other than the delayed rectification. In an experimental series of 18 muscles studied during the months of September and October (see the next section) the initiation of the development of the AP appeared at 7 to 9 days after denervation (for a transection of the sciatic at the level of the hip). The successive stages were also delayed. The data of this series, which extended over a period of 7 to 12 days after denervation, did not show overshooting APs. The timing of the individual experiments showed great heterogeneity in the stages attained at a given time after denervation, and in 86% of the muscles, the AP recorded in the different fibers of any one muscle distributed over two or three different stages of development.

The threshold for the AP in its various stages was at approximately −40 mV, and the E_m had to be held at more than −80 mV to obtain a full response.

In all the fibers studied, irrespective of the experimental series and stage, the time-to-peak of the AP was approximately 30 msec. The velocity of rise of the AP varied thus from less than 1 V/sec to approximately 1.5 V/sec. This is much slower than the values observed in the frog SMF, which at 6°C reached a rate of rise of 25 V/sec (Miledi et al., 1971).

The denervatory AP was dependent on the presence of Na^+ in the bathing medium and sensitive to TTX as in the frog (Miledi et al., 1971). This sensitivity to TTX was very marked from the initial stage: The responses were readily blocked by TTX at a concentration of 10^{-7} g/liter in the saline. The effect of TTX was not completely reversed after 1 hr of bathing and washing with normal saline.

The Timing of the Development of the Denervatory
AP as a Function of the Distal Nerve Stump Length

The experiments to determine if the course of development of the denervatory AP in the SMF depended on the length of the nerve stump left distal to the site of transection, were performed during the months of September and October (spring). The animals were kept at 18° to 22°C during the period of denervation. Because of the great heterogeneity mentioned in the preceding section, the experiments were conducted on the basis of comparing at one time both *pyriformis* muscles of one animal which had been denervated simultaneously by sections at different levels of the sciatic. One of the muscles was denervated through the usual dorsal approach at the level of the hip and the contralateral muscle was denervated more proximally, sectioning the sciatic trunk close to its emergency from the vertebral column, via a lateral transabdominal approach.

This gave a difference in length between both distal stumps of 1.2 cm in the mean (range: 0.7 to 1.7 cm), and a mean length for the short stump of 1.5 cm (range: 1.3 to 1.8 cm). These measurements were made after isolating both muscles with their nerve stumps.

The comparison of the stages of development of the denervatory APs between the "short" and the "long" stump muscles of nine successfully studied pairs of *pyriformis* showed that in eight the "short" stump muscle had a distribution of stages of development displaced towards a more ad-

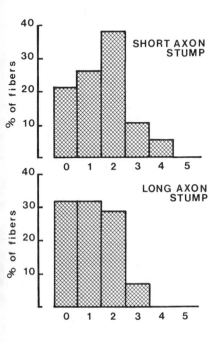

FIG. 3. Distribution of the stages of development of the denervatory AP in the SMF "short" and "long" stump muscles (September to October series). Total number of fibers in each group: 42 and 31, respectively.

vanced process. Moreover, in five of the pairs, the fibers of the "short" stump muscles showed APs which had reached stages that had not been attained by the APs in the corresponding "long" stump muscles. In Fig. 3 we have summarized the distribution of stages of denervatory AP development observed in the nine "short" and the nine "long" stump muscles. As can be seen, the frequency of the various stages is different for both groups. In the first group, stage 2 is the most frequently observed, whereas in the "long" stump group stages 1 and 0 do predominate.

These observations indicated that the length difference between stumps (1.2 cm) produced a 1 to 2 days difference in the stage of development of the APs.

DISCUSSION

The general electrophysiological features of the SMF in the *pyriformis* muscle of the toad *B. arenarum* H. and their denervatory AP do not seem to differ markedly from that known for the frog SMF (Stefani and Steinbach, 1969; Miledi et al., 1971). Nevertheless the time after denervation at which the AP appears seems to be shorter in the toad than in the frog (Miledi et al., 1971; Stefani and Steinbach, 1972; Miledi and Spitzer, 1974). Possibly, this change in the timing represents a greater velocity in the process which leads to this denervatory phenomenon, though no definite conclusion can be arrived at.[1]

A rather interesting observation can be made of the high sensitivity of the denervatory AP to TTX, from its initial stage of development, and the increasing rate of rise of the AP at constant time to peak. These data indicate that the different stages in the development of this AP are probably due to a progressive increase in the density of TTX-sensitive Na channels in the SMF membrane.

In the rat skeletal muscle the denervatory decrease of sensitivity to TTX of the AP (Redfern and Thesleff, 1971) represents a dedifferentiation to ontogenetically more primitive states, as it is the rule for denervatory changes in general. This is shown in that case by the fact that fetal rat skeletal muscle (Harris and Marshall, 1973) and rat myotubes in culture (Kidokoro, 1973) also have APs resistant to TTX. We did not find in the literature data that might indicate that the denervatory AP in the SMF of amphibia also represents such a dedifferentiation.

---

[1] There are mainly two reasons for this. First, in most of the frog experiments no statements on the length of the distal axon stump were published; nevertheless most probably this length was approximately the same as in our case (see Elul et al., 1970; Stefani and Steinbach, 1972). Second, in the toad we find marked changes of timing according to the period of the year and this is not mentioned by the authors who studied this denervatory phenomenon, though studies on other denervatory changes mention such variability (Harris and Miledi, 1972; Mallart and Trautman, 1973).

The difference of 1 to 2 days in the timing of the development of the denervatory AP for a mean 1.2-cm length difference between distal nerve stumps, observed in our experiments, is somehow great. This should be interpreted as due to the relationship of the phenomenon with some material traveling down the axons at a rather slow transport rate of the order of 1 cm/day. Partlow et al. (1972) studied isolated frog sciatic nerves at 22°C, and have seen such slow rates for enzymes related to mitochondria; but they determined still slower transport rates for other enzymes which they related to what is called the "slow" axoplasmic flow. Thus the phenomenon studied by us would be dependent on something disappearing from the distal axon stump at a velocity that still corresponds to a "fast" axoplasmic flow, as it has been postulated in the case of the denervatory changes of the AP in rat muscle fibers (Harris and Thesleff, 1972) and the mechanism of fibrillation (Luco and Eyzaguirre, 1955).

Some Considerations on Neuromuscular Trophism

The dependence of the timing of denervatory changes in general on the length of the axon stump (see Guth, 1968; Drachman, 1974) is a strong argument in support of the idea that there must exist some trophic substance or substances of presynaptic origin intervening in the regulation of the postsynaptic muscle. It is hard to imagine that denervations which interrupt the impulse conduction, could induce differing stages of inactivity of the postsynaptic muscle, which could explain the timing differences just because they are performed at various levels of the peripheral nerve. By the way, it might be worthwhile to stress at this point that what is usually called "muscle activity" (Lømo and Rosenthal, 1972) or "usage" (Drachman, 1974) as a factor capable of preventing or reversing the results of denervation, has to be carefully defined in each case, since Gruener et al., (1974) showed reduction in the denervatory supersensitivity to acetylcholine of muscle by subthreshold mechanical stimulation.

The shortcoming of the experiments on the relationship between denervatory changes and distal axon stump length is that they do not allow differentiation between acetylcholine (ACh) or some other substance as the possible regulatory agent, called the trophic substance, since the disappearance of the spontaneous and evoked ACh release are also dependent on the distal axon stump length (Birks et al., 1960; Harris and Miledi, 1972).

With respect to the question of whether ACh per se may cope with the whole responsibility of the trophic control exerted by the presynaptic structure, either through the depolarization and activation produced by the transmitter or through an yet unknown biochemical action, the experiments of organ culture where the presence of ACh in the medium did not prevent the spread of the ACh receptors (Miledi, 1960) speak strongly against identifying the transmitter as the trophic substance.

Experiments using substances that prevent the ACh release or block its postsynaptic action with production of denervatory-like changes (Drachman, 1974), have been taken as an argument in favor of ACh being the trophic substance. But this approach cannot exclude the simultaneous inhibition of the release and/or postsynaptic action of substances other than the transmitter. Recently Miledi and Spitzer (1974) did not find development of denervatory APs in frog SMF which had been pharmacologically "denervated" with botulinum toxin. They calculated that the ACh liberated at the neuromuscular junction was reduced in these experiments to 1/200 of the normal amount, and concluded that some other substance repressing the development of the AP was still being released.

The application of colchicine and related drugs to the nerve trunk with the apparition of denervatory-like changes has provided pertinent data regarding this point. Hofmann and Thesleff (1972), Albuquerque et al. (1973), and others used colchicine and showed that there was no major impairment of the physiological activity, and the data appeared to exclude postsynaptic inactivation and lack of ACh as critical factors. But Cangiano (1973) and Lømo (1974) have shown direct effects of colchicine on postsynaptic muscle in these kinds of experiments, curtailing somewhat the initial expectations.

In summary, we feel that results such as those presented here, showing a dependence of the timing of denervatory phenomena on the length of the distal axon stump, are one of the strongest arguments in favor of the idea of the existence of a trophic substance or substances originated at the presynaptic structure. A number of other data (which are not fully explained by changes in the liberation of ACh) join in indicating the necessity of searching what Drachman (1974) called "mysterine," in accordance with the exhortation of Guth (1968).

SUMMARY

The innervated slow muscle fibers of the *m. pyriformis* in the toad *B. arenarum* H. show general electrical properties similar to those of the frog such as the inability to generate APs. They, like frog fibers, develop the all-or-none response after denervation.

In summer months the initial stage of the development of the denervatory AP can be recognized after 5 to 6 days of surgical denervation, when a distal axon stump of 1 to 1.5 cm is left. In SMF denervated for longer periods, a more developed AP is recorded; 9 to 11 days after denervation the AP reaches a peak with an overshoot of 10 mV. This timing varies with the period of the year.

The denervatory AP is blocked in 0 mM Na^+ saline and by TTX (10^{-7} g/liter) already in its initial stage. The time to peak keeps constant as the AP develops, while the rate of rise increases up to a maximum of 1 to 2

V/sec. The appearance and progressive increment in density of Na channels in the SMF membrane has to be postulated to explain this data.

The timing of the development of the denervatory AP depends on the length of the distal axon stump. For a 1- to 1.5-cm longer distal axon stump a 1- to 2-day delay in that development was observed. This suggests the dependence of the development of the denervatory AP of the disappearance of a trophic substance flowing down the axon at a velocity of 1 cm/day.

ACKNOWLEDGMENTS

We are grateful to Dr. E. Stefani for introducing us to the subject area and for advice in the initial stages of this work. We thank Dr. J. H. Moreno and also Dr. O. D. Uchitel for their valuable criticism of the manuscript.

This work was supported by grant numbers 3326/72 and 6048/73 of the Consejo Nacional de Investigaciones Científicas y Técnicas (CONICET), Argentina. Dr. Epstein is a Career Scientist and Dr. Bekerman has a Special Contract from the CONICET.

REFERENCES

Albuquerque, E. X., Warnick, J. E., Tasse, J. R., and Sansone, F. M. (1972): Effects of vinblastine and colchicine on neural regulation of the fast and slow skeletal muscles of the rat. *Exp. Neurol.*, 37:607–634.

Belmar, J., and Eyzaquirre, C. (1966): Pacemaker site of fibrillation potentials in denervated mammalian muscle. *J. Neurophysiol.*, 29:425–441.

Birks, R., Katz, B., and Miledi, R. (1960): Physiological and structural changes at the amphibian myoneural junction, in the course of nerve degeneration. *J. Physiol.*, 150:145–168.

Burke, W., and Ginsborg, B. L. (1956): The electrical properties of the slow muscle fiber membrane. *J. Physiol.* 132:586–598.

Cangiano, A. (1973): Acetylcholine supersensitivity: the role of neurotrophic factors. *Brain Res.*, 58:255–259.

Drachman, D. B. (1974): The role of acetylcholine as a neurotrophic transmitter. *Ann. NY Acad. Sci.*, 228:160–176.

Elul, R., Miledi, R., and Stefani, E. (1970): Neural control of contracture in slow muscle fibers of the frog. *Acta Physiol. Lat. Am.*, 20:194–226.

Gruener, R., Baumbach, N., and Coffee, D. (1974): Reduction of denervation supersensitivity of muscle by submechanical threshold stimulation. *Nature*, 248:68–69.

Guth, L. (1968): "Trophic" influences of nerve on muscle. *Physiol. Rev.*, 48:645–687.

Harris, A. J., and Miledi, R. (1972): A study of frog muscle maintained in organ culture. *J. Physiol.*, 221:207–226.

Harris, J. B., and Marshall, W. W. (1973): Tetrodotoxin-resistant action potentials in new born rat muscle. *Nature New Biol.*, 243:191–192.

Harris, J. B., and Thesleff, S. (1972): Nerve stump length and membrane changes in denervated skeletal muscle. *Nature New Biol.*, 236:60–61.

Hofmann, W. W., and Thesleff, S. (1972): Studies on the trophic influence of nerve on skeletal muscle. *Eur. J. Pharmacol.*, 20:256–260.

Kidokoro, Y. (1973): Development of action potentials in a clonal rat skeletal muscle cell line. *Nature New Biol.*, 241:158–159.

Kuffler, S. W., and Vaughan Williams, E. M. (1953): Small-nerve junctional potentials. The distribution of small motor nerves to frog skeletal muscle and the membrane characteristics of the fibres they innervate. *J. Physiol.*, 121:289–317.

Li, C. L., Shy, G. M., and Wells, J. (1957): Some properties of mammalian skeletal muscle fibres with particular reference to fibrillation potentials. *J. Physiol.*, 135:522–535.

Lømo, T. (1974): Neurotrophic control of colchicine effects on muscle? *Nature*, 249:473–474.

Lømo, T., and Rosenthal, J. (1972): Control of Ach sensitivity by muscle activity in the rat. *J. Physiol.*, 221:493–513.

Luco, J. and Eyzaguirre, C. (1955): Fibrillation and hypersensitivity to Ach in denervated muscle: effect of length of degenerating nerve fibers. *J. Neurophysiol.*, 18:65–73.

Mallart, A., and Trautmann, A. (1973): Ionic properties of the neuromuscular junction of the frog: effects of denervation and pH. *J. Physiol.*, 234:553–567.

Miledi, R. (1960): The acetylcholine sensitivity of frog muscle fibres after complete or partial denervation. *J. Physiol.*, 151:1–23.

Miledi, R., and Spitzer, N. C. (1974): Absence of action potentials in frog slow muscle fibres paralysed by botulinum toxin. *J. Physiol.*, 241:183–199.

Miledi, R., Stefani, E., and Steinbach, A. B. (1971): Induction of the action potential mechanism in slow muscle fibres of the frog. *J. Physiol.*, 217:737–754.

Muchnik, S., Ruarte, A. C., and Kotsias, B. A. (1972): On the mechanism of denervatory electrical activity of single muscle fibers as tested in vivo with Tetrodotoxin. *Acta Physiol. Lat. Am.*, 22:24–28.

Nicholls, J. G. (1956): The electrical properties of denervated skeletal muscle. *J. Physiol.*, 131:1–12.

Partlow, L. M., Ross, C. D., Motwani, R., and McDougal, D. B., Jr. (1972): Transport of axonal enzymes in surviving segments of frog sciatic nerve. *J. Gen. Physiol.*, 60:388–405.

Redfern, P., and Thesleff, S. (1971): Action potential generation in denervated rat skeletal muscle. II. The action of Tetrodotoxin. *Acta Physiol. Scand.*, 82:70–78.

Schmidt, H., and Tong, E. Y. (1973): Inhibition by actynomicin D of the denervation induced action potential in frog slow muscle fibres. *Proc. R. Soc. Lond. Biol.*, 184:91–95.

Stefani, E., and Schmidt, H. (1972*a*): A convenient method for repeated intracellular recording of action potentials from the same muscle fibre without membrane damage. *Pfluegers Arch.*, 334:276–278.

Stefani, E., and Schmidt, H. (1972*b*): A "trophic" nerve influence independent of neuromuscular transmission: inhibition of action potentials in denervated frog slow fibres. *Pfluegers Arch.*, 335:127.

Stefani, E., and Steinbach, A. B. (1969): Resting potential and electrical properties of frog slow muscle fibres. Effect of different external solution. *J. Physiol.*, 203:383–401.

Stefani, E., and Steinbach, A. N. (1972): Trophic effect of nerve on electrical properties of frog slow muscle fibres. In: *Res. Publ. Ass. Nerv. Ment. Dis., Vol. 50: Neurotransmitters*, edited by I. J. Kopin, pp. 241–254. Williams and Wilkins, Baltimore.

Electrobiology of Nerve, Synapse, and Muscle,
edited by J. P. Reuben, D. P. Purpura, M. V. L. Bennett,
and E. R. Kandel. Raven Press, New York © 1976

Redundancy and Noise in the Nervous System: Does the Model Based on Unreliable Neurons Sell Nature Short?

Theodore Holmes Bullock

*Department of Neurosciences, School of Medicine, and Neurobiology Unit,
Scripps Institution of Oceanography, University of California, San Diego,
La Jolla, California 92037*

The purpose of this chapter is to go beyond the facts. First, I will point out how little we know and then I will argue that much of this is less relevant to the question than has been implied. Finally, I will speculate far beyond the meager residue—in the direction of an affirmative answer to the title question.

This is not inappropriate in this place, for the man we honor in this volume did much to teach me—sometimes indirectly, sometimes by example—to pay attention to phenomena ("mere" phenomenology) even before they are understood in respect to mechanism. The "mechanisms" are themselves mere phenomenology at their level. Reductionism is choosing the level where one stops explaining and appeals to magic.

One of the impressive phenomena of nature is the relatively high reliability of many achievements of the nervous system. Witness the pianist, the acrobat, and the typist—and your own achievement at this moment as a reader. The fact that many achievements, like my tennis serve, are not conspicuous for this feature does not negate it. When we see "27" we rarely read 26 or 28 or any other number unless our vision is poor (low signal-to-noise ratio at the receptor). Anytime I cannot demonstrate the predicted electric discharge of the weakly electric fish that Harry Grundfest introduced me to 20 years ago, I can be sure the unreliability is in my instruments, not the fish. Unpredictable behavior is more likely to be complex behavior than fundamentally capricious. (Is that a calumny or a compliment to the complexities of whimsy of *Capra,* the goat?) By reliability we mean the degree to which a subsystem operates as it should, given its function, for example, the degree to which a photoreceptor responds to light nonerratically. Reliable is not the same as deterministic; a device may be unreliable for its function due to excessive, deterministic interference. Predictability is only a measure of reliability after certain conditions are met, including the device having a reasonable dynamic range and the investigator having an understanding of the code and how to recognize a disturbance.

The standard explanation of this relatively high reliability of performance is that the nervous system uses high redundancy of individually noisy, unreliable nerve cells. This is an attractive, plausible idea and I shall not argue that it is altogether wrong; quite to the contrary, I *believe* it is right to some degree, in some places. But, as I have pointed out elsewhere (Bullock, 1970), it is essentially impossible to test this idea or obtain evidence not equally compatible with the model of a complex system of relatively low redundancy, low unwanted noise, and high reliability.

The evidence for redundancy and for unwanted noise is quite different but in each case quite unsatisfactory, beset by an ambiguity of terms, and subject to alternative interpretation. Even apart from the nature and meaning of the evidence, it is another matter, essentially subjective and still more unsatisfactory, to assess the prevalence of these characteristics in the brain.

REDUNDANCY

Redundancy is repetition that in the ideal case would be superfluous. It is that part of a communication or a system that could be eliminated without loss of essential information or performance if it were not for discrete non-linearities or noise. In a system of nerve cells, two kinds of redundancy can be looked for—partial and complete redundancy of neurons, with intergrades. There is much evidence of overlap of receptive fields among afferent neurons and to that extent, of partial redundancy. To the extent that the overlap is significantly incomplete, the neurons can also be regarded as unique. Even if the receptive fields overlap completely, the neurons cannot be called redundant if their output connections are not identical. My guess is that fully equivalent neurons are rare, with some exceptions (e.g., perhaps some neurosecretory cells). Even if equivalence were to be demonstrated, redundancy in the above sense does not necessarily follow since the system may need many independent samples of the environment to detect weak signals in noisy stimuli coming from the external world.

One argument that might be construed to favor relatively high redundancy is the indirect result of a type of model of the higher levels of the brain represented by that of John (1972). He calls the model the statistical configuration theory. It is based largely on averaged evoked potentials and the widespread distribution of some features of their form that are characteristic of certain stimuli. The view is that masses of neurons operate in a probabilistic way to form configurations of activity in very large numbers of not sharply defined constellations. John considers that an essential feature of his model is its denial of specific localization for the configurations of activity representing the response to specific stimuli. He implies a high degree of equivalence among masses of neurons. Equivalence has three main aspects: input connectivity, output connectivity, and intrinsic properties or transfer function. If any one of them is significantly different, the cells are not equivalent. The evidence cited by John does not make a compelling case for essential equivalence of large numbers of neurons. Configurations of spatio-temporally patterned activity, best described probabilistically, are just what would be expected with either the model of quite unreliable cells or that of relatively reliable, complex units. Such a system can have extensive overlap of the input and output fields of neurons, hence ambiguous and multimodal units, within a framework that could even be highly specified (Bullock, 1975). The alternative models are not sufficiently specified as yet to permit statements excluding either one on the basis of the observed properties of these configurations.

NOISE

Since we are talking about system operation rather than statistical structure of trains of events, noise is used here in its dictionary sense of unwanted action that interferes with desired signals. We should recognize the sharp difference between this dictionary usage and another current usage that refers to a stochastic sequence ("whiteness"). In the first meaning, noise is determined by the state of the receiver (sleep, attention) and depends on the usefulness, regardless of the character; any unwanted sequence is regarded as noise whether it is a hiss, a whistle, or a voice. In the second meaning, noise is determined by the state of the sender (filter settings) and depends on the statistical character regardless of the use; any quasirandom sequence is regarded as noise whether it is unwanted interference or a high resolution signal. The first meaning overlooks the difficulty of knowing what may be of value to a receiver; the second overlooks the difficulty of avoiding the common English sense, as in "signal-to-noise ratio." In each of seven dictionaries consulted, six scientific and one general, the first meaning is the principal or only one given (International Dictionary of Physics and Electronics, 1961; Thewlis's Encyclopedic Dictionary of Physics, 1962; Besancon's Encyclopedia of Physics, 1966; Meetham's Encyclopedia of Linguistics, Information and Control, 1969; Jordain's Condensed Computer Encyclopedia, 1969; Webster's Third New International Dictionary, 1965; see also, Walters in the Handbook of Electroencephalography, Vol. 4B, 1973). Throughout this chapter, noise is used in the sense of unwanted interference.

The main evidence cited in the literature that neurons are noisy is the variability of response to repetition of the same stimulus, either as a single-unit spike response or as compound, evoked, field potential of a population of neurons. Fluctuation of response at threshold comes close to satisfying the definition but at best proves that there is some noise; the unit cannot be called noisy unless this fluctuation is significant by some functional criterion relative to the normal dynamic range. The reason most response fluctuation, especially above threshold, only comes close, at best, to justifying the term noise is that in most preparations there are several possibilities for alternative interpretation. The fluctuation may be a sign of some significant change of state of the responding system, which is a whole organism. The fluctuation may be in a parameter, for example, number of spikes, that is irrelevant to the code carrying the signal, just as voice intonation and volume may be irrelevant to the spoken numeral "27." Other alternatives are developed in Bullock (1970).

Some of the evidence for "noise" in the literature is not relevant to the present discussion because it is based on a different definition. Nevertheless, it has been mistaken for support for the model of a brain of redundant, unreliable units. Adey's contribution (1972), entitled "Organization of Brain Tissue: Is the Brain a Noisy Processor?" adduces evidence that it is, from spike and brain wave data, on the stochastic structure definition. For example, he shows that EEG amplitudes have a Gaussian distribution, that interspike intervals in single units can have a pseudorandom distribution, that spikes in two units are often quite independent, that unit spikes are often temporally unrelated to the EEG, and the EEG in two places is often independent. Of course all of these findings are compatible with the model of a complex, reliable system and do not indicate that the brain is noisy in the unwanted, or antisignal sense. Adey does not intend to say it is, although this conclusion has been read into his words. The criteria for the statistical definition say nothing about the value of the random series, either as signal or as interference with a desired signal. The prima donna regards applause as the precious signal for which she has labored, although the intervals between claps may approach randomness. The engineer is trained to hear a hiss that signals danger or that all is well in his engine, although the spectrum might approach "white noise." The sound from many typewriters, or even from one, may meet the criteria without any necessary errors in the written communications.

Noise in the sense used here depends on the functional value of the receiver. We should not use the term unless we are prepared to claim we know the codes and functions of the system and can recognize its signals. There is likely to be more than one message in the same neuron at the same time, as when a person says one thing with words, something more with intonation, and still more with body language. Until we can defend that claim, it is safer and more heuristic to call unexplained fluctuation "unexplained fluctuation" instead of noise.

Some apparently meaningless stochastic fluctuation, such as the jitter of interspike intervals in ongoing trains of nerve impulses, would seem to be a compelling candidate for the designation "noise" in the neurons. However, there is both theoretical and experimental reason to propose that such jitter may have been selected as a desirable property. In a pulse code that, if highly regular, could be distorted into unwanted phase locking with input trains (Von Neuman, 1956; Perkel et al., 1964; Roberge, 1969; Stein, 1970; Bullock, 1970) jitter can avoid this and assure smoother, monotonic control of input. Some digital information processing devices introduce "dither" to extend by one or several orders of magnitude the useful dynamic range available with summing. Here we see in the time domain, the same principle we noted earlier in the spatial domain, when apparent redundancy turned out not to be superfluous but useful in detecting weak stimuli.

Another type of argument that may be taken to support unreliability and noise in the neurons is the antilocalizationist model of masses of neurons operating in floating, statistical configurations of very large numbers. We cited above, in connection with redundancy, the model of John (1972). This model is probabilistic and expressly depends on extensive spatial averaging, but in fact it does not require that neurons are particularly noisy or unreliable or preferentially support such a view with evidence.

Quite apart from John's or any theory of the brain, there is much evidence that central neurons commonly receive many independent nerve impulse trains, hence a stochastic input. The output of a typical neuron, after the intermediation of synaptic potentials, electrotonic spread, with time and space constants, and confluence of dendrites onto the spike initiation zone is also a train of impulses. Even without active noise, the processes that determine firing threshold and the recovery cycle of the spike require that the instantaneous output be described probabilistically. That is, if the neuron's pulse code be considered discretely, it is essentially a probabilistic device. It may nevertheless be relatively highly reliable. Because it integrates many input impulses and emits a smaller number of output impulses, it can be said to sum and average. The point is that the evidence for these characteristics says nothing about reliability and noise, although the terminology and the statistical treatment is often taken to imply the model of redundant, unreliable elements, as Walter (1968) pointed out.

CONCLUSIONS

However plausible the idea of a brain operating reliably with highly redundant, unreliable elements, it is difficult to test the idea or to adduce evidence for it that is not equally compatible with the opposite view. The latter is only opposite in emphasis or degree. It recognizes the abundant overlap and hence partially redundant, partially unique neurons. It recognizes the inherently probabilistic character of spike initiation and the expectation of at least thermal noise in threshold fluctuation and quantal transmitter release in presynaptic fluctuation. Other sources of apparent randomness may be even more important; the question at issue is not the existence but the relative importance of the aggregate of these factors compared to the changes in output that reliably follow changes in input.

In contrast to the difficulty of establishing in a given case that unexplained fluctuation is truly noise and not useful jitter or change of state with biologically significant meaning, it is easier to establish in many particular cases that reliability of response is higher than previously expected. Bishop (1933) found that much of the variability of cortical evoked potentials to electric shock of the optic nerve could be reduced by controlling the phase of the EEG at which the stimulus was given; there are cyclic changes in excitability of the cortex, several per second. MacDonald (1964) found a similar way to reduce variability of cortical evoked potentials to the physiologic stimuli of a click or flash, by a different contingency related to the EEG. If the stimulus is given only after a rest period plus at least 50 msec of EEG within some amplitude bounds, the response fluctuation is greatly diminished. Electroreceptors in electric fish specialized for evaluating the intensity of weak pulses of high-frequency content may exhibit little fluctuation within the normal working range (Bullock, 1970; Scheich et al., 1973). Neurons can be quite reliable. It seems wiser to investigate each case of a wide variability of response to look for causes of the variation, than to call it noise and assume it is unreliable and maladaptive "slop."

Similarly, the difficulty of proving the complete equivalence and true redundancy of neurons is in contrast with the relative ease of establishing nonequivalence. When advances in anatomy or physiology subdivide a population of cells on the basis of connectivity or type of response, apparent redundancy is reduced. This is the one-way direction of increased understanding of each part of the nervous system. Even when an advance has reduced the number of seemingly equivalent cells to those in a narrow column, as in the so-called orientation columns of cells in the visual cortex, it is still possible that new criteria may subdivide still further. In this case one wonders about differences in response dynamics or in permutations of stimulus preferences such as stripe width, optical disparity, intensity, contrast, and movement sensitivity.

SUMMARY

It is argued that an alternative view is more heuristic than the model of the nervous system with relatively high redundancy of relatively noisy neurons. These terms are defined. The difficulties of establishing true redundancy and noise are emphasized. Variation in neuronal activity, even when conforming to criteria of randomness, should be called unexplained fluctuation and be examined for adaptive significance and causal explanation. The designation noise should be reserved for the case in which one is prepared to define the normal functions and signals with which the noise interferes. My belief is that some parts of the brain operate with relatively little and others with much noise; sorting these out is more useful than sweeping generalizations. My belief is that fully equivalent neurons are not a prominent feature of the brain but neurons with large overlap in input or output fields are — therefore partly redundant, partly not. The value of such overlap may not be solely to average out internal noise but to an important degree to aid in detecting and resolving input signals for the given region of the nervous system.

ACKNOWLEDGMENTS

I would like to acknowledge research grants from the National Science Foundation and the National Institute of Neurological Diseases and Stroke of the National Institutes of Health.

REFERENCES

Adey, W. R. (1972): Organization of brain tissue: Is the brain a noisy processor? *Int. J. Neurosci.,* 3:271–284.

Bishop, G. H. (1933): Cyclic changes in excitability of the optic pathway of the rabbit. *Am. J. Physiol.,* 103:213–224.

Bullock, T. H. (1970): The reliability of neurons. *J. Gen. Physiol.,* 55:563–584.

Bullock, T. H. (1974): Comparisons between vertebrates and invertebrates in nervous organization. In: *The Neurosciences A Third Study Program,* edited by F. O. Schmitt and F. G. Worden, pp. 343–346. M.I.T. Press, Cambridge, Massachusetts.

Bullock, T. H. (1975): In search of principles in neural integration: Are there rules in the combination of elements in neural circuits? In: *Simpler Networks: An Approach to Patterned Behavior and Its Foundations* (Essays in Memory of D. M. Maynard, Neurobiologist and Educator), edited by J. Fentress. Raven Press, New York (*in press*).

John, E. R. (1972): Switchboard versus statistical theories of learning and memory. Coherent patterns of neural activity reflect the release of memories and may mediate subjective experience. *Science,* 177:850–864.

McDonald, M. (1964): A system for stabilizing evoked potentials obtained in the brain stem of the cat. *Med. Electron. Biol. Engng.,* 2:417–423.

Perkel, D., Schulman, J., Bullock, T. H., Moore, G. P., and Segundo, J. P. (1964): Pacemaker neurons: Effects of regularly spaced synaptic input. *Science,* 146:61.

Roberge, F. A. (1969): Paradoxical inhibition: A negative feedback principle in oscillatory systems. *Automatika,* 5:407.

Scheich, H., Bullock, T. H., and Hamstra, R. H., Jr. (1973): Coding properties of two classes of afferent nerve fibers: High-frequency electroreceptors in the electric fish, *Eigenmannia. J. Neurophysiol.,* 36:39–60.

Stein, R. B. (1970): The role of spike trains in transmitting and distorting sensory signals. In: *The Neurosciences: A Second Study Program,* edited by F. O. Schmitt. Rockefeller University Press, New York.

Von Neumann, J. (1956): Probability logic and synthesis of reliable organisms from unreliable components. In: *Automata Studies,* edited by C. E. Shannon and J. McCarthy. Princeton University Press, Princeton, New Jersey.

Walter, D. O. (1968): The indeterminacies of the brain. *Perspect. Biol. Med.,* 11:203.

Electrobiology of Nerve, Synapse, and Muscle,
edited by J. P. Reuben, D. P. Purpura, M. V. L. Bennett,
and E. R. Kandel. Raven Press, New York © 1976

Principles Relating the Biophysical Properties of Neurons and Their Patterns of Interconnections to Behavior

E. R. Kandel, T. J. Carew, and J. Koester

Division of Neurobiology and Behavior, College of Physicians and Surgeons, Columbia University, New York, New York 10032

A fascinating feature of the structure of the nervous system is the degree of differentiation that is found among its various cells. For example, cells vary in their intrinsic firing patterns: some cells are silent, some are autoactive. The autoactive cells may fire regularly, or may generate bursts. This differentiation, which extends to the mechanisms of the action potential, the resting potential and afterpotential, is implied in the concept of identified cells: the existence of unique cells in invertebrates (and in some cases in vertebrates) that can be identified in every member of the species. The discovery of this remarkable degree of differentiation raises the question: What is its function? In invertebrates behavioral analyses can help answer this question. Because invertebrates have relatively few nerve cells, one can causally relate specific cells to a given behavior, and investigate how a cell's unique biophysical properties are expressed in the behavior in which it participates. In this chapter we will try to illustrate that, just as cellular analyses can increase one's understanding of mechanisms underlying behavior, so can an understanding of behavior increase one's understanding of the functional significance of a cell's biophysical properties.

In our attempts to relate the properties of nerve cells to behavior, we have utilized the abdominal ganglion of the marine mollusk *Aplysia californica*. We at first thought this animal to be a rather sluggish brute, and expected that its abdominal ganglion would have a very restricted behavioral role. But as we got to know the animal better we found that its behavioral repertoire is rather extensive and that a variety of behaviors are controlled by the abdominal ganglion. In fact, this single ganglion regulates all four types of effector systems controlled by any nervous system: (1) somatic motor, (2) visceral motor, (3) neuroglandular, and (4) neuroendocrine.

Taking advantage of this rich behavioral repertoire, we have tried to determine what principles relate the biophysical properties of cells and their patterns of interconnections to various classes of behavior. But before considering this issue it is essential that we first discuss the criteria whereby behavioral responses can be categorized. Although there is agreement among psychologists that behavior is best studied in terms of overt responses — movement of muscles and secretions of glands — there is little agreement on how to divide the spectrum of behavior into elementary behavioral units that can be used as building blocks for more complex behavior.

Among the various schemes that have been used to classify behavior, we think that one of the simplest, most useful, and also the best defined, is that which is based on differences in the stimulus–response characteristics of a behavioral response: the manner in which the intensity and pattern of the sensory stimulus controls the amplitude and pattern of the motor response. Based on this distinction one can delineate at the extreme of a behavioral spectrum two broad categories: (1) *graded responses* and (2) *all-or-none responses* (Sherrington, 1906). Examples of graded responses are the flexion withdrawal of the cat or monkey and the pupillary response of man. Here the amplitude of the response is a function of the intensity of the stimulus and the pattern of response is largely determined by the temporal pattern of the stimulus (see, for example, Sherrington, 1906; Lloyd, 1957). At the other extreme are steep stimulus–response relationships. Examples of stereotypic all-or-none responses are swallowing, vomiting, sneezing, and orgasm (see, for example, Doty, 1968; Morris, 1957). Here the response amplitude and pattern are relatively independent of the strength and pattern of the stimulus. The stimulus primarily acts as a trigger to release an all-or-none stereotypic response. Once the eliciting stimulus reaches threshold it produces a full response that often outlasts the stimulus. Further increments in stimulus strength do not produce greater increments in the amplitude or form of the response.

These two behavioral categories — graded responses and all-or-none responses — describe the common (and perhaps the most objective) feature of what have been called *reflex acts* on the one hand and *fixed acts* on the other (Barlow, 1968; Kandel, 1976). It is also useful to distinguish between elementary behavioral responses (fixed acts and reflex acts) consisting of a single episode in a single motor pathway, and complex behavioral responses (fixed-action patterns and reflex patterns) consisting of recurring episodes or motor patterns involving more than one motor pathway (for discussion see Kandel, 1976). In the case of elementary behavior the distinction between a reflex and a fixed act can be made by reference to their stimulus–response characteristics. Thus the stimulus–response curve for a simple graded reflex act has a gradual slope, whereas that of an all-or-none fixed act resembles a step function (Fig. 1). An additional dimension is introduced in the case of complex behavior, where both amplitude and sequence of components can vary. In a reflex pattern the amplitude and sequence vary in a graded manner whereas in a fixed action pattern they tend to be stereotypic.

We have previously focused on a graded reflex in the course of studying

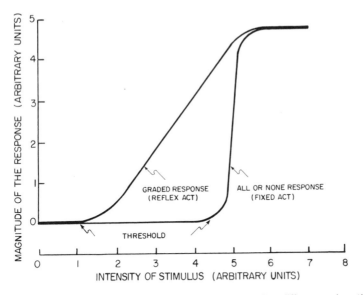

FIG. 1. Schematic input–output relationship illustrating the difference in stimulus–response characteristics between graded reflex responses and all-or-none fixed acts.

mechanisms of behavioral modifications (see, for example, Castellucci et al., 1970; Carew and Kandel, 1973a; Kandel et al., 1976). In this chapter we will focus on mechanisms underlying stereotypy — on the neural machinery that generates a step function (or a steep input–output relationship). The presence of such a step function suggests that suprathreshold stimuli trigger a pre-programmed motor "tape" (Hoyle, 1964). The stimulus does not guide or control the behavior to the same degree as in a simple graded response. Beyond threshold there are features in the pattern or intensity of the output that are not apparent in the input. The mechanism which results in the stereotypic nature of the output pattern (its characteristic amplitude or sequence) is often referred to as a *central program*.

In considering stereotypic behaviors we will focus on two questions: (1) Where in the nervous system are the cellular loci for the central programs of the different fixed acts? (2) What are the mechanisms of these programs? Are the programs generated by cellular properties or by circuit properties?

We will consider four types of stereotypic behaviors generated by the abdominal ganglion. We will first describe a simple fixed act, inking, and compare that to a graded reflex, gill withdrawal. We will then consider a more complex fixed act, egg laying, and two fixed-action patterns (a phasic increase in heart rate and a respiratory pumping sequence). The behavioral analyses of several of the responses that we describe are incomplete and our inferences about them are tentative. We would therefore emphasize, at the outset, that some of the discussion of these findings is speculative. Our primary purpose in this chapter is to propose and begin to examine testable hypotheses relating specific types of neuronal properties to graded reflexes on the one hand and stereotypic all-or-none responses on the other.

A COMPARISON OF A FIXED ACT AND A REFLEX ACT: ALL-OR-NONE INKING AND GRADED GILL WITHDRAWAL

Mollusks have a respiratory space called the mantle cavity which houses the respiratory organ, the gill. In *Aplysia* the roof of this cavity is covered by a protective sheet, the mantle shelf, which contains at its center the residual shell and at its margin an ink or purple gland. Posteriorly the mantle shelf terminates in a fleshy spout, the siphon. A weak or moderate intensity tactile stimulus to the siphon of *Aplysia* elicits a graded defensive gill-withdrawal reflex (Fig. 2). If the stimulus that elicits this reflex is greatly increased to the point where it is noxious, it elicits, in addition to gill withdrawal, a massive inking response. The ink is ejected from acinar vesicles of the purple gland into the mantle cavity, from which it is expelled as a dark purple cloud by pumping movements of the mantle organs (Carew and Kandel, 1967*a*). Figure 2 compares the simultaneously obtained input–output curves for gill withdrawal and inking. Whereas gill withdrawal has a low threshold and is smoothly graded, inking has a high threshold and tends to

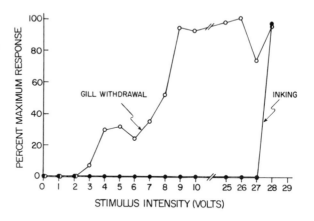

FIG. 2. Gill withdrawal and inking produced in intact, restrained animals by electrical stimulation of the siphon. Gill withdrawal was measured by means of a photo cell and inking by means of a spectrophotometer (for details of procedure, see Carew and Kandel, 1976a). The data are normalized by expressing each response as a percentage of the maximum response exhibited by the animal. Electrical stimuli (1.5-msec biphasic pulses, 6/sec for 800 msec) of increasing intensity were delivered to the siphon skin (once every 20 min) by means of platinum wires sewn into the skin. These curves are representative data from one of five such experiments. In all experiments the threshold for inking was higher than for gill withdrawal by at least an order of magnitude and the stimulus–response characteristic for inking was very steep compared to that for gill withdrawal.

be all-or-none. This relationship holds for graded increases in stimulus duration as well as for graded increases in stimulus intensity.

Thresholds

To determine what underlies the differences in threshold between inking and gill withdrawal, attention was focused on the motor neurons that control these behaviors (Carew and Kandel, 1973b; 1976a,b). Inking is mediated by three adjacent identified motor cells (cells $L14_A$, $L14_B$, and $L14_C$) that are interconnected by means of electrical synapses. Defensive gill withdrawal is mediated by six identified motor neurons which are not connected to one another by either chemical or electrical synapses (Kupfermann et al., 1974). For comparison to the ink-gland motor cells, we will concentrate on only one gill motor neuron, cell L7, which accounts for about 40% of the motor component of the gill-withdrawal reflex.

The difference in thresholds for these two behaviors is correlated with the cellular properties of the motor neurons. One critical difference is in their resting potentials. The gill motor cell L7 has a resting potential of about −35 to −40 mV and the ink-gland motor neurons have a resting potential of about −70 mV. The membrane potential at which spikes are generated is about the same in L7 and in the ink-gland motor cells. As a result a small excitatory postsynaptic potential (EPSP) will increase the firing rate of L7, whereas an EPSP has to be 30 mV to cause an ink motor neuron to fire. When hyperpolarizing current is injected into L7, to bring its membrane potential to the same level as that of the L14 cells, it is still activated by sensory input from the mantle organs at a lower stimulus strength than are the ink motor cells. Thus, in addition to having a lower resting potential than the ink-gland cells, L7 also receives a larger excitatory synaptic volley in response to a brief tactile or noxious stimulus.

Unlike gill withdrawal, inking is not effectively triggered by a single brief stimulus, but requires a more prolonged stimulus. This feature can also be explained by the properties of the motor cells. Whereas L7 responds to a steady train of depolarizing synaptic potentials with a train of spikes that is of nearly constant frequency throughout, with a slight tendency to adapt, the L14 cells respond to a train with an accelerating burst of spikes. There may be no spikes at all during the first 1 or 2 sec of the train. This property of the ink-gland motor neurons undoubtedly contributes to the high threshold for inking as a function of stimulus duration.

The burst tendency of the ink-gland motor cells determines the steep slope of the stimulus–response curves and may constitute the central program for inking. We have therefore analyzed the factors that contribute to converting the graded sensory input into an all-or-none accelerating burst output of the motor neurons.

Conversion of a Graded Sensory Input into an All-Or-None Motor Output

There are three possible loci in the neural circuit for inking at which a graded sensory input could be converted to an all-or-none motor output. The first is on the input side. With gradually increasing stimulus strength or duration there might be a very steep increase in the amplitude of the synaptic input to the motor cells. A second possible locus is the intrinsic response of the motor neuron to the synaptic input. A third possible locus is the ink-gland response to activation by the ink-gland motor cells.

The central program for inking does not seem to lie either in the sensory input to the L14 cells or in the effector organs of the ink gland. Thus, as the intensity or duration of the sensory stimulus is gradually increased to a level that generates all-or-none inking, the excitatory synaptic input recorded in the L14 cells increases in a smoothly graded manner at a time when the spike output of the cells is increasing in an almost step-like manner (Fig. 3A and B). Similarly, if one of the motor neurons is fired directly by injection of

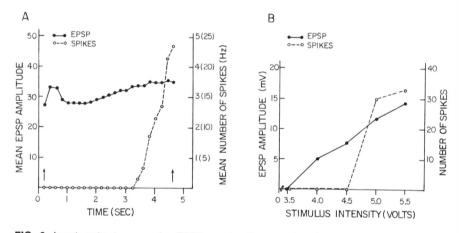

FIG. 3. Input–output curves for EPSPs and spikes produced in ink-gland motor cells. **A:** Effects of stimulus duration on EPSP amplitude and spike number. A train of electrical stimuli of constant intensity (2-msec pulses, 6/sec for 4.6 sec) was delivered to the connectives (*arrows*). Cell $L14_A$ was alternately hyperpolarized to a constant level ($N = 3$ runs), to permit measurement of EPSP amplitude, and at resting level ($N = 3$ runs), to permit spike generation. With the cell hyperpolarized, the mean amplitude of the EPSP was measured at 200-msec intervals (*solid circles*); and at resting potential, the mean spike number (*open circles*) was measured for comparable intervals (spike frequency indicated on ordinate in parentheses). Whereas the amplitude of the EPSP is rather constant with increasing duration (first decreasing, then gradually increasing), the spike number increases in a step-like fashion. **B:** Effects of stimulus intensity on EPSP amplitude and spike number. A train of electrical stimuli (2-msec pulses, 6/sec for 3 secs) of increasing intensity was delivered to the connectives, with cell $L14_A$ either hyperpolarized to a constant level to measure the EPSP amplitude (*solid circles*), or at resting potential to measure spike number (*open circles*). Whereas the amplitude of the EPSP increases gradually as a function of stimulus intensity, the spike number increases in a step-like fashion. Data are from a separate experiment from that shown in **A.**

depolarizing current, the amount of ink released increases in a graded manner as a function of the number of spikes in L14 (Fig. 4). It therefore seems likely that the steepness of the behavioral input–output curve for inking is largely attributable to a property of the spike-generating mechanisms of the L14 cells.

If the spike-generating properties of the motor cells account for the steep stimulus–response curves, then one would predict that as the strength or duration of the stimulus to the siphon is increased over a range that causes inking, the number of spikes in the ink-gland motor cells would suddenly increase very steeply. This, in fact, is what happens. Once the synaptic input reaches a certain threshold of intensity or duration, a burst of spikes is triggered in an almost step-like fashion (Fig. 5). In contrast, the spike frequency produced in the gill motor cell L7 increases much more gradually over the same stimulus range.

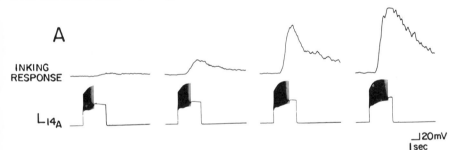

FIG. 4. A: Graded release of ink as a function of spike discharge in the ink-gland motor cell L14$_A$. *Top trace,* photocell record of the release of ink from purple gland. *Bottom trace,* intracellular recording from L14$_A$. Increasing depolarizing pulses in L14$_A$ produces progressively greater release of ink from the gland. In this and subsequent figures showing ink release, the latency of the response is exaggerated because the photocell records the ink after it has been released from the gland and drawn across the photocell in the perfusing stream (see Carew and Kandel, 1973*b;* 1976*a* for details). **B:** Graphic illustration of graded ink release as a function of spike number. In a separate experiment from that shown in **A,** cell L14$_A$ was depolarized with intracellular pulses of varying intensities producing a discharge with a varying number of spikes. The amount of ink released is expressed as a function of spike number. Data are normalized by expressing each amount of ink released as a percentage of the maximum ink response exhibited. The release of ink is graded across a fourfold increase in spike number.

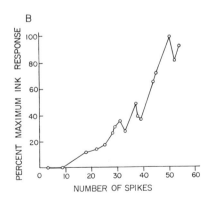

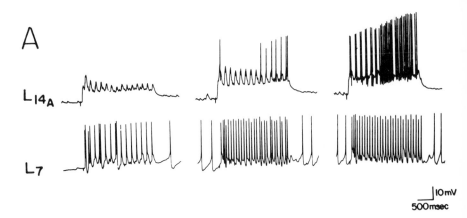

A

L14ₐ

L7

10 mV
500 msec

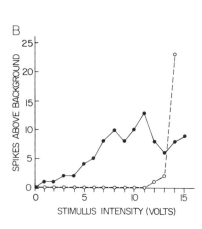

B

FIG. 5. Comparison of spike output of gill and ink-gland motor cells from trains of synaptic input of increasing intensity. **A:** Intracellular records from ink-gland motor cell L14$_A$ (*top trace*) and gill motor cell L7 (*bottom trace*) during trains of stimuli (6/sec for 2.5 sec) of increasing intensity to the connectives. The ink-gland motor cell has a higher threshold for activation than L7 but once threshold for activation is reached the ink-gland motor cell exhibits an accelerating burst which reaches a higher frequency than seen in L7. **B:** In a separate experiment from that shown in **A,** a quantitative comparison of the ink-gland motor cell's (*open circles*) and L7's (*filled circles*) response to trains of stimuli to the connectives was made. The spike output from L7 was graded as a function of increasing stimulus intensity, finally reaching a plateau, whereas the ink-gland motor cell showed a much higher threshold and then abruptly surpassed L7's response.

Two mechanisms seem to account for the steep input–output curve for the ink-gland motor cells, one a circuit property and the other a cellular property. The circuit property that contributes to the steepness of this curve is the electrical coupling among the motor cells (Fig. 6). When one cell fires, it produces an electrotonic PSP in each of the other two cells which may cause the other cells to fire, in turn producing electrotonic PSPs in the first cell. This tendency for positive feedback is enhanced during repetitive firing because the spikes become broader, presumably due to a gradual build-up of inactivation of the spike-generating currents. Given the low-pass filter characteristics of electrical synapses (Bennett, 1966) longer spikes result in an increase in electrotonic PSP amplitude (Berry, 1972). Enhancement of positive feedback by repetitive firing can contribute to the steep input–output curves for increasing stimulus strength or duration.

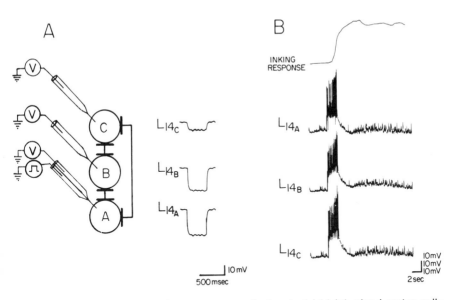

FIG. 6. Electrical coupling and common synaptic input of L14 ink-gland motor cells. **A:** Electrotonic coupling among ink-gland motor cells. A hyperpolarizing current pulse was injected into cell L14$_A$ and the change in membrane potential it produced was recorded in all three ink-gland motor cells (as diagrammed at left). The coupling between L14$_A$ and L14$_B$ is usually greater than the coupling between either cell and L14$_C$. **B:** Firing pattern in response to synaptic input. Synchrony of firing pattern is attributable to two factors: (1) electrical coupling **(A)**; and (2) identical synaptic input. *Top trace:* photocell record of ink released from ink gland. Bottom three traces are intracellular records from L14$_A$, L14$_B$, and L14$_C$. A strong train of stimuli (6/sec for 2.5 sec) was delivered to the connectives producing an accelerating spike discharge in the ink-gland motor cells and the release of ink from the gland. Following the train of stimuli, large synchronous PSPs occur in the motor cells for several seconds.

The cellular properties that contribute to the steepness of the spike-frequency–stimulus-duration curve for the ink-gland motor neurons are the high resting potential and the presence of fast-K$^+$ conductance channels (Connor and Stevens, 1971; Neher and Lux, 1971; Connor, 1975). Suggestive evidence for a fast-K$^+$ conductance was provided by experiments in which constant depolarizing current pulses were injected into an ink-gland motor cell (Figs. 7 and 8). When a train of near-threshold pulses is injected, the amplitudes of the potential changes gradually increase. These changes in amplitude occur only near threshold. Because these changes occur in the absence of external sodium and calcium it seems likely that they are caused by a gradual inactivation of a fast-K$^+$ current. Preliminary voltage-clamp studies (Byrne et al., *in preparation*) support this interpretation and indicate that the fast-K$^+$ channels are essentially free of inactivation in the resting cell because of the high membrane potential. Thus a strong depolarizing stimulus (such as a train of EPSPs) that approaches threshold is first shunted by the activation of the fast-K$^+$ conductance channels. If the depolarization is maintained, however, the fast-K$^+$ channels inactivate (see also Daut, 1973).

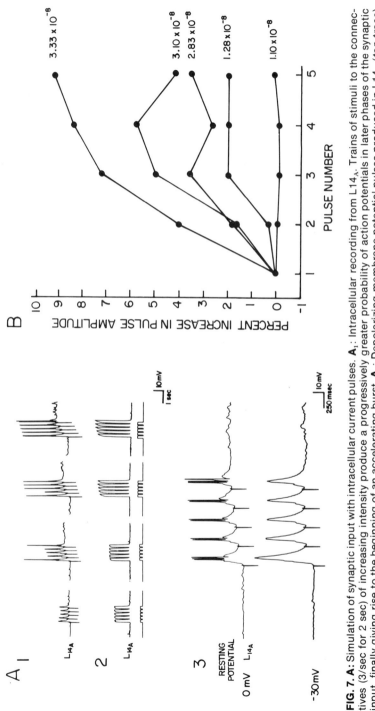

FIG. 7. A: Simulation of synaptic input with intracellular current pulses. **A₁:** Intracellular recording from $L14_A$. Trains of stimuli to the connectives (3/sec for 2 sec) of increasing intensity produce a progressively greater probability of action potentials in later phases of the synaptic input, finally giving rise to the beginning of an accelerating burst. **A₂:** Depolarizing membrane potential pulses produced in $L14_A$ (*top trace*) resulting from injection of 200 msec constant current depolarizing pulses (*bottom trace* = current monitor) of increasing intensity, which simulate the temporal pattern (3/sec for 2 sec) of the synaptic input in **A₁**. With increased current strength the membrane potential pulse increases in size during the train. **A₃:** The top trace is a fast sweep record of the last trace of **A₁** showing the acceleration of spikes in the late phase of the burst. In the bottom trace the ink-gland motor cell has been hyperpolarized to reveal the underlying synaptic potentials. Identical stimulation produces EPSPs which decrement, ruling out EPSP facilitation as a mechanism of the burst. **B:** Increase in membrane potential pulse amplitude in ink-gland motor cells as a function of intensity of current pulses. Trains of constant current pulses of increasing intensities (indicated at the right of each curve; current is expressed in amps) were delivered to $L14_A$ and the amplitude of the electrotonic pulse produced was measured. Data are normalized by expressing the pulse amplitude for each pulse in each train as a percentage of the

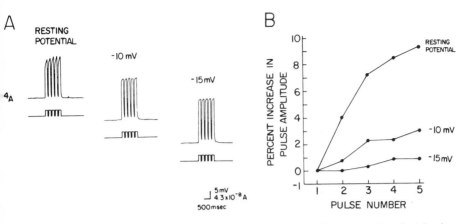

FIG. 8. Voltage dependency of depolarizing pulse increase. **A:** *Top trace* of each pair of records is an intracellular recording from $L14_A$; *bottom trace* is a monitor of independent current electrode. With the ink-gland motor cell at resting potential, repeated constant current intracellular depolarizing pulses produce a progressive increase in the amplitude of the membrane potential pulse. When the ink-gland motor cell is hyperpolarized 10 mV below resting potential, the increase in pulse amplitude from identical pulses as before is greatly reduced. When the ink-gland cell is further hyperpolarized to 15 mV below resting potential, increase in pulse size is almost completely abolished. **B:** Graphic representation of data shown in **A.**

Normally, complete inactivation would be achieved in a few hundred milliseconds, but a train of brief synaptic depolarizations (such as those that trigger inking in these experiments) and the consequent burst of action potentials, would contain periods of partial repolarization especially during the afterpotentials of the spikes, that might allow enough removal of inactivation to prolong the time course for full inactivation up to a few seconds. Such a gradual inactivation of the fast-K^+ conductance channels could contribute to the lack of spikes at the beginning of the train and the accelerating burst tendency at the end, which the ink-gland motor cells show in response to a steady train of EPSPs (Fig. 9). Other possible mechanisms which might contribute to this antiaccommodation process in the ink-gland motor cells are a gradual build-up of inactivation of delayed rectification or a delayed increase of a slow inward current (Nakamura et al., 1965; Eckert and Lux, 1974).

In summary, our data suggest that the locus of the central program for inking resides in the unusual properties of the ink gland motor cells. As a corollary, the differences in shape between the stimulus–response curves for inking and the gill-withdrawal reflex may be explained largely by the differences in intrinsic properties of the motor cells. The high resting potential of the ink-gland cells contributes to the high threshold for inking as a function of stimulus intensity. The steep stimulus–response curve can be attributed to the fact that the motor neurons take a graded input and convert it into an all-or-none output. Only a small change in amplitude or

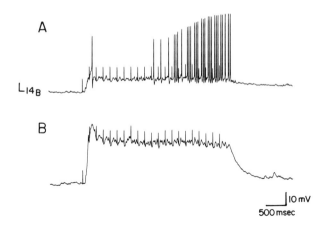

FIG. 9. EPSPs underlying the accelerating burst in ink-gland motor cells. Intracellular record from ink-gland motor cell L14$_B$. **A:** A train of stimuli to the connectives (6/sec for 3 sec) produces an accelerating burst of spikes in L14$_B$. **B:** An identical train of stimuli is delivered to the connectives with L14$_B$ hyperpolarized to prevent spiking and allow examination of the EPSPs underlying the discharge. EPSP facilitation cannot account for the accelerating burst because the EPSPs do not grow larger but rather they show slight decrement. In **A** and **B**, small spike-like deflections are stimulus artifacts.

duration of synaptic input is necessary to drive these cells from threshold to maximum firing rate.

AN ALL-OR-NONE NEUROENDOCRINE FIXED ACT: EGG LAYING

Another behavior in *Aplysia* which might be classified as an all-or-none fixed act is egg laying. Since the behavioral stimuli that trigger egg laying are unknown, it has not yet been possible to describe the stimulus–response curve for this behavior. Nevertheless, informal observations of *Aplysia* kept in the laboratory indicate that the different egg masses laid by a given individual vary in size over a rather restricted range. This suggests that egg laying probably has a rather steep stimulus–response curve.

Egg laying is triggered by two symmetrical clusters of neuroendocrine cells called the bag cells, which are located at the rostral margins of the abdominal ganglion (Fig. 10). In the mature animal each cluster contains about 300 cells. The bag cells release a hormone that causes contraction of muscle in the ovotestis, resulting in the expulsion of the several hundred thousand eggs which make up the egg mass (Kupfermann, 1972; Coggeshall, 1970). Kupfermann and Kandel (1970) found that stimulation of the connectives from the head ganglia caused the bag cells to fire in a long (about 40 min) decelerating burst (Fig. 11). During the burst all the cells in a cluster invariably fired in tight synchrony. Indirect evidence suggests that this is due to the fact that the cells within each cluster are electrically coupled to each other. The number of stimuli necessary to initiate the burst was variable, and once triggered, the time course of the burst was essentially insensitive to further stimulation. Because of the stereotyped burst

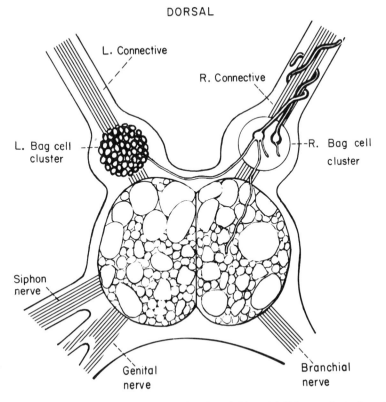

DORSAL

L. Connective

R. Connective

L. Bag cell
cluster

-R. Bag cell
cluster

Siphon
nerve

Genital
nerve

Branchial
nerve

FIG. 10. Diagram of abdominal ganglion, showing right and left bag cell clusters. Two cells are schematically shown in the right cluster in order to illustrate the relationship of the bag cell processes to the connective and the main part of the ganglion (from Coggeshall, cited in Kupfermann and Kandel, 1970).

pattern, and the highly synchronous nature of firing of the bag cells (Fig. 12) it seems reasonable to assume that the bag cell clusters release a relatively fixed amount of hormone each time they are activated.

The available evidence suggests that the motor program for the long-lasting repetitive discharge in the neurosecretory cells resides in the cells themselves. For example, the burst capability is unaffected when the bag cells are isolated from the rest of the abdominal ganglion. But it is not yet known whether the ability to generate the prolonged burst is due to reverberation of activity between the neuroendocrine cells (by means of their electronic connections) or, more likely, to endogenous properties of the cells' membranes which cause them to fire repetitively to a brief stimulus.

In both egg laying and inking the motor program resides in the effector cells. This is most efficient if the effector cells are used in only one way and for only one behavior. Another locus for a central program might be required in more complex visceromotor or somatic motor systems where motor cells are used for different behaviors. With that idea in mind we

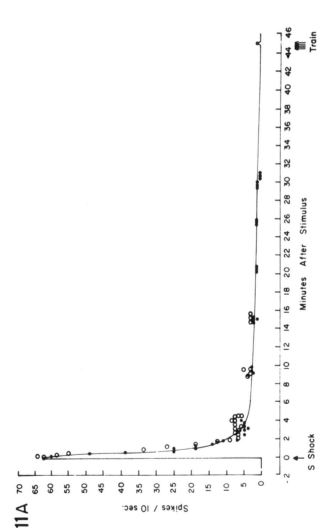

11A

FIG. 11. Bag cell spike activity elicited by connective stimulation. **A:** Time course of sustained discharge in a single cell recorded from two different bag cell preparations. Both discharges were elicited by a single shock applied to a connective. **B:** Time course of two sustained discharges elicited in the same bag cell preparation following repetitive stimulation of a connective. *Closed circles* indicate the time course of the earlier discharge; *open circles* indicate a discharge elicited 2 hr later. Attempts at eliciting a sustained discharge at several intervals during the 2-hr period between discharges were unsuccessful (Kupfermann and Kandel, 1970).

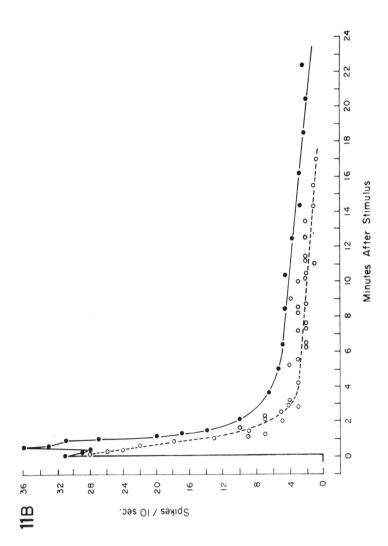

11B

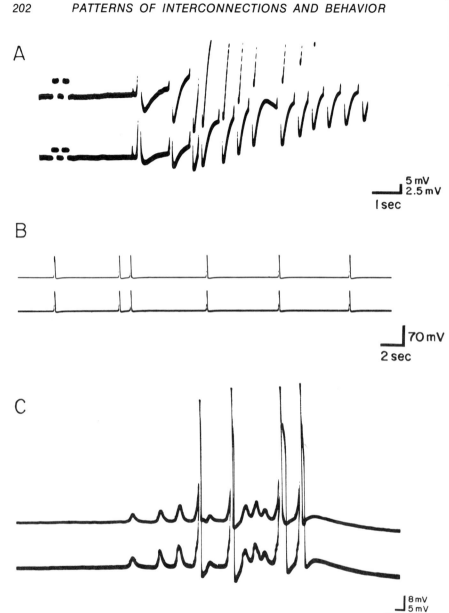

FIG. 12. Simultaneous recordings from two bag cells in the same cluster. **A:** High-gain recording to illustrate the initiation of discharge following a single stimulus. **B:** Low-gain recording of same two cells several minutes later to show they are still firing in perfect synchrony. **C:** Simultaneous recordings from two bag cells illustrates the close parallel of spikes and graded potentials of cells in the same cluster. Bag cells were firing in bursts and were activated by a shock applied to a connective several minutes prior to the recording (Kupfermann and Kandel, 1970).

examined two additional behaviors which tend to occur in an all-or-none fashion: (1) a phasic increase in heart rate; and (2) a respiratory pumping movement consisting of a complex contraction of the mantle organs and parapodia, associated with inhibition of heart beat.

A SIMPLE VISCEROMOTOR FIXED-ACTION PATTERN: PHASIC INCREASE IN HEART RATE

Brief, phasic increases in heart rate may be recorded in the semi-intact preparation (Koester et al., 1974). Under conditions with the heart pumping against an artificial resistive load, the phasic heart rate increases are often associated with an increase in cardiac output (Dieringer and Koester, *unpublished*). No detailed input–output curves have been determined for this behavior because the stimulus that triggers the phasic heart rate increase is not known. But preliminary observations indicate that this increase in heart rate typically varies over a rather narrow range. Moreover, the behavior involves at least two motor systems, one controlling heart rate and the other vasomotor tone, so it seems reasonable to classify it as a fixed-action pattern.

The motor components of this behavior are controlled by the abdominal ganglion. Seven motor neurons have been described (Mayeri et al., 1974) which account for a major portion of the motor control of the cardiovascular system (Fig. 13). There are two heart inhibitors (LD_{HI} cells) and three vasoconstrictors (LB_{VC} cells) that constrict the abdominal aorta and gastroesophageal artery. There are also two types of heart excitatory motor neurons: LD_{HE}, a cell which has a brief, phasic effect on heart rate, and RB_{HE}, which has tonic, more lasting effects on heart rate. None of the cardiovascular motor neurons are interconnected with each other.

During the phasic increase in heart rate and cardiac output the heart excitor (RB_{HE}) is excited and the heart inhibitors (LD_{HI}) are inhibited (Fig. 14). A single, multiaction cell mediates these actions (Koester et al.,

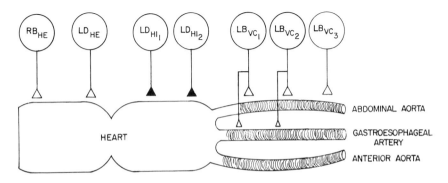

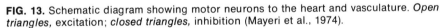

FIG. 13. Schematic diagram showing motor neurons to the heart and vasculature. *Open triangles,* excitation; *closed triangles,* inhibition (Mayeri et al., 1974).

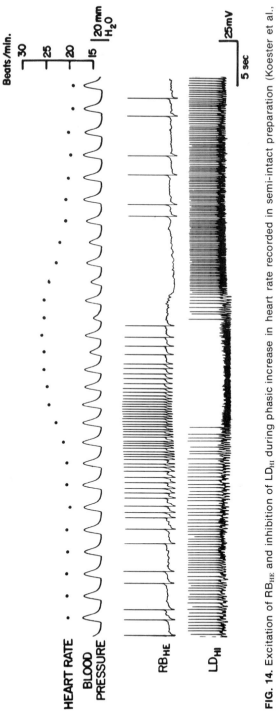
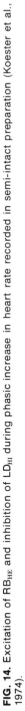

FIG. 14. Excitation of RB_{HE} and inhibition of LD_{HI} during phasic increase in heart rate recorded in semi-intact preparation (Koester et al., 1974).

1974). This neuron, cell L10, excites RB_{HE}, inhibits the LD_{HI} cells, and also inhibits the vasoconstrictors (Fig. 15A,B). Figure 15C summarizes these actions. The behavioral functions of this multiaction cell are not restricted to a single motor pathway. L10 acts on the heart excitatory and inhibitory motor pathway as well as on the vasoconstrictor motor cells. Thus, L10 serves as a command cell (Kennedy and Davis, 1976) coordinating the activity of three different motor pathways.

The finding that a single cell affects all of these motor pathways raises two questions: (1) Can the activity of L10 by itself produce the fixed act? (2) If so, how is the central program of the fixed act normally generated?

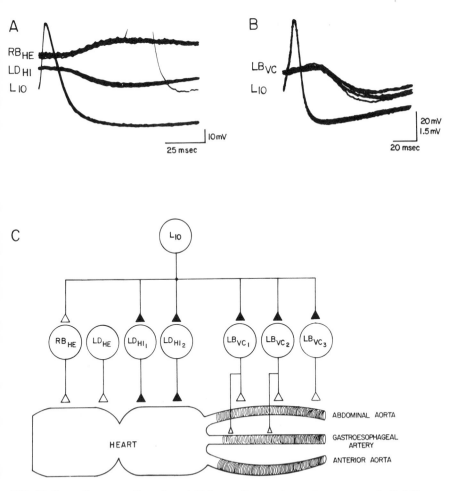

FIG. 15. Synaptic connections from L10 to cardiovascular motor neurons. **A, B:** L10 produces in EPSP in RB_{HE} and IPSPs in LD_{HI} and LB_{VC}. **C:** Schematic diagram summarizing connections made by L10 to cardiovascular motor neurons. *Open triangles*, excitation; *closed triangles*, inhibition (Koester et al., 1974).

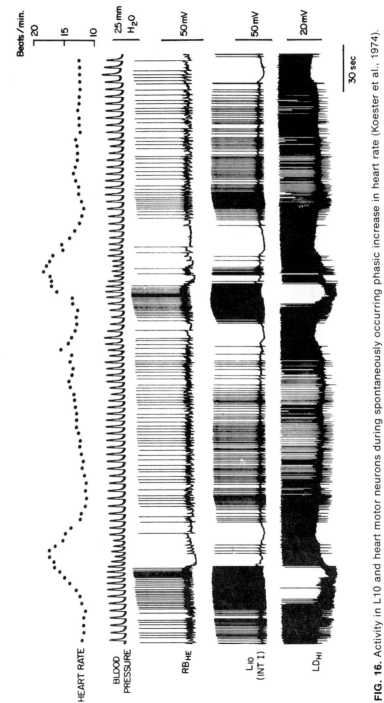

FIG. 16. Activity in L10 and heart motor neurons during spontaneously occurring phasic increase in heart rate (Koester et al., 1974).

What triggers L10 into activity and what is responsible for the time course of its firing?

In the semi-intact preparation, each phasic increase in heart rate produces a burst of spikes in L10 (Fig. 16). That the burst in L10 is causally related to the change in heart rate can be shown by two observations: (1) firing L10 with a current pulse produces a similar motor effect (Fig. 17); and (2) hyperpolarizing the follower cell RB_{HE} during a spontaneous L10 burst eliminates the heart acceleration (Koester et al., 1974). Thus the activity of L10 generates the fixed-action pattern: it increases heart rate and causes vasodilation. The connections of L10 to the cardiac and vascular motor neurons are invariant, which explains the stereotypic pattern of response. Moreover, L10 fires at certain preferred frequencies which explains why the amplitude of the response, although not fixed, nevertheless occurs in characteristic steps.

To see how the central program for this fixed-action pattern is generated we examined the synaptic input to L10 and found it to be almost entirely inhibitory. L10 tends to fire spontaneously in either a steady, pacing mode, or in brief, high-frequency bursts. Although the inhibitory input can modulate L10's firing pattern to some degree, the bursts which occur in L10 are the product of a burst-generating mechanism endogenous to L10's membrane. This can be shown by changing the frequency of the burst by passing polarizing current (*unpublished*), or by resetting the rhythm of a series of regularly occurring bursts (Fig. 18). Similar bursting patterns are observed when the abdominal ganglion is completely isolated from the periphery

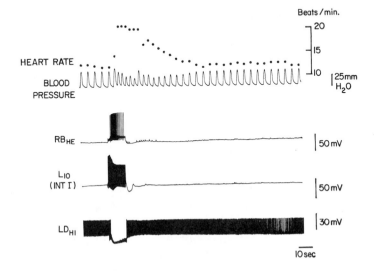

FIG. 17. Phasic increase in heart rate produced by firing L10 with an intracellular current pulse. Spike activity in L10 produced excitation of RB_{HE} and inhibition of LD_{HI} (Koester et al., 1974).

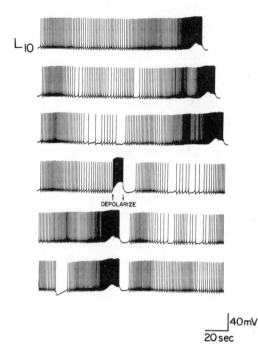

FIG. 18. Resetting of L10's bursting rhythm. Sequence of these continuous traces, recorded in the isolated ganglion, is from top to bottom. The top three traces show the normal interburst interval for L10 spontaneous bursts recorded in this preparation. Midway through the next interval a burst was produced in L10 by injecting an intracellular current pulse. The subsequent interburst intervals were about the same duration as the earlier ones, but the bursting rhythm was shifted about 180° out of phase with the original rhythm.

and from the rest of the central nervous system. Thus these patterns can be generated in the absence of peripheral feedback. They represent a centrally generated motor program. The fixed-action pattern results from the burst-generating properties of L10.

A COMPLEX VISCEROMOTOR FIXED-ACTION PATTERN: RESPIRATORY PUMPING MOVEMENTS

A fourth stereotypic behavior which has been observed in *Aplysia* is a complex respiratory pumping action which consists of a phasic, coordinated contraction of gill, siphon, mantle shelf, and parapodia, accompanied by inhibition of heart beat (Koester et al., 1974; Kupfermann et al., 1974; Perlman, 1975). This behavior enhances respiration by rapidly exchanging the fluid in the gill and in the mantle cavity. Preliminary behavioral observations (Hening and Grundfest, *unpublished*) indicate that stimuli that trigger this behavior affect primarily its *frequency* of occurrence, and have less effect on its *amplitude*. In addition, the response is fairly constant in form. Because of its apparent stereotypy, we consider this behavioral sequence a fixed-action pattern.

With the exception of parapodial contraction (which is controlled by the pedal ganglia) all of the motor components of respiratory pumping are located in the abdominal ganglion. The central command acts on at least 13 excitatory motor neurons to the respiratory complex (the gill, siphon, and mantle shelf) as well as on the seven cardiovascular motor neurons (Koester et al., 1974; Kupfermann et al., 1974; Perlman, 1975). None of these 20 motor cells are connected to one another. The central command acts directly on these motor cells to trigger: (1) respiratory pumping, (2) inhibition of heart rate, and (3) decreased vasomotor tone (Fig. 19).

The synaptic input to these motor cells has been attributed to an unidentified cluster of higher order interneurons which is called Interneuron II (Kandel et al., 1967; Waziri and Kandel, 1969; Koester et al., 1974; Kupfermann et al., 1974). The mechanism of burst generation in the Interneuron II cluster is not yet understood. However, as with L10, Interneuron II makes invariant connections to its motor cells. Interneuron II also shows bursts in the isolated ganglion similar to those seen in the intact animal. Thus peripheral feedback is also not important for the fixed-action patterns driven by Interneuron II. The phasic increase in heart rate and cardiac

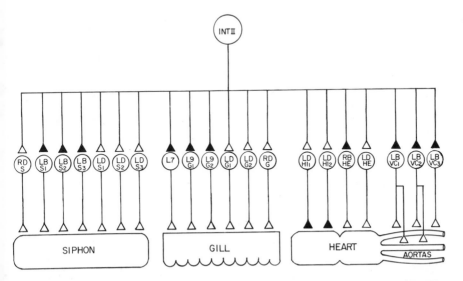

FIG. 19. Schematic diagram showing the connections made by Interneuron II to the motor neurons to siphon, gill, heart, and aortas (*open triangles,* excitation; *closed triangles,* inhibition). The net effect of these connections during Interneuron II activity is gill and siphon contraction, heart inhibition, and decreased vasoconstrictor activity. Unpublished evidence indicates that Interneuron II is a cluster of cells which fire synchronously (Byrne and Koester, *unpublished*).

output and respiratory pumping also share another feature in common. The motor program is located presynaptic to the final motor pathways which generate the behaviors. This type of organization may result from the fact that the motor neurons involved are used to control a variety of different behaviors.

SUMMARY

The recent extensions of cellular techniques to the study of behavior has made it possible to examine the relationship between different patterns of cellular interconnections and behavior. We have attempted to examine these relationships in the abdominal ganglion where parts of the neural circuitry underlying several behavioral responses have now been analyzed. To correlate these patterns of connection with behavior we have divided the various responses controlled by the ganglion into two general classes, graded and all-or-none, based on differences in the stimulus–response characteristics. We have further subdivided each of these classes into elementary and complex. Thus, elementary fixed acts consist of single episodes in a single effector system and tend to be all-or-none in amplitude. Complex fixed-action patterns involve recurring episodes or more than one effector system; as a result both sequence (form) and amplitude are free to vary. Fixed-action patterns tend to be stereotypic in form (in the sequence of components); their amplitudes, although not all-or-none, tend to occur in certain characteristic steps.

Although we have found this distinction useful, we would emphasize the preliminary nature of our studies. We have so far only analyzed the detailed behavioral input–output relationships for two of the five behaviors we have reviewed (gill withdrawal and inking). In the other three cases (egg laying, phasic increases in heart rate, and respiratory pumping) we have inferred aspects of the input–output curve from known features of the behavior. This is an obvious weakness in the behavioral data.

Figure 20 summarizes the results from the four all-or-none behaviors we have studied and indicates some of the tentative conclusions we have reached in our search for principles relating types of neural circuitry to classes of behavior. The first principle concerns the *locus for central programs*. In inking and egg laying, essential features of the central program for the fixed act reside in the motor cells. But motor cells are most likely to be the locus of a program if they are limited in function to one behavioral act. Some motor cells, as those of the circulatory and respiratory system, are used in different behavioral sequences and for both reflex acts and central commands. Here the motor program for the fixed act does not reside at the level of the motor cell but is moved centrally. This is a simple example of centralization of function.

A second principle concerns the *interconnections between motor neurons*.

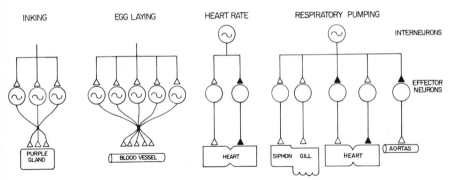

FIG. 20. Schematic diagram showing the patterns of neural organization used for the generation of four all-or-none behaviors. The ~ symbol represents the site where the all-or-none properties of the behaviors are thought to reside.

Motor neurons that are involved in only one all-or-none behavior—inking and egg laying—are coupled electrically, whereas motor cells that drive multiple independent behaviors (both graded and all-or-none) are not. Why are the ink-gland and egg-laying motor cells coupled, whereas the motor neurons to the heart, aortas, or respiratory complex are not? One possible function for the electrical coupling in the ink motor cells and the bag cells is that these cells always function as a single unit; the coupling assures synchronous activation[1] (Bennett, 1966). An additional and perhaps more important reason for tight electrical coupling is that it may provide an effective means (although not the only means) for the generation of an all-or-none motor program.

A third principle relates to the *mechanism of the central program*. Although their loci differ, the central programs of the four stereotypic behavioral responses in *Aplysia* that we have analyzed share features in common. The programs do not require feedback from the periphery for their timing or maintenance. This is not surprising; similar findings have been made previously in a number of other systems (for review see Wilson, 1970; Grillner, 1975; Kennedy and Davis, 1976). What is interesting is that, of the three central programs that have been most extensively analyzed (inking, egg laying, and increased heart rate), none of the mechanisms for generating the central program seems to rely on either chemical synaptic connections or complex circuit properties. Rather, the mechanisms seem

---

[1] There are alternative mechanisms for synchrony, which do not rely on electrical coupling. This can be seen in the neural circuit controlling the cardiovascular system, where the two LD_{HI} cells and the three LB_{VC} cells also seem to represent a functional unit. They seem always to receive identical synaptic input, and to be synchronously active. Yet the members of these two groups (LD_{HI} and LB_{VC}) are not electrically (or chemically) connected to each other. They also are not involved in the generation of all-or-none fixed acts.

to reside either in the membrane characteristics of the critical cells involved, in the electrotonic connections between them, or in a combination of both features.

An interesting distinction is often made in the ability to behaviorally modify reflex and fixed acts. Reflex acts are modifiable in both form and frequency of occurrence. By contrast, the form of fixed acts is not modifiable. The only feature that is usually modified is the frequency of occurrence. *This distinction is consistent with the notion that the chemical connections between nerve cells may be particularly important for achieving plasticity in the form of response, whereas the electrical connections between cells generating the central program and the intrinsic membrane properties of these cells may be particularly important for maintaining stereotypy of the form of the response* (Kandel, 1976).

In conclusion, we would like to outline two new directions that can now be investigated. First, how are the various fixed and reflex acts of a nervous system coordinated? What determines their sequence and the priority of their expression? Here we can begin to examine the possible cellular mechanisms underlying behavioral choice (Hull, 1934; Tinbergen, 1951; Eibl-Eibesfeldt, 1970; Davis et al., 1974). We have begun to examine this problem by looking at two antagonistic central commands: phasic increases and decreases in heart rate. Whereas the phasic increase is mediated by L10, the phasic decrease is mediated by Interneuron II. The selection of behaviors in this case is determined at the level of the command element

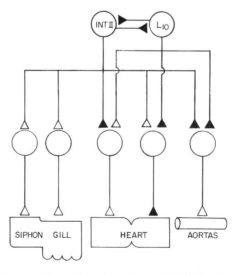

FIG. 21. Schematic diagram illustrating the reciprocal inhibition between L10 and Interneuron II, and the major connections they make to motor neurons that innervate cardiovascular and respiratory systems (*open triangles*, excitation; *closed triangles*, inhibition).

and achieved by mutual inhibition. The two command elements (Interneuron II and L10) reciprocally inhibit each other (Kandel, Frazier and Wachtel, 1969) so that only one and not the other fixed-action pattern can be expressed (Fig. 21). The principle encountered here is similar to the reciprocal pattern of innervation described by Sherrington (1906) for antagonistic reflex responses.

Finally, one might consider how analyses of these simple fixed acts might lead one to understand more complex fixed-action patterns such as those involved in escape, feeding, and copulating. An attractive possibility is that the neural circuits for elementary fixed acts, such as those that we have considered here, might serve as basic building blocks or circuit modules that can be combined much as different components in an electronic circuit are combined. Complex behavior might then simply be generated by different combinations of elementary neural modules. The challenge, however, is not only to develop hypotheses but also to test them. Fortunately, the preparations and techniques to undertake such a task are now at hand.

ACKNOWLEDGMENTS

We thank Drs. Vincent Castellucci, Irving Kupfermann, and Alden Spencer for critically reading an earlier draft of this manuscript.

This work was supported by a Research Scientist Award 5-K05 MH 18558–09 to E.R.K., a Foundation Fund for Research in Psychiatry Fellowship 71–524 to T.J.C., and NSF Grant BMS74–18410 and NIH Grants 2 ROI NS 12744–02 and ROI MH 26212–02.

REFERENCES

Barlow, G. W. (1968): Ethological units of behavior. In: *Central Nervous System and Fish Behavior*, edited by D. Ingle, pp. 217–232. University of Chicago Press, Chicago.

Bennett, M. V. L. (1966): Physiology of electrotonic junctions. *Ann. NY Acad. Sci.*, 137:509–539.

Berry, M. S. (1972): A system of electrically coupled small cells in the buccal ganglion of the pond snail *Planorbis corneus. J. Exp. Biol.*, 56:621–637.

Carew, T. J., and Kandel, E. R. (1973a): Acquisition and retention of long-term habituation in *Aplysia:* Correlation of behavioral and cellular processes. *Science*, 182:1158–1160.

Carew, T. J., and Kandel, E. R. (1973b): Mediation of inking behavior in *Aplysia californica* by an identified neuron in the abdominal ganglion. *Fed. Proc.*, 32(3).

Carew, T. J., and Kandel, E. R. (1976a): Inking in *Aplysia californica:* I. The neural circuit of an all-or-none behavioral response (*unpublished*).

Carew, T. J., and Kandel, E. R. (1976b): Inking in *Aplysia californica:* II. The central program for inking (*unpublished*).

Castellucci, V., Pinsker, H., Kupfermann, I., and Kandel, E. R. (1970): Neuronal mechanisms of habituation and dishabituation of the gill-withdrawal reflex in *Aplysia. Science*, 167:1745–1748.

Coggeshall, R. E. (1970): Cytologic analysis of the bag cell control of egg laying in *Aplysia. J. Morphol.*, 132:461–485.

Connor, J. A. (1975): Neural repetitive firing: A comparative study of membrane properties of crustacean walking leg axons. *J. Neurophysiol.,* 38:922–932.

Connor, J. A., and Stevens, C. F. (1971): Voltage clamp studies of a transient outward membrane current in gastropod neural somata. *J. Physiol.,* 213:21–30.

Daut, J. (1973): Modulation of the excitatory synaptic response by fast transient K^+ current in snail neurones. *Nature [New Biol.],* 246:193–196.

Davis, W. J., Mpitsos, G. J., and Pinneo, J. M. (1974): The behavioral hierarchy of the mollusk *Pleurobranchaea.* I. The dominant position of the feeding behavior. *J. Comp. Physiol.,* 90:207–224.

Doty, R. W. (1968): Neural organization of deglutition. In: *Handbook of Physiology, Section 6: Alimentary Canal,* 4:1861–1902.

Eibl-Eibesfeldt, I. (1970): *Ethology: The Biology of Behavior.* Holt, Rinehart, and Winston, New York.

Grillner, S. (1975): Locomotion in vertebrates: Central mechanisms and reflex interaction. *Physiol. Rev.,* 55:247–304.

Hoyle, G. (1964): Exploration of neuronal mechanisms underlying behavior in insects. In: *Neural Theory and Modelling,* edited by R. F. Reiss, pp. 346–376. Stanford University Press, Stanford, California.

Hull, C. L. (1934): The concept of habit-family-hierarchy and maze learning. Part 1. *Psychol. Rev.,* 41:33–54.

Kandel, E. R. (1976): *The Cellular Basis of Behavior.* Freeman Press, San Francisco.

Kandel, E. R., Brunelli, M., Byrne, J., and Castellucci, V. (1976): A common presynaptic locus for the synaptic changes underlying short-term habituation and sensitization of the gill-withdrawal reflex in *Aplysia. Symposium on Quantitative Biology XL: The Synapse.* Cold Spring Harbor Symposium, Cold Spring Harbor, New York.

Kandel, E. R., Frazier, W. T., and Wachtel, H. (1969): Organization of inhibition in abdominal ganglion of *Aplysia.* I. Role of inhibition and disinhibition in transforming neural activity. *J. Neurophysiol.,* 32:496–508.

Kandel, E. R., Frazier, W. T., Waziri, R., and Coggeshall, R. E. (1967): Direct and common connections among identified neurons in *Aplysia. J. Neurophysiol.,* 30:1352–1376.

Kennedy, D., and Davis, W. J. (1976): Principles of organization of invertebrate motor systems. In: *Handbook of the Nervous System,* Vol. I, edited by E. R. Kandel. American Physiological Society, Bethesda, Maryland (*in press*).

Koester, J., Mayeri, E., Liebeswar, G., and Kandel, E. R. (1974): Neural control of circulation in *Aplysia.* II. Interneurons. *J. Neurophysiol.,* 37:476–496.

Kupfermann, I. (1972): Studies on the neurosecretory control of egg laying in *Aplysia. Am. Zool.,* 12:513–519.

Kupfermann, I., Carew, T. J., and Kandel, E. R. (1974): Local, reflex and central commands controlling gill and siphon movements in *Aplysia. J. Neurophysiol.,* 37:996–1019.

Kupfermann, I., and Kandel, E. R. (1970): Electrophysiological properties and functional interconnections of two symmetrical neurosecretory clusters (bag cells) in abdominal ganglion of *Aplysia. J. Neurophysiol.,* 33:865–876.

Lloyd, D. (1957): Input-output relation in a flexor reflex. *J. Gen. Physiol.,* 41:297–306.

Lux, H. D., and Eckert, R. (1974): Inferred slow inward current in snail neurons. *Nature,* 250:574–576.

Mayeri, E., Koester, J., Kupfermann, I., Liebeswar, G., and Kandel, E. R. (1974): Neural control of circulation in *Aplysia.* I. Motoneurons. *J. Neurophysiol.,* 37:458–475.

Morris, D. (1957): "Typical intensity" and its relation to the problem of ritualization. *Behavior,* 11:1–12.

Nakamura, Y., Nakajima, S., and Grundfest, H. (1965): Analysis of spike electrogenesis and depolarizing K inactivation in electroplaques of *Electrophorous electricus L. J. Gen. Physiol.,* 49:321–349.

Neher, E., and Lux, H. D. (1971): Properties of somatic membrane patches of snail neurons under voltage clamp. *Pfluegers Arch.,* 322:35–38.

Perlman, A. (1975): Neural control of the siphon in *Aplysia.* Ph.D. dissertation, New York University.

Sherrington, C. S. (1906): *The Integrative Action of the Nervous System.* Yale University Press, New Haven.

Tinbergen, N. (1951): *The Study of Instinct.* Clarendon Press, Oxford, England.
Waziri, R., and Kandel, E. R. (1969): Organization of inhibition in abdominal ganglion of *Aplysia.* III. Interneurons mediating inhibition. *J. Neurophysiol.,* 32:520–539.
Wilson, D. M. (1970): Neural operations in arthropod ganglia. In: *The Neurosciences: Second Study Program,* edited by F. O. Schmitt, pp. 397–409. Rockefeller University Press, New York.

Electrobiology of Nerve, Synapse, and Muscle,
edited by J. P. Reuben, D. P. Purpura, M. V. L. Bennett,
and E. R. Kandel. Raven Press, New York © 1976

Development of Specific Sensory-Evoked Synaptic Networks in CNS Tissue Cultures

Stanley M. Crain

Departments of Neuroscience and Physiology, and the Rose F. Kennedy Center for Research in Mental Retardation and Human Development, Albert Einstein College of Medicine, Bronx, New York 10461

ACTION POTENTIALS OF DORSAL ROOT GANGLION CELLS IN CULTURE

Electrophysiologic studies of dorsal root ganglia (DRG) isolated in tissue culture were initiated in 1952 during the course of my predoctoral work in the Department of Neurology at Columbia University. Harry Grundfest and Fred Mettler provided inspiration, stimulation, guidance, and support during the early years while methods were being developed to record the bioelectric activities of these cultured neurons. In collaboration with Margaret Murray and Edith Peterson, in the tissue culture laboratory at Columbia, we were able to demonstrate for the first time, in 1953, that DRG neurons could maintain the capacity to generate and propagate characteristic action potentials even after months of isolation in culture (Crain et al., 1953). Grundfest's strong encouragement and kind assistance with electronic instrumentation greatly facilitated subsequent intracellular recordings from these cultured DRG neurons (Figs. 1,2; Crain, 1954a,b, 1956; see also Crain, 1973, 1976; cytologic correlates in Peterson and Murray, 1956).

In addition to showing normal membrane resting and action potentials, intracellular recordings from cultured chick embryo spinal sensory ganglion cells also demonstrated several interesting types of repetitive spike patterns. Immediately after impalement, "injury discharges" could often be recorded (before the membrane sealed up around the shaft of the impaling microelectrode). The repetitive spike bursts that occur during such periods involve gradual membrane depolarization following each spike leading to triggering of the next one (Fig. 1C_1), similar to patterns recorded from spontaneously contracting cardiac and skeletal muscle fibers *in vitro* (Fig. 1A and B), except for the large differences in time scale. Aside from these transient injury discharges, the membrane potential of cultured spinal sensory ganglion cells generally remained stable unless excited by electric stimuli (Crain, 1956; Scott et al., 1969).

Many of the ganglion cells in explants of whole chick spinal ganglia de-

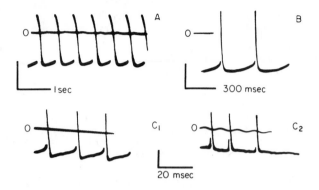

FIG. 1. Intracellularly recorded membrane resting and action potentials of spontaneously contracting, cultured chick embryo cardiac **(A)** and fetal rat skeletal **(B)** muscle fibers compared with repetitive activity of cultured chick embryo spinal sensory ganglion cell recorded immediately following injury associated with microelectrode impalement (**C₁**). Note similarity in basic pattern—involving gradual depolarization following each spike which leads to triggering of the next one—in spite of large differences in time scale. Record **C₂** shows absence of depolarizing prepotential between repetitive spikes in another ganglion cell where impulses are *propagating toward* the recording site from a peripherally excited neurite, rather than being *generated* directly in the soma region (see Fig. 2). Amplitude calibrations: 50 mV. *Note:* in Figs. 1–3 upper sweep in each record indicates baseline potential obtained before impalement (0) and, in some cases, also time-calibrating signals and stimulus current data (Fig. 2). (From Crain, 1954a, 1965.)

velop extraordinarily complex arborizing neurites in culture (Levi and Meyer, 1938). Gross electric stimulation of such neuritic arborizations may lead to sequential propagated invasions of the impaled perikaryon by impulses arriving from several neurites with substantially different conduction times from the sites of impulse origin (Fig. 1C₂). These repetitive spikes arise *abruptly* from the resting potential level, in contrast to the gradual depolarization preceding each spike when the impulse is generated directly in the soma region (see Fig. 1C₁ and C₂). The latter (injury discharge) spike pattern can also be systematically produced by passing small depolarizing currents across the ganglion cell membrane (Fig. 2). The frequency of these repetitive spike responses can be graded from under 100/sec to more than 300/sec by careful control of the depolarizing current intensity, at least during intervals up to 20 msec.

It is ironic that the first attempt to record intracellularly from cultured CNS neurons failed to demonstrate any evidence of synaptic potentials (Hild and Tasaki, 1962), whereas long-lasting depolarizing potentials resembling excitatory postsynaptic potentials have actually been detected in cultures of spinal sensory ganglion cells where synapses are not ordinarily encountered *in situ*. A complex discharge sequence has been evoked in some cultured chick embryo ganglion cells (Crain, 1971) consisting of an early spike potential followed by a long-duration depolarization (Fig. 3A₁ and B₁), and often a second or third spike occurred during the rising phase of

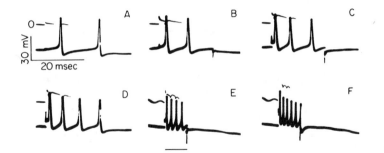

FIG. 2. Repetitive activity of cultured chick embryo spinal sensory ganglion cell evoked during passage of depolarizing current (20-msec duration) across soma membrane by direct application through the intracellular recording electrode. Upper sweep in each record indicates onset and magnitude of stimulating current during these membrane potential measurements, increasing from less than 10^{-10} to about 3×10^{-9} A in records **A** to **E**. Termination of 20 msec stimulus duration is indicated by shock artifact in lower sweep of records **B,C,E,** and **F,** and by gap during final spike in records **A** and **D.** A bridge circuit was used to balance out most of the artifact produced in the voltage recording by this mode of stimulation. Note increase in frequency of spike discharges from less than 100 to approximately 300 per sec. Gradual depolarization occurs preceding each spike (except for initial spike bursts elicited at high current intensity). Note similarity to soma injury-discharge patterns (Fig. $1C_1$), in contrast to effect of sequential invasion of propagated impulses (Fig. $1C_2$). (From Crain, 1973.)

this depolarization, with latencies of 8 to 20 msec (Fig. $3A_{2-4}$ and B_2). The duration of these postspike depolarizing potentials ranged from about 50 to several hundred milliseconds and they were graded in amplitude (Fig. 3B). This complex pattern of repetitive spike and slow-wave responses following a single brief electric stimulus is in sharp contrast to the pattern observed in cells where peripherally initiated propagated impulses sequentially invade the soma (see Fig. 3 versus $1C_2$).

It is tempting to interpret this long-lasting postspike depolarizing potential recorded in some cultured sensory ganglion cells as an excitatory postsynaptic potential generated in the impaled perikaryon after an impulse, initially evoked in the cell body, propagates through recurrent collateral pathways leading back to junctions on the same perikaryon. This simple interpretation is based on Nakai's (1956) direct cinematographic observations of the growth of recurrent collaterals in dissociated ganglion cells in culture, where some neuritic branches are seen to loop back (over distances of hundreds of microns) and to *terminate* on their perikarya of origin. Recent electron microscopic demonstrations of axosomatic synaptic junctions in cultures of chick embryo spinal sensory ganglia (Miller et al., 1970) may, indeed, provide the ultrastructural basis for the above interpretations, but the evidence is still only circumstantial and needs to be proved by correlative cytologic and electrophysiologic analyses of the same identified cells in culture.

Although synapses have not been detected in previous ultrastructural

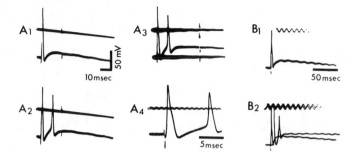

FIG. 3. Long-duration depolarizing potential (resembling excitatory postsynaptic potential) following early spike response evoked by single stimulus in cultured spinal sensory ganglion cells (from 9-day chick embryo; 1 month *in vitro*). (**A₁,B₁**): Intracellular recordings from cells in two different cultures. Note second spike which occurs during rising phase of this depolarizing potential (**A₂₋₄, B₂**). (**A₃**): Similar response to that in **A₂**, but superimposed on a control record obtained by reversing the polarity of the stimulating electrodes. (**B₂**): Similar response to that in **B₁**, but superimposed on a repetitive response similar to **A₂**. Note increased amplitude of postspike depolarization following the latter response. The stimulating electrodes were located 200 to 300 μm from the impaled perikaryon. (A 1-msec calibrating square pulse follows the spike in records **A₁₋₃**.) (From Crain, 1971.)

studies of spinal ganglia *in situ* (Andres, 1961; Tennyson, 1970) and *in vitro* (Bunge et al., 1967), light-microscopic evidence has demonstrated that recurrent collaterals from ganglion cells axons often *appear* to fuse with their *own* perikarya in normal sensory ganglia, *in situ* (i.e., *Paraphytenbildung* or *Fensterapparat:* Scharf, 1958). The bioelectric discharge patterns of cultured sensory ganglion cells described above suggest, then, that these recurrent collaterals may be functionally significant and, under certain conditions, may lead to excitatory axosomatic synaptic feedback within individual neurons of this type. Alternatively, functional synapses may form *between* DRG neurons under certain conditions *in vitro,* as suggested by intracellular microelectrode analyses in cultures of dissociated chick DRG cells (Fischbach and Dichter, 1974; Peacock et al., 1973). Contamination of DRG cultures by sympathetic ganglion cells could provide still another source of synaptic junctions in all of these experiments.

ENHANCED AFFERENT SYNAPTIC FUNCTIONS IN SPINAL CORD-GANGLION EXPLANTS FOLLOWING NGF-INDUCED DRG HYPERTROPHY

Cytologic Aspects

The next stage in our studies of DRG neurons in culture involved explantation of fetal rodent spinal cord cross sections (0.5–1 mm thick) with attached pairs of DRGs. These tissues were grown on collagen-coated coverglasses in Maximow depression slide chambers. The nutrient medium included 33% human placental serum, 53% Eagle's minimum essential medium, 10% chick embryo extract, and 600 mg% glucose (Crain and Peterson, 1963, 1964; Peterson et al., 1965). The cultures were incubated at 34° to 35°C in lying-drop position. Twice a week they were washed in Simms' balanced salt solution (BSS) and fed a drop of nutrient fluid. Initial electrophysiologic studies of 14-day fetal rodent cord-DRG explants demonstrated that synaptically mediated cord responses could be evoked by DRG stimuli within the first week after explantation of these "presynaptic" embryonic tissues (Crain and Peterson, 1967). Although some DRG-evoked cord networks could be maintained for months in culture, we were concerned that a substantial fraction (up to 90%) of the DRG neurons in 13- to 14-day fetal rodent cord-ganglion explants atrophied or degenerated during the first few days in our control culture medium (Fig. 4A versus B). Addition of nerve growth factor at explantation, in concentrations ranging from 10^{-8} to 10^{-5} g/ml (i.e., 1 to 1,000 biologic units/ml) led to a higher survival rate of DRG neurons (Crain and Peterson, 1974a), in addition to the characteristic dose-dependent enhancement of neuritic outgrowth (Levi-Montalcini, 1958; Levi-Montalcini and Angeletti, 1968). Vastly increased neuronal survival occurred in higher concentrations of NGF (100 to 1,000 units/ml) concomitant with more abundant neuritic outgrowths from the DRG cells, as in cultures of NGF-"hypertrophied" mouse sympathetic ganglia (Crain et al., 1964). These *in vitro* effects resembled the remarkable selective hypertrophy of sensory dorsal root ganglia and sympathetic ganglia in 7- to 10-day chick embryos *in vivo* within 3 to 4 days after daily injection of μg quantities of NGF (Levi-Montalcini, 1958). At the higher NGF levels, massive DRGs containing many hundreds of neuron perikarya developed during the first week *in vitro* and often remained densely packed in close proximity to the spinal cord tissue (Fig. 4C). This is in sharp contrast to the sparse, irregular array of several dozen DRG neuron perikarya (rarely more than 100) in control cultures (Fig. 4B) which generally "migrate" about 0.5 to 1 mm away from the cord (Peterson et al., 1965), retaining characteristic dorsal root connections (Crain and Peterson, 1974b; Peterson and Crain, 1972). The NGF-stimulated DRG neurons continued to mature during the following weeks in culture even though no additional NGF was introduced beyond that included in the medium at explantation. Some of the DRGs actually became comparable in volume to their associated spinal cord segment (see Figs. 4A and C). Examination of the living cultures, at high magnification, indicate that the enlarged DRGs were composed of many layers of healthy neuron perikarya, and normal neuronal and supporting cell morphology has been observed in preliminary histologic analyses at the light- and electron-microscope level (Peterson et al., 1974; and *in preparation*).

These experiments are consonant with the earlier demonstrations that NGF is necessary for the survival and development of dissociated sensory

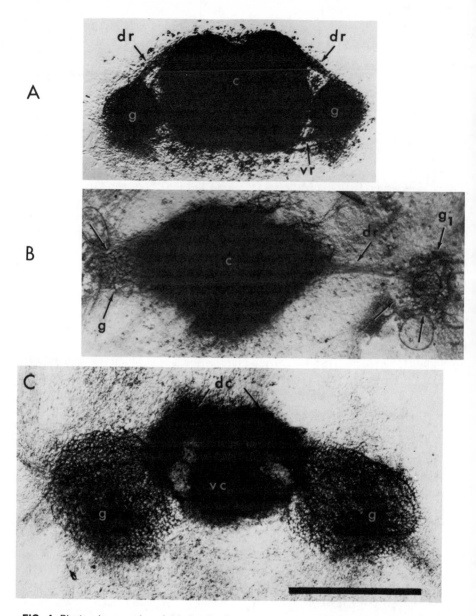

FIG. 4. Photomicrographs of 14-day fetal mouse spinal cord explants (cross sections) with attached dorsal root ganglia (DRG); living unstained cultures. **A:** Shortly after explantation (1 day *in vitro*). Note size of DRGs (g) relative to cord tissue (c); also dorsal and ventral roots (dr, vr). **B:** One month in normal culture medium. Many of the ganglion cells degenerated during the first few days *in vitro*, leaving a relatively small (thin) array of DRG neurons (g) which have matured and retained characteristic (myelinated) dorsal root (dr) connections to the cord (see also comparable cultures after 2 to 6 months *in vitro;* Crain and Peterson, 1974b: Figs. 5 and 8). Note that both DRGs are of similar size, although only one DRG (g₁) shows the characteristic "migration" away from the cord. Most

ganglion cells in culture (Levi-Montalcini and Angeletti, 1963; Varon et al., 1973). Our present data show moreover that NGF may play an essential role, at least at a critical developmental stage, in determining the survival of fetal rodent sensory ganglion cells, even when they remain within an organized ganglion, in close association with the normal array of supporting cells. Most of the NGF-stimulated DRG cells can then mature and be maintained for months in culture. Further controls will be required to clarify the degree to which the NGF-enlarged DRG represent a real hypertrophy or simply a closer approximation to their *in situ* counterparts. In addition to NGF-induced DRG "hypertrophy," the dorsal regions of the associated spinal cord segment appeared to develop unusual enlargements which became increasingly prominent. Preliminary observations indicate that these dorsal cord regions contain far more abundant arrays of densely packed axons which, as they become myelinated during the second and third weeks *in vitro,* can be traced to, and appear in continuity with, the entering dorsal roots of the ganglion (Fig. 4C).

Electrophysiologic Aspects

Correlative electrophysiologic experiments have been carried out on these fetal mouse cord-DRG explants to determine whether the NGF-stimulated growth and development of DRG neurons leads to enhancement of organized synaptic relationships with spinal cord neurons or whether the additional neuritic bundles and arborizations are merely unregulated growth processes leading to "dead ends" or to aberrant functional connections (as occurs in some types of NGF-stimulated sympathetic ganglion cells *in situ,* e.g., Olson, 1967).

Extracellular recordings were made with Ag–AgCl electrodes via micropipettes (3 to 5 μm tips) filled with isotonic saline, using high input impedance preamplifiers and a 4-channel oscilloscope (passband from 0.2 Hz to 10 kHz). An Ag–AgCl wire in the periphery of the bath served as a grounded reference electrode. Electric stimuli (0.1 to 0.5 msec) were applied through pairs of similar pipettes with 10 μm tips, and stimulating currents ranged up to 50 μA. The culture coverglass was transferred from the Maximow slide to a larger closed chamber that was mounted on an inverted

---

of the other control cultures showed even lower survival of DRG neurons (see text). **C:** Another cord-DRG explant after 1 month in same culture medium, but NGF was added at explantation (1,000 BU/ml). Note remarkable enlargement of DRGs (g) relative to initial size at explantation **(A)** and in contrast to control culture. **B:** Many hundreds of ganglion cells form densely packed clusters close to the cord. (Major DRG volume increase has been reached by second week *in vitro*.) Relatively dense appearance of dorsal cord (dc) is due to large numbers of myelinated axons which represent central branches of DRG neurons (see text). Dense region in ventromedial cord (vc) is due primarily to a "necrotic core" which generally develops in both treated and control explants. Scale **(A–C):** 1 mm. (From Crain and Peterson, 1974a).

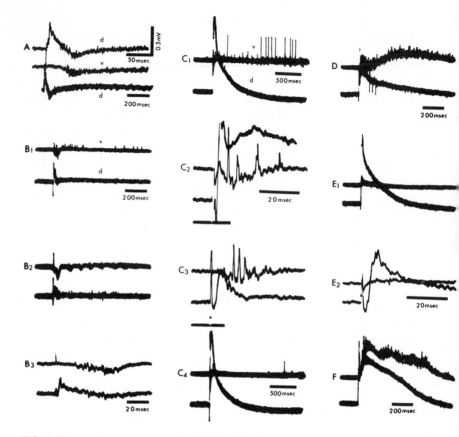

FIG. 5. Enhanced responses evoked in dorsal regions of fetal mouse spinal cord explants by stimuli applied to NGF-hypertrophied DRG. **A:** Control culture, 4 weeks *in vitro* (see Fig. 4B). Early-latency negative slow-wave potential (resembling "PAD"—see text) is evoked in dorsal cord (d) by single DRG stimulus (via focal 10 μm tip electrode), and is followed by a positive slow-wave concomitant with a high-frequency spike barrage (dorsal cord response is shown at slower sweep rate on lowest record). Ventral cord response (v) begins after longer latency and involves primarily a positive slow-wave and spike barrage. **B₁:** Smaller PAD elicited in dorsal cord (d) of another control explant (2 weeks *in vitro*); ventral cord response (v) again consists of a primary positive slow-wave and a repetitive spike barrage. **B₂,₃:** After introduction of strychnine (10^{-6} M), ventral cord discharge becomes larger and more complex, but PAD is relatively unchanged, although it is now followed by long-lasting spike barrage. At faster sweep rate (**B₃**), PAD is seen to begin shortly after DRG stimulus, whereas ventral cord response shows longer latency (as in **A**). **C₁:** Similar explant, 2 weeks *in vitro*, but NGF added at explantation (1,000 BU/ml). PAD-like potential evoked in dorsal cord (d) by single stimulus to NGF-hypertrophied DRG (see Fig. 4C) is much larger in amplitude and longer in duration (cf. **A** and **B₁**), whereas ventral cord response (v) is similar to control pattern. **C₂:** Early latency, sharp rising phase, and complexity of PAD response are seen at faster sweep rate. **C₃:** Tenfold reduction of DRG stimulus intensity evoked smaller but still prominent PAD and ventral cord discharge now begins after longer latency, during falling phase of PAD (as in **A** and **B₃**). **C₄:** Larger DRG stimulus (as in **C₁**) again elicits characteristic large PAD just before drug application. **D:** Introduction of bicuculline (10^{-5} M) leads to marked decrease in amplitude of PAD concomitant with onset of convulsive negative slow-wave and repetitive-

microscope (Crain, 1973, 1976). Microelectrodes were positioned in the tissue with micromanipulators and recordings were made in 0.5 ml of BSS (pH about 7.2; temperature, 35°).

In control cultures, application of a focal stimulus close to the DRG or dorsal root (via a 10 μm electrode) often evokes a small negative slow-wave potential in the dorsal regions of the spinal cord, with a rapid rising phase and a slower falling phase (Fig. 5A and B). The amplitude and duration of this potential are quite variable, ranging up to about 0.5 mV and 100 msec, depending upon the stimulus intensity, geometry of the cellular array, and proximity of the stimulating and recording electrodes to the excitable neuronal elements. This negative slow-wave response appears after a latency of 2 to 3 msec when the stimulus is applied to the DRG perikarya or to the dorsal root (Fig. 5A and B_3). [No clear-cut evidence of these dorsal cord potentials was obtained in our earlier studies of 14-day fetal rat cord-DRG explants during development in normal media (Crain and Peterson, 1967).] Simultaneous recordings in the ventral regions of the spinal cord segment generally show longer-latency (>5 to 10 msec) responses, often including a positive slow-wave potential (ca. 100 msec) and a spike barrage of variable complexity (Fig. 5A and B).

Application of similar stimuli to NGF-hypertrophied DRGs evoked comparable negative slow-wave responses in the dorsal cord, with similar latency and sharp rising phase, but the amplitude and duration were now remarkably larger (Fig. 5C). The cord potentials often reached 2 mV in response to a single large DRG stimulus, and a prominent negative slow wave could be evoked even after 10-fold reduction in stimulus strength to these low-threshold neurons (Fig. $5C_3$ and E_2). Furthermore, the duration of the DRG-triggered dorsal cord responses was often more than 500 msec (Fig. 5C), far longer-lasting than generally observed in control cultures. Single stimuli applied to peripheral branches of NGF-stimulated DRG cells, as much as 2 to 3 mm beyond the explant zone, were also effective, and elicited responses comparable to those in Fig. $5C_3$ and E_2, but with longer latencies (ca. 5 to 10 msec).

The temporal patterns of the dorsal cord potentials evoked by stimula-

---

spike discharge in ventral cord (v). E_1: After transfer to 10^{-3} M GABA, large PAD response is restored (see C_4) in contrast to almost complete block of ventral cord discharge. E_2: Tenfold reduction of DRG stimulus intensity still evokes relatively large PAD (see C_3, in BSS). F: Return to bicuculline (10^{-5} M) leads to partial depression of PAD and appearance of secondary longer-lasting negative slow-wave in dorsal cord, concomitant with onset of huge negative slow-wave and oscillatory discharge in ventral cord. Note: In this and subsequent figures, time and amplitude calibrations and specification of recording and stimulating sites apply to all succeeding records, until otherwise noted; in these extracellular recordings, upward deflection indicates negativity at focal electrode, and onset of stimuli is indicated by first sharp pulse or break in baseline of each sweep (third sweep in records $C_{2,3}$ shows stimulus signal directly). Unless otherwise specified, all recordings were made in Simms' balanced salt solution (BSS). (From Crain and Peterson, 1974a).

tion of NGF-hypertrophied DRGs *in vitro* contain components that are remarkably similar to those characteristic of the primary afferent depolarization (PAD) response in mammalian spinal cord *in situ* (Eccles, 1964). The PAD-like component recorded with extracellular microelectrodes in the cord explants appears to be a field potential produced by summated EPSPs generated following DRG activation of dorsal cord circuits (see below). The weak PAD-like response generally observed with focal DRG stimulation in control cultures may be due partly to the lower density of excitable DRG neurons developing in the absence of added NGF, and also to less extensive (or less effective) synaptic connections of each DRG cell with cord neurons. In contrast to the dramatic enhancement of the "PAD" potentials in the dorsal cord of NGF-treated explants no substantial alterations in the response patterns of *ventral* cord regions have been observed (see Fig. 5A and C).

Marked temporal facilitation of PAD responses in explants occurs following brief application of 100/sec DRG volleys, at low stimulus strength, resembling characteristic facilitation of PADs evoked by repetitive afferent stimuli *in situ* (Eccles, 1964). Furthermore, whereas strychnine showed relatively little effect on PAD potentials in dorsal cord [even at concentrations (ca. 10^{-5} M) which greatly enhanced complex long-latency spike-barrage and slow-wave discharges in both dorsal and ventral cord (see Fig. 5B$_2$ versus B$_1$)], bicuculline and picrotoxin (10^{-5} M) produced marked attenuation of the PADs concomitant with onset of convulsive discharges, especially in ventral cord regions (Fig. 5D and F). On the other hand, after introduction of 10^{-3} M GABA into the culture bath the PAD responses in dorsal cord were generally maintained or even *augmented* (Fig. 5E), in contrast to the rapid and sustained depression of almost all detectable synaptically mediated discharges in ventral cord regions as well as long-latency discharges in dorsal cord (Fig. 5E). GABA-enhancement of PADs occurred in control as well as in NGF-treated cord explants and was especially marked during brief 100/sec DRG volleys. Generation of the PADs by Ca^{2+}-dependent, synaptic transmitter release is suggested by the rapid and complete block of PAD potentials after increasing the Mg^{2+} concentration from 1 to 10 mM, whereas spikes could still be directly evoked (Crain, 1974a, 1975, 1976).

Although the PADs recorded in our explants probably include field potentials due to summated EPSPs in dorsal cord interneurons triggered by DRG collaterals, the marked selective attenuation of these responses in bicuculline and picrotoxin suggests that a major component is generated by GABA-mediated EPSPs, possible at DRG terminals as *in situ* (Barker and Nicoll, 1973; Benoist et al., 1974; Davidoff, 1972). (Attempts are being made to obtain more direct evidence for this interpretation by selective recordings from dorsal root fibers during generation of these PAD potentials in dorsal cord regions of the explants.) Depolarization of DRG terminals (by these GABA interneurons triggered by DRG collaterals) presumably decreases both the amplitude of the presynaptic action potential and quantity of transmitter released, and this presynaptic inhibition provides a potent regulatory mechanism which depresses the central excitatory actions of many primary afferent fibers in the mammalian CNS (Eccles, 1964; Wall, 1964; see Curtis et al., 1971). Analyses of dorsal and ventral cord responses to selective single and paired stimuli applied to various neural elements in these cord-DRG explants provide additional evidence that the observed PADs are associated with inhibitory mechanisms (Crain, in preparation). The longer-latency negative slow-wave and oscillatory potentials elicited by DRG stimuli in bicuculline probably represent summated postsynaptic potentials synchronously and sequentially activated after interference with GABA-mediated IPSPs of cord neurons involved in these complex network responses (Crain, 1974a, 1975; Crain and Bornstein, 1974; Zipser et al., 1973). Introduction of 10^{-3} M GABA, on the other hand, may block convulsive network discharges by enhancing GABA-mediated IPSPs of cord neurons as well as GABA-mediated EPSPs (or other depolarization) of DRG terminals.

This study demonstrates, for the first time, that at least some of the abundant additional neurites which develop after exposure of fetal DRG cells to NGF can proceed to make characteristic longterm synaptic relationships with *specific* types of spinal cord neurons. The data also indicate that responses resembling "primary afferent depolarization" can be generated in organized spinal cord-DRG explants with remarkable mimicry of these specialized synaptic network functions *in situ*. Moreover, if further analyses of the greatly enhanced PAD-like potentials in spinal cord explants in response to the unusually large input from NGF-hypertrophied DRGs do, indeed, demonstrate their relationship to presynaptic inhibitory functions, this may be evidence of an intrinsic CNS regulatory system, involving development of compensatory (homeostatic) inhibitory circuits proportional to the magnitude of the excitatory synaptic input (Crain, 1974b, 1976).

DEVELOPMENT OF SPECIFIC SENSORY-EVOKED SYNAPTIC NETWORKS IN MEDULLA EXPLANTS AFTER INNERVATION BY "DORSAL COLUMN" FIBERS

After showing that DRG neurons could establish characteristic functional synaptic networks in dorsal regions of cord explants, we proceeded to prepare model systems suitable for analyzing further development of central DRG neurites up the neuraxis. Our earlier electrophysiologic studies showed that complex synaptic interactions can, indeed, develop between neurons in explants of fetal rodent spinal cord and brainstem tissues after growth of neurites across gaps of 0.5 to 1 mm, but no signs of

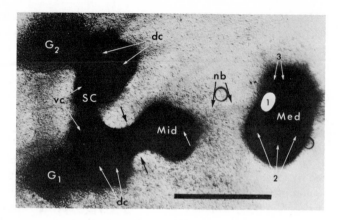

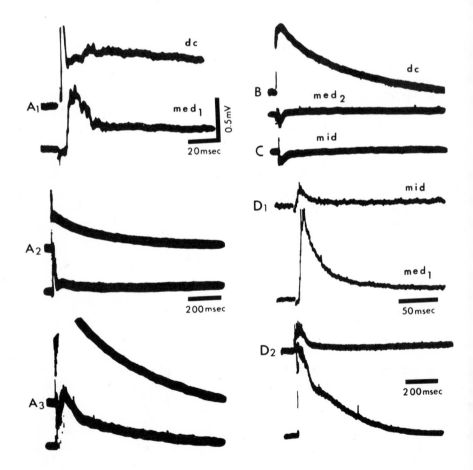

selective synaptic connections between *specific* types of neurons were detected (Crain et al., 1968; Crain and Bornstein, 1972; Crain, 1974b, 1976). Prior to explantation of fetal cord-DRG explants (Fig. 4A), a midline section of the spinal cord cross section was made from the central canal through the dorsal cord and meninges; in the younger fetuses only the meninges required cutting since dorsal closure of the cord was not yet completed. This ensured outgrowth of CNS neurites and glial cells, including DRG fibers which have passed through the cord, comparable to dorsal column axons. Previous studies showed that "peripheral-type" neurites (invested by Schwann cells) will not invade separate CNS explants (Peterson et al., 1965; Bunge and Wood, 1973). Fetal mouse brainstem explants were carefully positioned near the dorsal edge of the cord cross sections (Fig. 6; Crain and Peterson, 1975). Tissues from various regions of the medulla and midbrain were presented to the cord explant, including complete cross sections through the medulla at the level of the cuneate and gracilis nuclei (Fig. 7).

PAD-like potentials similar to those evoked in dorsal cord explants have now been detected in small regions of medulla explants connected to cord with NGF-hypertrophied DRGs. The medulla PADs evoked by single DRG stimuli ranged up to 1 mV and arose after longer (ca. 3 to 10 msec) latencies (Figs. 6,7). The large amplitude of these PADs indicates that relatively large numbers of DRG terminals probably make synaptic connections with "target" neurons in the medulla explants. In cord-DRG cultures without added NGF, where only a few dozen neurons may survive (Fig. 4B), dorsal cord PADs were often much smaller than these medulla PADs, in spite of the abundant dorsal cord neurons available for establishing sensory

---

FIG. 6. Negative slow-wave potentials resembling PADs evoked in spinal cord and brainstem explants by DRG stimuli (14-day fetal mouse tissues; 14 days in culture). Photomicrograph shows spinal cord cross section (SC) with attached dorsal-root ganglia ($G_{1,2}$); dorsal edge of one-half of cord is "fused" to midbrain (Mid) explant (*black arrows*); thinly spread array of neurites and glial cells have formed a bridge (nb) to the medulla (Med) explant (barely visible at this low magnification). Midline section of dorsal cord (see text) resulted in lateral displacement of dorsal horns and DRGs at either end of ventral cord (vc). Scale 1 mm. A_1: Simultaneous recordings of PADs in dorsal cord (dc: *lower left arrow*) and medulla (Med: site 1) in response to single DRG stimulus (G_1). Note abrupt onset and long duration of these potentials; also longer latency of medulla response. A_2: Same at slower sweep rate. A_3: Brief 100/sec DRG volley (at smaller, near-threshold stimulus strength) elicits much larger and longer-lasting PADs in both cord and medulla. **B**: Large DRG_1 stimulus evoked only small positive slow-wave responses in other regions of medulla explant (Med_2); dorsal cord PAD is still large. Microelectrode mapping showed no signs of medulla PADs in response to DRG stimuli, except in zone indicated in white around site 1, and none in entire midbrain (Mid) explant (e.g., at *white arrow:* record **C**). D_1: After adding 10^{-3} M GABA, PAD in medulla (Med_1) shows marked increase in amplitude and duration (as in Fig. 7B), and it can now also be evoked in adjacent region "3"; polarity of midbrain response (Mid) has now become negative, though still relatively small. D_2: Brief 100/sec DRG volley elicits still larger and longer-lasting PAD in medulla "target zone" (Med_1). (From Crain and Peterson, 1975.)

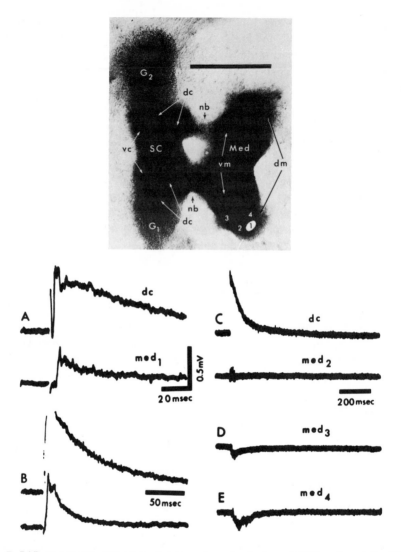

FIG. 7. PAD responses evoked in dorsal region of spinal cord (SC) and medulla (Med) explants (complete cross sections) by DRG stimuli (14-day fetal mouse tissues; 14 days in culture). Medulla cross section is at level of cuneate and gracilis nuclei [dorsal closure has not yet occurred at this fetal stage so that the dorsal medulla tissues (dm) are laterally displaced]. Note bridges (neurites and glia) that have formed between dorsal edge of cord (dc) and ventral edge of medulla (vm) explants in two regions (nb); DRGs ($G_{1,2}$) are located more laterally in this explant (see Fig. 6), further away from ventral cord (vc). Scale: 1 mm. **A:** Simultaneous recordings of PADs in dorsal cord (dc: *lower left arrow*) and dorsal medulla (Med: site 1) in response to single DRG_1 stimulus. **B:** After adding 10^{-3} M GABA, PADs at this site in medulla (Med_1) and in dorsal cord are augmented (as in Fig. 6D). **C:** Large DRG_1 stimulus evokes only spike burst at site 2 in medulla (Med_2) and small positive slow-wave responses at $Med_{3,4}$ **D,E:** Systematic mapping of entire medulla explant showed no signs of PADs in response to DRG stimuli except in small zone indicated in white around Med_1 (ca. 0.1 × 0.2 mm), even during GABA exposure. (Mapping was not attempted in this culture with stimuli to DRG_2.) (From Crain and Peterson, 1975.)

synaptic networks with ingrowing DRG neurites (Crain and Peterson, 1974a, 1975). Introduction of 10^{-3} M GABA generally augmented the brainstem and dorsal cord PADs (Figs. 6D and 7B), whereas various cord-evoked brainstem network discharges were seriously depressed, as were ventral cord responses. Moreover, in cases where a midbrain explant was positioned between the cord and medulla, prominent DRG-evoked PADs were detected only in the latter explant, even when it was located more than 1 mm distal to the interposed midbrain tissue (Fig. 6A). Weak PADs could, however, be detected in some midbrain regions, especially when medulla target neurons were relatively distant (Fig. 6C and D) or absent. By use of this "pharmacologic marker" technique, we have been able to carefully map more than 12 DRG-cord-brainstem cultures, and in most cases PADs were sharply localized to one or two small zones (ca. 100 to 300 μm) in each medulla explant. In six cultures where cross sections of the entire medulla at the level of the cuneate and gracilis nuclei were presented to the DRG-cord explant, with controlled orientation, prominent PADs were evoked only in the *dorsal* medulla regions (Fig. 7), precisely where dorsal column sensory fibers normally terminate and lead to PADs *in situ* (Eccles, 1964; Wall, 1964; Andersen et al., 1964a,b; Davidson and Southwick, 1971). Similar results were obtained in cultures where the medulla cross section was rotated 90° to 180° with respect to its orientation to the cord explant in Fig. 7 (Crain, 1976).

These *in vitro* experiments demonstrate that DRG neurites, after passing through spinal cord tissue, can grow across a homogeneous collagen-film substrate and, in mimicry of dorsal column fibers *in situ,* established characteristic functional synaptic networks with programmed target neurons in brainstem explants, even in the presence of a variety of alternative CNS neurons with abundant synaptogenic receptor sites (see also Olson and Bunge, 1973). Furthermore, although the initial neuritic and glial spinal cord outgrowth in relation to these nearby medulla explants was comparable to that extending towards nontarget CNS tissues, preliminary analyses in suitably arrayed cultures suggest that prominent fascicles of "dorsal column fibers" may become organized towards the target neuron zones in the medulla (Crain and Peterson, 1975, and in preparation; Crain, 1976). The remarkable degree of characteristic pharmacologic sensitivity and regional specificity of these sensory-evoked spinal cord and brainstem networks provides the basis for a powerful new model system to analyze mechanisms underlying formation and development of specific synaptic connections in the mammalian CNS (Sperry, 1965) which are now accessible for more direct studies under rigidly controlled physicochemical conditions in culture.

CONCLUDING REMARKS

Electrophysiologic studies of neural tissue cultures have thus developed from the "pipedream stage" in 1950 to a well-established experimental method which has recently begun to be utilized in many laboratories throughout the world. Our initial bioelectric experiments with cultured DRG neurons at Columbia have led to the development of a powerful model system for correlative cytologic and physiologic studies of the central as well as peripheral nervous system. As fetal CNS and PNS explants are analyzed more intensively, it becomes increasingly clear that the organotypic functional properties of these isolated tissues can develop *in vitro* with remarkable mimicry of their *in situ* counterparts. Chemical specificities and regional specializations of complex synaptic networks develop under well-ordered "self-organizing" programs *in vitro* (Crain, 1974*b*, 1976). CNS culture models should provide valuable systems for further analyses of important molecular control mechanisms which regulate development and functional organization of the brain.

ACKNOWLEDGMENTS

This work was supported by research grants from the National Institute of Neurological and Communicative Neurologic Disorders and Stroke (B-945R, while the author was located in the Department of Neurology, College of Physicians and Surgeons, Columbia University; NS-06545 and NS-08770 after transfer to Einstein). This work has also been supported by the Alfred P. Sloan Foundation and a Kennedy Scholar Award to Dr. Crain. The cultures were prepared by Edith R. Peterson in the nerve tissue culture laboratories at the College of Physicians and Surgeons and in the Kennedy Center at Einstein.

Purified NGF (7S form) was kindly provided by Dr. Eric M. Shooter (see Varon et al., 1967), and our assay with DRG cultures (Levi-Montalcini, 1958) indicated a potency of about 1 biologic unit (BU) per 10^{-8} g.

REFERENCES

Andersen, P., Eccles, J. C., Schmidt, R. F., and Yokota, T. (1964*a*): Slow potential waves produced in the cuneate nucleus by cutaneous volleys and by cortical stimulation. *J. Neurophysiol.*, 27:78–91.

Andersen, P., Eccles, J. C., Schmidt, R. F., and Yokota, T. (1964*b*): Depolarization of presynaptic fibres in the cuneate nucleus. *J. Neurophysiol.*, 27:92–106.

Andres, K. H. (1961): Untersuchungen Uber den Feinbau von Spinalganglion. *Z. Zellforsch.*, 55:1–48.

Barker, J. L., and Nicoll, R. A. (1973): The pharmacology and ionic dependency of amino acid responses in the frog spinal cord. *J. Physiol.*, 228:259–278.

Benoist, J. M., Besson, J. M., and Boissier, J. R. (1974): Modifications of presynaptic inhibition of various origins by local application of convulsant drugs on cat's spinal cord. *Brain Res.*, 71:172–177.

Bunge, R. P., and Wood, P. (1973): Studies on the transplantation of spinal cord tissue in the rat. I. The development of a culture system for hemisections of embryonic spinal cord. *Brain Res.*, 57:261–276.

Bunge, M. B., Bunge, R. P., Peterson, E. R., and Murray, M. R. (1967): A light and electron microscope study of long-term organized cultures of rat dorsal root ganglia. *J. Cell Biol.*, 32:439–466.

Crain, S. M. (1954a): Electrical activity in tissue cultures of chick embryo spinal ganglia. Univ. Microfilms, Ann Arbor, No. 10,785. Ph.D. thesis.

Crain, S. M. (1954b): Action potentials in tissue cultures of chick embryo spinal ganglia. *Anat. Rec.*, 118:292.

Crain, S. M. (1956): Resting and action potentials of cultured chick embryo spinal ganglion cells. *J. Comp. Neurol.*, 104:285–330.

Crain, S. M. (1965): Nervous and muscle tissues *in vitro:* Electrophysiological properties. In: *Cells and Tissues in Culture*, Vol. 2., edited by E. N. Willmer, pp. 335–339, 344–347, 422–431. Academic Press, New York.

Crain, S. M. (1971): Intracellular recordings suggesting synaptic functions in chick embryo spinal sensory ganglion cells isolated *in vitro*. *Brain Res.*, 26:188–191.

Crain, S. M. (1973): Microelectrode recording in brain tissue cultures. In: *Methods in Physiological Psychology*, Vol. 1, *Bioelectric Recording Techniques: Cellular Processes and Brain Potentials*, edited by R. F. Thompson and M. M. Patterson, pp. 39–75. Academic Press, New York.

Crain, S. M. (1974a): Selective depression of organotypic bioelectric activities of CNS tissue cultures by pharmacologic and metabolic agents. In: *Drugs and the Developing Brain*, edited by A. Vernadakis and N. Weiner, pp. 29–57. Plenum Press, New York.

Crain, S. M. (1974b): Tissue culture models of developing brain functions. In: *Studies on the Development of Behavior and the Nervous System*, Vol. 2, *Aspects of Neurogenesis*, edited by G. Gottlieb, pp. 69–114. Academic Press, New York.

Crain, S. M. (1975): Development of complex synaptic functions in 'simple' neuronal arrays in culture. In: *'Simple' Nervous Systems*, edited by P. N. R. Usherwood and D. R. Newth, pp. 67–117. Edward Arnold Ltd., England.

Crain, S. M. (1976): *Neurophysiologic Studies in Tissue Culture*. Raven Press, New York.

Crain, S. M., and Bornstein, M. B. (1972): Organotypic bioelectric activity in cultured reaggregates of dissociated rodent brain cells. *Science*, 176:182–184.

Crain, S. M., and Bornstein, M. B. (1974): Early onset in inhibitory functions during synaptogenesis in fetal mouse brain cultures. *Brain Res.*, 68:351–357.

Crain, S. M., and Peterson, E. R. (1963): Bioelectric activity in long-term cultures of spinal cord tissues. *Science*, 141:427–429.

Crain, S. M., and Peterson, E. R. (1964): Complex bioelectric activity in organized tissue cultures of spinal cord (human, rat and chick). *J. Cell. Comp. Physiol.*, 64:1–15.

Crain, S. M., and Peterson, E. R. (1967): Onset and development of functional interneuronal connections in explants of rat spinal cord-ganglia during maturation in culture. *Brain Res.*, 6:750–762.

Crain, S. M., and Peterson, E. R. (1974a): Enhanced afferent synaptic functions in fetal mouse spinal cord-sensory ganglion explants following NGF-induced ganglion hypertrophy. *Brain Res.*, 79:145–152.

Crain, S. M., and Peterson, E. R. (1974b): Development of neural connections in culture. *Ann. NY Acad. Sci.*, 228:6–34.

Crain, S. M., and Peterson, E. R. (1975): Development of specific sensory-evoked synaptic networks in fetal mouse cord-brainstem cultures. *Science*, 188:275–278.

Crain, S. M., Benitez, H., and Vatter, A. E. (1964): Some cytologic effects of salivary nerve-growth factor on tissue cultures of peripheral ganglia. *Ann. NY Acad. Sci.*, 118:206–231.

Crain, S. M., Peterson, E. R., and Bornstein, M. B. (1968): Formation of functional interneuronal connections between explants of various mammalian central nervous tissues during development *in vitro*. In: *Ciba Foundation Symposium, Growth of the Nervous System*, edited by G. E. W. Wolstenholme and M. O'Connor, pp. 13–31. Churchill, London.

Crain, S. M., Grundfest, H., Mettler, F. A., and Flint, T. (1953): Electrical activity from tissue cultures of chick embryo spinal ganglia. *Trans. Am. Neurol. Assoc.*, 78:236–239.

Curtis, D. R., Duggan, A. W., Felix, D., and Johnston, G. A. R. (1971): Bicuculline, an antagonist of GABA and synaptic inhibition in the spinal cord of the cat. *Brain Res.* 32:69–96.

Davidoff, R. A. (1972): The effects of bicuculline on the isolated spinal cord of the frog. *Exp. Neurol.*, 35:179–193.

Davidson, N., and Southwick, C. A. P. (1971): Amino acids and presynaptic inhibition in the rat cuneate nucleus. *J. Physiol.*, 219:689–708.

Eccles, J. C. (1964): *The Physiology of Synapses*. Springer-Verlag, Berlin.

Fischbach, G. D., and Dichter, M. A. (1974): Electrophysiologic and morphologic properties of neurons in dissociated chick spinal cord cell cultures. *Develop. Biol.*, 37:100–116.

Hild, W., and Tasaki, I. (1962): Morphological and physiological properties of neurons and glial cells in tissue culture. *J. Neurophysiol.*, 25:277–304.

Levi, G., and Meyer, H. (1938): Présentation de cultures d'un nombre restreint d'éléments nerveux avec quelques considerations sur les rapports d'interdépendence entre les neurones. *C.R. Assoc. Anat.*, 33:312–328.

Levi-Montalcini, R. (1958): Chemical stimulation of nerve growth. In: *Symposium on the Chemical Basis of Development*, edited by W. D. McElroy and B. Glass, pp. 646–664. Johns Hopkins Press, Baltimore, Md.

Levi-Montalcini, R., and Angeletti, P. U. (1963): Essential role of the nerve growth factor in the survival and maintenance of dissociated sensory and sympathetic embryonic nerve cells *in vitro. Develop. Biol.*, 7:653–659.

Levi-Montalcini, R., and Angeletti, P. U. (1968): Biological aspects of the nerve growth factor. In: *Ciba Found. Symposium, Growth of the Nervous System*, edited by G. E. W. Wolstenholme and M. O'Connor, pp. 126–147. Churchill, London.

Miller, R., Varon, S., Kruger, L., Coates, P. W., and Orkand, P. M. (1970): Formation of synaptic contacts on dissociated chick embryo sensory ganglion cells *in vitro. Brain Res.*, 24:356–358.

Nakai, J. (1956): Dissociated dorsal root ganglia in tissue culture. *Am. J. Anat.*, 99:81–130.

Olson, L. (1967): Outgrowth of sympathetic adrenergic neurons in mice treated with a nerve-growth factor (NGF). *Z. Zellforsch.*, 81:155–173.

Olson, M. J., and Bunge, R. P. (1973): Anatomical observations on the specificity of synapse formation in tissue culture. *Brain Res.* 59:19–33.

Peacock, J. H., Nelson, P. G., and Goldstone, M. W. (1973): Electrophysiologic study of cultured neurons dissociated from spinal cords and dorsal root ganglia of fetal mice. *Develop. Biol.* 30:137–152.

Peterson, E. R., and Crain, S. M. (1972): Regeneration and innervation in cultures of adult mammalian skeletal muscle coupled with fetal rodent spinal cord. *Exp. Neurol.* 36:136–159.

Peterson, E. R., and Murray, M. R. (1956): Regeneration and development of sensory neurons in vitro. *Neuropathol. Exptl. Neurol.*, 15:288–292.

Peterson, E. R., Crain, S. M., and Murray, M. R. (1965): Differentiation and prolonged maintenance of bioelectrically active spinal cord cultures (rat, chick and human). *Z. Zellforsch.*, 66:130–154.

Peterson, E. R., Masurovsky, E. B., and Crain, S. M. (1974): Enhanced survival and selective 'hypertrophy' of dorsal root ganglia after exposure of fetal rodent spinal cord-ganglion explants to nerve growth factor. *J. Cell Biol.*, 63:265a.

Scharf, J. H. (1958): Sensible ganglien. In: *Handbuch der Mikroskopischen Anatomie*, edited by W. Bargmann, pp. 336–352. Springer, Berlin.

Scott, B. S., Engelbert, V. E., and Fisher, K. C. (1969): Morphological and electrophysiological characteristics of dissociated chick embryonic spinal ganglion cells in culture. *Exp. Neurol.*, 23:230–248.

Sperry, R. W. (1965): Embryogenesis of behavioral nerve nets. In: *Organogenesis*, edited by R. L. DeHaan and H. Urpsrung, pp. 161–186. Holt, Rinehart, and Winston, New York.

Tennyson, V. M. (1970): The fine structure of the developing nervous system. In: *Developmental Neurobiology*, edited by W. A. Himwich, pp. 47–116. Charles C Thomas, Springfield, Ill.

Varon, S., Nomura, J., and Shooter, E. M. (1967): The isolation of the mouse nerve growth factor protein in a high molecular weight form. *Biochem. J.*, 6:2202–2209.

Varon, S., Raiborn, C., and Tyszka, E. (1973): *In vitro* studies of dissociated cells from newborn mouse dorsal root ganglia. *Brain Res.*, 54:51–63.

Wall, P. D. (1964): Presynaptic control of impulses at the first central synapse in the cutaneous pathway. *Progr. Brain Res.*, 12:92–118.

Zipser, B., Crain, S. M., and Bornstein, M. B. (1973): Directly evoked "paroxysmal" depolarizations of mouse hippocampal neurons in synaptically organized explants in longterm culture. *Brain Res.*, 60:489–495.

Electrobiology of Nerve, Synapse, and Muscle,
edited by J. P. Reuben, D. P. Purpura, M. V. L. Bennett,
and E. R. Kandel. Raven Press, New York © 1976

Higher Olfactory Projections

Fumiaki Motokizawa

*Department of Physiology, Gunma University, School of Medicine, Maebashi,
Gunma, Japan*

In general, sensory afferent impulses generated in a sensory receptor
reach the cerebral cortex after a thalamo-cortical relay. The cortical area is
a final sensory projection and constitutes the primary sensory cortex. However the olfactory system does not obey such a general pattern of sensory
projection; the prepyriform cortex, which is widely called the primary olfactory cortex, does not receive olfactory projections from the thalamus
according to present knowledge, but receives direct afferent fibers from the
olfactory bulb. Moreover, it has not yet been determined whether or not
the prepyriform cortex is a final olfactory cortex. O'Leary (1937) introduced the term "primary olfactory cortex" in the sense that the prepyriform
cortex is the first cortical station in the olfactory pathway. Cajal (1955)
notes that the prepyriform cortex and some other areas adjacent to it
represent a cortical center of olfactory sensation. According to Lorente de
Nó (1949), it is not cortex but a subcortical center comparable to the
geniculate bodies, etc. Without regard to this problem, tertiary or higher-
order olfactory projections have rarely been the subject of experimental
analysis. This chapter is primarily a summary of results obtained in this
laboratory with the electrophysiological technique in studies of determination of the olfactory areas in the subcortex as well as in the neocortex of
cats.

MESENCEPHALIC PROJECTIONS

Much electrophysiological evidence indicates that the brain stem reticular
formation is the site of a remarkable convergence and interaction of het-
erogenous afferent impulses. Excepting the olfactory system, afferents of
almost all sensory modalities project to their relay nuclei in the brainstem
or pass through the brainstem to the primary sensory cortex.

In trigeminally deafferented encéphale isolé cats immobilized with
gallamine triethiodide, an EEG arousal response was elicited by odor
stimulation both in the neocortex and in the hippocampus with occurrence
of the induced waves in the olfactory bulb and the prepyriform cortex
(Motokizawa and Furuya, 1973). Electrical stimulation of the olfactory bulb

also elicited an EEG arousal response as odor stimulation. The difference between responses produced by the two types of olfactory stimulation was in the constancy of reproducibility. In the case of electrical stimulation both intensity and duration of the response were fairly invariable for each stimulation, whereas they were unstable and the EEG became unresponsive to repetitive stimulation over several times in the case of odor stimulation. In a high cerveau isolé preparation, in which the brain stem was transsected at the cephalic border of the mesencephalon, neither odor stimulation nor electrical stimulation of the olfactory bulb converted the resting EEG into an arousal pattern, though an arousal effect of the nonspecific thalamic system remains intact. This indicates that the mesencephalic reticular formation plays an important role in producing EEG arousal to olfactory stimulation.

Such indirect evidence for an olfactory projection to the mesencephalic reticular formation was substantiated by recording unitary discharges and field potentials from the mesencephalon (Motokizawa, 1974a). Out of 167 units isolated from 40 cats, the spontaneous activity of 97 units (58%) were clearly influenced by odor stimulation, but 70 units (42%) were unresponsive. The response type was mainly a prolonged acceleration or a reduction of the firing rate. [Percentages being 66% (64 units) and 34% (33 units), respectively.] The olfactory response of reticular units was induced almost equally from any part of the nostrils. There were no apparent differences in the responsiveness to acetic acid, amyl acetate, clove oil, and xylene. Figure 1 shows sample records in which two pairs of odor substances were examined in two different neurons, respectively. Both responsive and unresponsive units were distributed widely in the mesencephalic reticular formation and the central grey matter, i.e., there were no preferential localizations of any particular type of responsive unit. Electrical stimulation of the olfactory bulb also modified unit reticular activities, and evoked field mass potentials from the mesencephalic reticular formation. Three types of olfactory responses, as described above, were all abolished by lesion of the medial forebrain bundle.

From these results, it is likely that olfactory impulses are equal to those of other sensory modalities in driving the ascending and descending actions of the reticular formation. It is not likely, however, that olfactory impulses project to the mesencephalic reticular formation in accordance with the general route of the sensory projection to it. Because the medial forebrain bundle receives many and diverse inputs (Millhouse, 1969) it may not be involved in the specific olfactory pathway.

THALAMIC PROJECTIONS

An anatomical study shows that the amygdaloid complex, a part of which receives centripetal fibers from the olfactory bulb, connects with the thalamus in cats (Valverde, 1963).

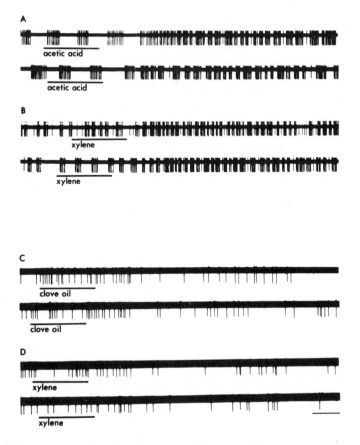

FIG. 1. Olfactory responses of reticular units. Upper and lower traces in each set of records show reticular unit responses to odor introduced into ipsilateral and contralateral nostrils. Odors were presented alternately into bilateral nostrils at intervals of 10 min. **A** and **B:** Same unit and increase in firing rate equally to acetic acid and xylene. **C** and **D:** Same unit and decrease to clove oil and xylene. Downward deflection, positive. Time mark: 0.5 sec.

In our experiment the olfactory input to the thalamus was studied electrophysiologically in low cerveau isolé cats (Motokizawa, 1974*b*). This preparation is especially useful in experiments on olfactory functions of the central nervous system because an involvement of the trigeminal system in olfactory responses to odor stimuli is excluded by the decerebration. The distribution of field potentials evoked by electrical stimulation of the olfactory bulb was examined throughout the thalamus with stereotaxically oriented macroelectrodes. When the thalamus was explored monopolarly, a reference electrode being placed on the temporal muscle, the field potentials could be recorded from the whole thalamus. The shape, polarity and amplitude of these potentials were quite uniform (Fig. 2A and D). With

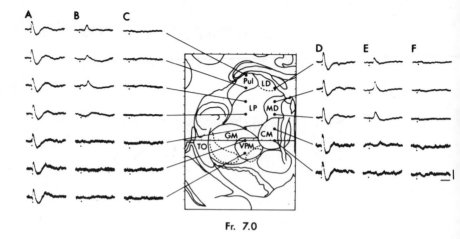

Fr. 7.0

amyl acetate

FIG. 2. Olfactory responses in the thalamus. **A–F:** Example of distribution of field potentials to olfactory bulb shock at +7 mm in the frontal plane. Calibration: 100 µV, 50 msec. CM, n. centrum medianum; GM, corpus geniculatum laterale; LD, n. lateralis dorsalis; LP, n. lateralis posterior; MD, n. medialis dorsalis; Pul, pulvinar; TO, tractus opticus; VPM, n. ventralis postero-medialis. **G:** Unit response to amyl acetate. Downward deflection, positive. Time scale: 1 sec.

bipolar recording the thalamic areas responsive to olfactory stimuli were highly restricted to the dorsomedial, dorsolateral, and posterolateral nuclei and the pulvinar (Fig. 2B and E). The problem of deciding whether evoked potentials, which are recorded in a depth of the brain upon sensory stimulation, are due to local activity at a tip of the recording electrode or electrical spread from remote, active areas was studied in detail on somatically evoked potentials in different areas of the hypothalamus (Rudomin et al., 1965; Rudomin et al., 1965; Malliani et al., 1965). On the basis of criteria for the decision established by these latter workers, the bipolarly recorded potentials in our study are judged to be due to local activity in the thalamic nuclei, whereas the monopolarly recorded potentials are due to spread from another active area. Latencies of these olfactory responses ranged from 10 to 30 msec. No potential changes were observed by stimulation of the olfactory bulb contralateral to a recording side (Fig. 2C and F).

The medial part of the dorsomedial nucleus, from which the most distinctive response was always obtained by olfactory bulb shock, was further explored with microelectrodes during odor stimulation (Fig. 2G). Percents of responsive and unresponsive units were roughly equal in 54 units. Thus it has been demonstrated that the olfactory system has also a thalamic projection as is the case for other sensory systems.

CORTICAL PROJECTIONS

Efferent connections of the dorsomedial nucleus of the thalamus to the frontal lobe have been demonstrated both anatomically (Khalifeh et al., 1965) and physiologically (Wells, 1966). Since our results as described above show a definite olfactory input to the dorsomedial nucleus, olfactory projections to the cerebral cortex were studied in the next series of experiments. Evoked potentials were recorded from the pial surface of the cerebral cortex including not only the frontal cortex but also all other cortical areas following electrical stimulation of the olfactory bulb or lateral olfactory tract in pre- or mid-pontine pretrigeminal cats (Motokizawa, 1974c). Some of the results are illustrated in Fig. 3. Three kinds of evoked potentials were observed: (1) biphasic negative-positive potentials in the

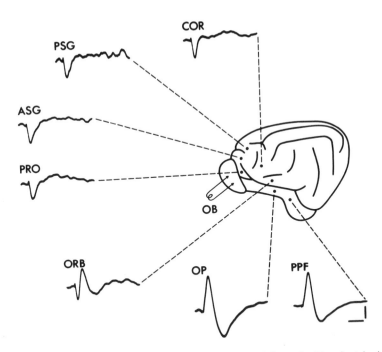

FIG. 3. Distribution in the frontal region of cortical potentials evoked by electrical stimulation of the olfactory bulb (OB). Each record shows a representative response from detailed mapping of responses in the corresponding gyrus. Positivity at the active electrode is designated by a downward deflection. Calibration: 1 mV for the olfactory peduncle (OP) and the prepyriform cortex (PPF), 0.2 mV for others, 25 msec. ASG, g. sigmoideus anterior; COR, g. coronalis; ORB, g. orbitalis; PRD, g. proreus; PSG, g. sigmoideus posterior.

prepyriform cortex; (2) positive-negative potentials in the orbital gyrus; (3) monophasic positive potentials from the rest of the cortex. Latencies of these potentials were relatively fixed at 3 msec at all recording sites. When paired stimuli were presented, the positive components to the second of the pair in the orbital gyrus and cortical areas other than the prepyriform cortex augmented between conditioning-test intervals of 20 and 200 msec. These showed very similar recovery characteristics to the negative waves in the prepyriform cortex. On the other hand the recovery characteristic of the negative component in the orbital gyrus was quite different and its amplitude considerably reduced between these intervals. Intravenous administration of pentobarbital sodium abolished both the negative and positive components in the orbital gyrus, but there was an obvious difference in the dosage between them; 5 mg/kg for the former and 20 mg/kg for the latter. Topical application of KCl to the cortical surface reduced the negative component in the orbital gyrus, whereas the positive components in all cortical areas except the prepyriform cortex remained intact. In the prepyriform cortex both the negative and positive waves disappeared simultaneously. At all recording sites intracortical distributions of the evoked potentials were checked with microelectrodes. The negative component in the orbital gyrus and both waves in the prepyriform cortex reversed their polarity in the depth of the cortex, while the positive components in all other areas remained unchanged throughout the cortical layer. These results indicate that the negative component in the orbital gyrus originates in the cortex under the electrode, whereas the positive components in all cortical areas other than the prepyriform cortex represent the negative wave originating at the prepyriform cortex and spreading by volume conduction.

It has been reported that the orbital gyrus receives vagal (Bailey and Bremer, 1938), splanchnic (Korn, 1969) and somatosensory (Korn et al., 1966) afferents. Also in our study such polysensory projections to this gyrus were confirmed in chloralose-anesthetized cats with intact brain. Furthermore, in order to determine whether these various inputs occupied the same cortical neuron pool, olfactory, trigeminal, and vagal responses were mutually interacted by pairing two inputs optionally selected from the three kinds of afferent sources. Blocking interactions were observed for all pairs of inputs by varying intervals between them.

CONCLUDING REMARKS

The foregoing series of experiments indicates that the olfactory system has the same pattern of afferent connections as other sensory systems. First, olfactory arousal is considered to be based on the general mechanism for producing arousal responses, namely, from modification of neuron activities of the mesencephalic reticular formation by olfactory impulses. Second, the olfactory system also projects to both thalamus and neocortex.

From the existence of the latter two projections, however, it cannot be concluded that the olfactory system also has a specific thalamocortical projection in common with all other specific sensory systems. Behavioral studies combined with lesions of each of the whole olfactory areas including the newly defined ones of the present study, as well as an odor discrimination studies at a single neuron level, will be necessary to reach a final conclusion on these matters.

REFERENCES

Bailey, P., and Bremer, F. (1938): A sensory cortical representation of the vagus nerve. *J. Neurophysiol.*, 1:405–412.

Cajal, S. R. (1955): *Studies on the Cerebral Cortex (Limbic Structures)*, translated by L. M. Kraft. Lloyd-Luke, London.

Lorente de Nó, R. (1949): Cerebral cortex: architecture, intracortical connections, motor projections. In: *Physiology of the Nervous Systems*, 3rd ed., edited by J. F. Fulton, pp. 288–312. Oxford Univ. Press, New York.

Khalifeh, R. R., Kaelber, W. W., and Ingram, W. R. (1965): Some efferent connections of the nucleus medialis dorsalis. *Am. J. Anat.*, 116:341–354.

Korn, H. (1969): Splanchnic projection to the orbital cortex of the cat. *Brain Res.*, 16:23–38.

Korn, H., Wendt, R., and Albe-Fessard, D. (1966): Somatic projection to the orbital cortex of the cat. *Electroenceph. Clin. Neurophysiol.*, 21:209–226.

Malliani, A., Rudomin, P., and Zanchetti, A. (1965): Contribution of local activity and electric spread to somatically evoked potentials in different areas of the hypothalamus. *Arch. Ital. Biol.*, 103:119–135.

Millhouse, O. E. (1969): A Golgi study of the descending medial forebrain bundle. *Brain Res.*, 15:341–363.

Motokizawa, F. (1974a): Electrophysiological studies of olfactory projection to the mesencephalic reticular formation. *Exp. Neurol.*, 44:135–144.

Motokizawa, F. (1974b): Olfactory input to the thalamus: Electrophysiological evidence. *Brain Res.*, 67:334–337.

Motokizawa, F. (1974c): Olfactory response field in the fronto-orbital cortex of cats. *J. Physiol. Soc. Japan*, 36 (*in press*).

Motokizawa, F., and Furuya, N. (1973): Neural pathway associated with the EEG arousal response by olfactory stimulation. *Electroenceph. Clin. Neurophysiol.*, 35:83–91.

O'Leary, J. L. (1937): Structure of the primary olfactory cortex of the mouse. *J. Comp. Neurol.*, 67:1–31.

Rudomin, P., Malliani, A., Borlone, M., and Zanchetti, A. (1965): Distribution of electrical responses to somatic stimuli in the diencephalon of the cat, with special reference to the hypothalamus. *Arch. Ital. Biol.*, 103:60–89.

Rudomin, P., Malliani, A., and Zanchetti, A. (1965): Microelectrode recording of slow wave and unit responses to afferent stimuli in the hypothalamus of the cat. *Arch. Ital. Biol.*, 103:90–118.

Valverde, F. (1963): Amygdaloid projection field. In: *Progr. Brain Res., Vol. 3: The Rhinencephalon and Related Structures*, edited by W. Bargman and J. P. Schade, pp. 20–30. Elsevier, Amsterdam.

Wells, J. (1966): The pathway from the dorsomedial thalamus to the frontal lobe. *Exp. Neurol.*, 14:338–350.

Electrobiology of Nerve, Synapse, and Muscle,
edited by J. P. Reuben, D. P. Purpura, M. V. L. Bennett,
and E. R. Kandel. Raven Press, New York © 1976

Membrane Properties of the Transverse Tubular System of Amphibian Skeletal Muscle

Shigehiro Nakajima and Joseph Bastian*

Department of Biological Sciences, Purdue University, West Lafayette, Indiana 47907

Muscle has a contractile element and an intracellular membranous system. The membranous system regulates the activity of the contractile machinery. The details of this regulatory activity are still largely unknown. The ignorance has mainly originated from the fact that the intracellular membranous system—the sarcoplasmic reticulum (SR) and the transverse tubular system (T system)—is a relatively newly discovered structural entity.

Early in 1954 and 1955 Natori conducted experiments on "skinned muscle fibers," fibers from which the sarcolemma was stripped. He found that the "skinned fiber" produced slowly conducting potential changes and slowly propagating contractions upon electrical stimulation. These observations were made too early to enable Natori to interpret the findings in terms of functions of the intracellular membranous system. Nevertheless, the findings may well be related to some functions of SR or T system.

The first physiological experiments that were aimed at elucidating the function of the internal membranous system were carried out by Huxley and Taylor (1958). They depolarized a minute area of muscle surface by an externally applied micropipette and discovered that contraction was elicited only when the location of the stimulus coincided with the place where the internal membranous system existed. This finding strongly suggested that the physiological role of the membranous system was to transmit electrical information from the surface into the interior of the fiber, thereby bringing about a rapid initiation of contraction. Recently, it has been elucidated that the structure that initially transmits the electrical information from the surface to the center is the T system, whereas the function of the SR is to receive information from the T system and to release calcium into the sarcoplasm (for reviews, see Ebashi and Endo, 1968; Huxley, 1971).

Because of the physiological importance of the T system, it has become necessary to know more about its membranous properties. The progress

---

* Present address: Department of Zoology, University of Oklahoma, Norman, Oklahoma 73069

has been rapid during the past few years. The purpose of this article is to summarize the recent progress, emphasizing the experiments in which we have been involved. Unless otherwise noted, the material discussed is the amphibian twitch muscle fibers.

PASSIVE ELECTRICAL PROPERTIES OF THE T SYSTEM

Electrical Capacity

Katz (1948) found that the value of the electrical capacity of muscle membrane measured at low frequency (5 μF/cm^2) is far greater than that of nerve or other biological membranes (about 1 μF/cm^2; Cole, 1968). Falk and Fatt (1964) partially solved this problem. They carefully analyzed the impedance of muscle membrane, and correlated the results with the structure. They showed that the impedance characteristics measured over the frequencies from 1 Hz to 10 kHz could be represented by the simple equivalent circuit shown in Fig. 1; C_M and R_M represent the capacity and resistance of the surface membrane, and C_e and R_e represent the input capacity and resistance of the T system. They assigned 2.6 μF/cm^2 to C_M and 4.1 μF/cm^2 to C_e (both values referred to the unit area of the surface). This model is called the "lumped model." It is obvious from this model that the apparent large capacity that Katz (1948) obtained was due to the fact that the capacity measured at low frequency would become approximately the sum of C_M and C_e.

After the publication of this classic work of Falk and Fatt (1964), three steps of methodological and theoretical developments have occurred: First is the introduction of the glycerol-treated muscle fibers; second is the devising of a more realistic electrical model of the T system (the distributed model), and third is an improvement in the technique of impedance measurement.

Gage and Eisenberg (1969a), following attempts by Howell and Jenden

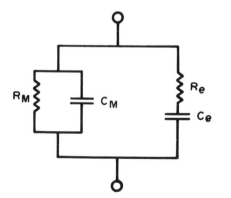

FIG. 1. Falk and Fatt's (1964) model of the membrane system of muscle fiber. R_M = resistance of the surface membrane. C_M = capacity of the surface membrane. R_e and C_e were thought to represent the properties of the internal membrane system.

(1967) and by Krolenko (1969) to solve a peculiar effect of glycerol on muscle (Fujino et al., 1961), have established a procedure to functionally disconnect the T system from the surface (the glycerol-treated fiber). [This treatment produces not only the disconnection of the T system but some other effects that decouple the excitation-contraction mechanism (Dulhunty and Gage, 1973)]. The procedure is to treat the muscle with a Ringer solution added with 400 mM glycerol for 1 hr and then to return the muscle to normal Ringer solution. By comparing the electric properties of the glycerol-treated fibers with normal fibers, Gage and Eisenberg (1969a) concluded that 2.2 $\mu F/cm^2$ was attributable to the surface capacity (C_M) and 3.9 $\mu F/cm^2$ to the input capacity of the T system (C_T) (both values referred to the unit surface area). These values are in good agreement with those of Falk and Fatt (1964). [The input capacity of the T system, C_T, corresponds to C_e of Falk and Fatt, and the value is referred to unit area of surface membrane. On the other hand, C_W (see below) is the capacity value referred to unit area of the T-system wall.]

In the lumped model, electrical properties of the T system were lumped together in spite of its distributed nature. It would be more realistic to regard the T system of each sarcomere as a disk consisting of fine meshes of tubules having the same density over the transverse section. This "distributed model" was first introduced by Falk and Fatt (1964), and solutions were given for the AC case. Subsequently, Adrian et al., (1969) and Schneider (1970) gave solutions for different conditions. Based on this model Adrian et al. (1969) calculated the values of the capacity of the surface membrane (C_M) and the wall of the T system (C_W) from the then known electrical properties of muscle fibers, assuming that $C_M = C_W$, and obtained the value of 1 $\mu F/cm^2$ for both C_M and C_W (referred to unit area of the respective membrane).

In the original impedance measurement Falk and Fatt (1964) carefully minimized stray capacities around the intracellular microelectrodes by shielding. Nevertheless, these stray capacities introduced serious errors at high frequency. Freygang et al. (1967) introduced another method of measuring membrane impedance. The most important feature of this method was that the output potential of the voltage measuring electrode was held virtually at the resting potential of the fiber by an operational amplifier, thus eliminating the current that would flow through the capacity between the inside and outside of the voltage electrode. However, it should be noted that this method introduced other drawbacks: (1) that the membrane is short-circuited by two microelectrodes; (2) that the signal to noise ratio becomes less; and (3) that both electrodes should have a perfect linear resistance.

Using this new method, Schneider (1970) measured the impedance carefully. He analyzed his data based on the two models of the T system (the lumped model and the distributed model) and found that theory fitted to the experimental data better if the distributed model was used. Furthermore, he found that when both C_M and C_W were about 1 $\mu F/cm^2$, the distributed model fitted best to the data. [It is noted that in his calculation no particular relation was assumed between C_M and C_W, whereas in Adrian et al.'s (1969) calculation $C_M = C_W$ was assumed.]

Recently, Valdiosera et al. (1974a–c) have carried out impedance measurements again, in essentially the same way as Schneider (i.e., Freygang et al.'s method), but with an extreme degree of accuracy. They discussed all possible sources of errors in Freygang et al.'s method. They emphasized the importance of the nonisopotentiality of the bathing solution. This error, as well as the interelectrode capacitative current, was reduced by shielding the current electrode with a conductive paint. Allowance was made for the three dimensional current flow inside the fiber. They analyzed their data on the lumped model, the distributed model, and a hybrid model (hybrid between the lumped and distributed models). They concluded that a better fit to the data was obtained by either the distributed model or the hybrid model than by the lumped model. Their values of C_M and C_W were 0.73 and 0.78 $\mu F/cm^2$ (Table VI of Valdiosera et al., 1974c) at the sarcomere length of 2.5 μm if the distributed model was adopted. These values became larger at the sarcomere length of 2.0 μm (1.26 and 1.13 for C_M and C_W). As can be expected, when the hybrid model was used, the value of C_M was increased (the extreme case of the hybrid model is the lumped model, and the value of C_M is as much as 2.6 $\mu F/cm^2$).

Hodgkin and Nakajima (1972a,b) investigated the passive electrical properties of the T system from a different approach. The essential feature of their approach was to see how high- and low-frequency capacities vary according to fiber diameter. They investigated this on normal and glycerol-treated muscle fibers. They found that the total low-frequency capacity of muscle membrane per unit surface area increased with fiber diameter. This result suggests that at low-frequency currents can spread freely into the center of the fiber through the T system. (The surface area is in direct proportion to the fiber diameter, whereas the membrane area of the T system is in proportion to the cross sectional area of the fiber. This is the reason why the total capacity per unit surface area increased in proportion with fiber diameter.) On the other hand, high frequency capacity (at about 1 kHz) did not change according to the diameter, suggesting that current at the high-frequency flows only through a peripheral portion of the fiber. Their analysis revealed that the distributed model with values $C_M = C_W = 0.9$ $\mu F/cm^2$ fitted well with the data. The value $C_M = 0.9$ was also obtained independently from the value of high-frequency capacity of the glycerol-treated fiber. It is interesting to note that both sets of measurements, one to see the frequency dependence of the impedance (Schneider, 1970; Valdiosera et al., 1974c) the other to see the diameter dependence of the impedance (Hodgkin and Nakajima, 1972b) yielded similar values for C_M and C_W.

The conventional technique of analyzing low-frequency capacity is to use voltage transients when current steps are applied to the membrane. Adrian and Almers (1974), however, have analyzed the membrane capacity from current transients when potential was suddenly changed. They showed that the capacity measured in this way corresponded to the membrane capacity provided that the conductance of the tubular wall is small. They observed that the capacity increased as diameter increased, and that the capacity did not change according to the ionic strength of the bathing medium, indicating that current flows deep in the T system under these conditions.

There are some unsolved problems concerning the capacity of muscle, which need future investigations.

1. In all the measurements described above the muscle fiber was treated as a cylinder having a smooth surface without foldings. However, since it is known that there are caveolae and foldings on the surface, the true value of the unfolded membrane capacity would be smaller than 1 $\mu F/cm^2$. Franzini-Armstrong and Dulhunty (1974) have recently reported that the presence of foldings and caveolae increase the surface area by as much as 80% at a sarcomere length of 2.4 μm. Mobley and Eisenberg (1975) reported that caveolae might increase the surface area by 47%. However, how much contribution the presence of caveolae (with various size of the opening) would make to the total capacity measured at slack length is not known. In another report Dulhunty and Franzini-Armstrong (1975; and *personal communication*) have suggested that the surface capacity, if the contribution of caveolae and foldings are substracted, would be about 0.8 to 0.9 $\mu F/cm^2$. Somewhat related to this is the finding of Valdiosera et al.'s (1974c) that the capacity at the sarcomere length of 2.0 μm is larger than that at 2.5 μm.

2. Between Adrian and Peachey (1973) on one hand and Valdiosera et al. (1974c) on the other, a disagreement exists about the value of access resistance (extra resistance located in the luminal fluid near the opening of the T system). According to the value of access resistance assigned, the value of the surface capacity would vary (the extreme case is Falk and Fatt's value of 2.6 $\mu F/cm^2$, where all the tubular luminal resistance is the access resistance).

3. All the models assume that the membrane capacity is a perfect capacitance. There is no evidence for or against the existence of imperfect capacitance (Cole, 1968) over the frequency range below 2 kHz. Muscles in some developmental stages or in tissue culture might be a good material to investigate this problem.

Conductance

The value of the electrical conductance of the T system membrane is difficult to determine because of large individual variations among fibers, possibly varying according to frog's conditions, species, seasons, etc.

Impedance studies of the kind that Schneider (1970) or Valdiosera et al. (1974b,c) carried out could not reveal the conductance value, since the impedance characteristics were very insensitive to changes of conductance.

By comparing the membrane conductances of normal and glycerol-treated muscle fibers, Eisenberg and Gage (1969) obtained a value of 0.247 mmho/cm^2 for surface conductance (G_M) and 0.055 mmho/cm^2 for the input conductance of the T system (G_T) (both referred to unit surface area); the latter value of G_T would correspond to G_W (the conductance of the T membrane referred to unit area of T membrane) of about 0.01 mmho/cm^2 on the distributed model. Hodgkin and Nakajima (1972b) analyzed the diameter dependency of membrane conductance, and revealed that G_M is about 0.11 mmho/cm^2 and G_W 0.03 mmho/cm^2. These values are very rough estimates. In the case of Eisenberg and Gage's estimation, it is possible that G_M was overestimated and G_W underestimated, since the values were derived on the assumption that the glycerol treatment did not change the ionic permeability. Hodgkin and Nakajima's values are dependent on the assumption that ionic permeabilities were the same in large and small fibers. Both are unproven assumptions. (It might be possible that while membrane capacity is independent of fiber size, ionic permeabilities vary according to diameter. Nevertheless, the fact that the distributed model that explained the behavior of muscle capacity also fitted the conductance data indicates that there is no marked difference in permeabilities between large and small fibers; Hodgkin and Nakajima, 1972a,b.)

Ionic Permeability of the Resting Membrane

Despite the uncertainty about the values of conductance, the qualitative aspects of ionic permeabilities are fairly well established. Hodgkin and Horowicz (1960a) studied the effects of a very quick change of external potassium concentration $[K]_0$ and chloride concentration $[Cl]_0$ on the membrane potential of single muscle fibers, and revealed a strange phenomenon. Potential changes accompanying sudden changes in $[Cl]_0$ were very quick (with a half-time of a fraction of a second) with little asymmetry between an increase and a decrease of $[Cl]_0$. On the other hand, potential changes due to changes in $[K]_0$ had an asymmetry: repolarization took place much slower than depolarization. Hodgkin and Horowicz (1960a) attributed the slowness of the repolarization to a washout process of K ions, which were retained in a special region of muscle fiber (now identified as the T system). The rapidity of potential changes accompanying changes in $[Cl]_0$ was thought to indicate that the chloride channels were located mainly in the surface membrane. The work by Eisenberg and Gage (1969) on the glycerol-treated fibers also indicated that chloride conductance of the T system was close to zero.

Nakajima et al. (1973) conducted experiments using glycerol-treated muscle fibers. They found that in these fibers a sudden increase or decrease in $[K]_0$ produced a rapid depolarization and a rapid repolarization in contrast to the case of normal fibers (Fig. 2). These results seem to constitute evidence for the idea that the slow K repolarization in normal fibers is due to a retention of K ions in the T system.

A summary of these results is that the resting K conductance is located in the T system as well as in the surface, whereas the Cl conductance is located mainly in the surface of the normal muscle fiber.

Luminal Conductance and Diffusion of Substance in the T System

As described above, the slow repolarization phase when $[K]_0$ is suddenly decreased, probably represents a wash-out process of potassium ions that were retained in the T system. Therefore, by analyzing the time course of the repolarization, the apparent diffusion constant of potassium inside the lumen of the T system could be calculated. When a single muscle fiber is immersed in a Na-free solution for some time, and then normal Ringer is suddenly introduced, the ability of the fiber to produce a twitch contraction recovers with a certain time course (Fig. 3; also Hodgkin and Horowicz, 1960b). The time course of the twitch recovery perhaps represents the diffusion of Na ions into the T system: as more and more Na ions enter the T system, greater portions of the T system become excitable resulting in an

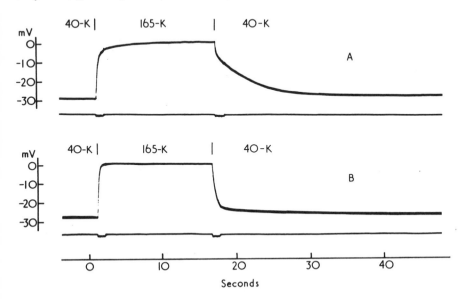

FIG. 2. Time courses of membrane potential in single fibers when $[K]_0$ was suddenly changed from 40 to 165 mM and back again to 40 mM. Chloride-free solutions were used throughout. The lower traces of each record indicate the flushes of solutions. **A:** normal fiber. **B:** glycerol-treated fiber. (From Nakajima et al., 1973.)

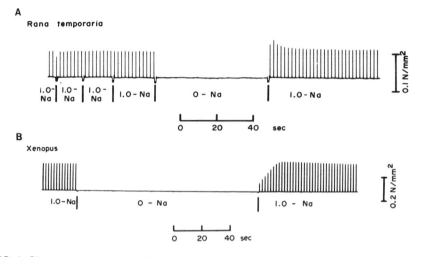

FIG. 3. Changes in isometric twitch tension produced by sudden changes in [Na]$_0$. There was a large individual variability in the recovery time course of twitch tension when normal Ringer was suddenly applied to a fiber that had been immersed in a Na-free solution. 1.0 Na means normal Ringer. 0 Na is a Na-free solution (Tris substituted). **A:** 60-μm radius fiber from *Rana temporania*. **B:** 76.5 μm radius fiber from *Xenopus laevis*. (From Nakajima et al., 1975.)

activation of more myofibrils that are located near the center. Therefore, if the time course of the twitch recovery and the relation between [Na]$_0$ versus twitch height are given, calculation of the apparent diffusion constant of Na inside the T system lumen is possible.

Nakajima et al. (1975) have calculated the apparent diffusion constant of K and Na inside the T-system lumen from the time courses of the above two phenomena. The values obtained were both about 1.5×10^{-6} cm^2/sec. This is about one order of magnitude less than the diffusion constants of Na and K in an aqueous solution; the latters are 1.2×10^{-5} cm^2/sec for Na and 1.8×10^{-5} cm^2/sec for K (0.1 M and 25°C). Since the T system forms a network inside the fiber, the tortuous geometry would decrease the apparent diffusion constant by a factor of 2.0 to 2.5 in the same manner as it affects the radial luminal conductance of the T system (Adrian et al., 1969; Schneider, 1970; Barry and Adrian, 1973). Even if this tortuosity factor is allowed for, our values are smaller than those in the free solution by a factor of about 4.

Electrical measurements, in agreement with the low values of apparent diffusion constants, have suggested that the specific conductance (G$_L$) of the luminal fluid of the T system is low. Thus, Schneider's (1970) impedance analysis revealed that the value of G$_L$ was about 3 mmho/cm. Hodgkin and Nakajima (1972*b*) gave 6 mmho/cm, Valdiosera et al. (1974*c*) obtained 5.4 mmho/cm, and Adrian and Almers' (1974) value was 4 mmho/cm for G$_L$. All of these values are less than the conductivity of Ringer fluid (about

12 mmho/cm) by a factor of 2 to 4. Also Endo (1966) reported that the speed of exchange of a fluorescence dye inside the T system was very slow.

It is possible to interpret the low values of the apparent diffusion constant and G_L as indicating the real slowness of ionic movement in the lumen. Another explanation would be to ascribe it to a more complex anatomy of the T system than envisaged from Peachey's (1965) paper. For example, the tubules may have a complex irregular course, or they may have an undulation in the longitudinal plane as well as in the transverse plane, or the lumen of the T system may have bottlenecks here and there. We hope structural studies will solve these questions in the future. [A recent study by Peachey (*personal communication*) with a high voltage electron microscope has revealed a fairly complex structure of the T system with frequent dead ends. Another recent development is that Eisenberg and his coworkers (*personal communication*) have devised a completely new model of the T system, starting from solving a differential equation which describes the current flows in each unit of T-system mesh and using difference equations derived from the flow of current at each node of the mesh. Analysis of the impedance data based on this new model has revealed that the conductance of the luminal fluid is roughly the same as that of Ringer fluid. In other words, the tortuosity factor is smaller than 1/2 or 1/2.5 in the new model. In agreement with this view, Gilai (1975) has recently reported that the value of G_L was about the same as the conductivity of the external fluid in scorpion muscle fibers, in which the T system shows a relatively simple cable structure without branches.]

Somewhat related to this problem is the controversy over the presence of access resistance. Access resistance (R_a) refers to an extra resistance in the tubular lumen near the opening of the T system. Adrian and Peachey (1973) conducted a computer modeling study of the action potential of muscle using the distributed model. They showed that when an access resistance (R_a) of about 150 $\Omega \cdot cm^2$ (referred to unit area of surface) was introduced, the calculated conduction velocity of action potential approached the experimentally determined value. Also the shape of the calculated action potential became more realistic, and a hump appeared at the beginning of the early afterpotential (Fig. 4). In fact we know that this kind of hump is often recorded experimentally. In Adrian and Peachey's model the effective radial resistance of the tubular fluid (R_L) is about 70 $\Omega \cdot cm^2$ (referred to unit surface area). Therefore the access resistance (150 $\Omega \cdot cm^2$) constitutes more than half of the total radial luminal resistance ($R_a + R_L$). Contrary to the result of Adrian and Peachey (1973), Valdiosera et al. (1974c) have shown that the access resistance, if there is any at all, would be about 20 $\Omega \cdot cm^2$, and R_L about 130 $\Omega \cdot cm^2$. Therefore, the results of both groups are in quantitative disagreement.

Recently, Franzini-Armstrong et al. (1975) have described the ultra-structure of the T system opening in detail. Their data suggest that each

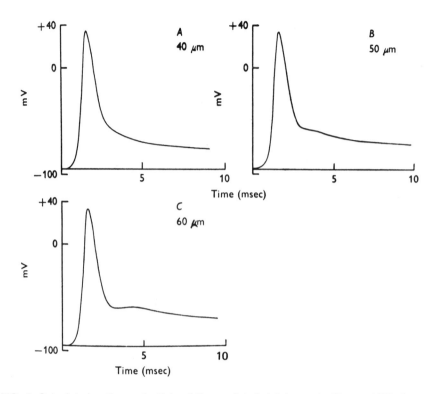

FIG. 4. Calculated action potentials of the model skeletal muscle fiber at 20°C. Access resistance of 150 $\Omega \cdot cm^2$ was assigned in all records. **A:** 40μm radius fiber. **B:** 50 μm radius fiber. **C:** 60 μm radius fiber. (From Adrian and Peachey, 1973.)

opening does not seem to produce a large hindrance to diffusion. This may mean that if a large access resistance really exists, it is not a consequence of narrowness of each opening site, but is due to scarceness of the opening. Unfortunately, we still do not know the exact spacing of the openings in the surface.

VOLTAGE-DEPENDENT PERMEABILITY CHANGES OF T SYSTEM

Na-Conductance Change

One of the most important questions in the physiology of the T system is whether an action potential occurs in the T system under physiological conditions, and if so, what is the physiological role of the action potential. The local stimulation experiments by Huxley and Taylor (1958) suggested that the transmission of surface depolarization along the T system was due to a decremental electrotonic conduction rather than to a regenerative process. However, as Huxley (1971) mentioned, this did not prove the absence of action potential in the T system under physiological conditions, since the highly localized depolarization of the surface membrane is a non-physiological means of stimulating the T system, and in 1967 it was still "an open question" (Huxley, 1971).

For some time there have been reports, which suggest the presence of some kinds of regenerative activities occurring either in the SR or in the T system (Natori, 1954; Strickholm, 1966; Sugi and Ochi, 1967; Costantin and Podolsky, 1967). Costantin (1970) and Costantin and Taylor (1971) carried out elegant experiments, and gave a definite answer to this question. They imposed square pulse depolarizations to the surface of single fibers bathed in 50% $[Na]_0$. When muscle fibers had been treated by tetrodotoxin, small depolarizations produced contraction of myofibrils near the surface membrane only, and larger depolarizations induced the contraction of all myofibrils as originally observed by Adrian et al. (1969). However, when tetrodotoxin was not applied, the situation sometimes was reversed; when a near-threshold depolarization was applied, axially located myofibrils contracted, while peripherally located ones did not. Under the experimental conditions of Costantin (1970) and Costantin and Taylor (1971), the surface membrane was voltage clamped, whereas the T system near the axis was not. Thus, the T system near the axis produced action potential freely. This triggered the contraction of axially located myofibrils, whereas the T system near the surface was well clamped, and remained subthreshold for activation. Thus, the observations by Costantin (1970) and Costantin and Taylor (1971) constitute good evidence for the presence of action potential in the T system.

Bastian and Nakajima (1972, 1974) have conducted experiments to determine: (1) whether an action potential of the T system is triggered under physiological conditions (i.e., whether the action potential in the surface membrane can trigger an action potential in the T system); and (2) the physiological roles of the T-system action potential (i.e., to what extent the T-system action potential contributes to the mechanical output of normal contraction).

In order to answer these questions it was necessary to apply the double sucrose gap method of the Julian, Moore, and Goldman (1962) type to single muscle fibers. With the double sucrose gap technique we can work on a short segment of muscle fiber (the artificial node), which is electrically virtually isolated from other parts of the fiber by pure sucrose solutions. Although we failed to apply the sucrose gap technique to muscle fibers of frog, we later found that muscle fibers from *Xenopus* were more suitable for this purpose (Nakajima and Bastian, 1974).

When an action potential occurs in the artificial node under the sucrose gap, it will freely shorten and pull other resting parts of the fiber. We could record the twitch contraction as a change of force by a tension transducer attached to one end of the fiber. From the wave form of the force change, and from the mechanical frequency response of resting single fibers, we could recover the original wave form of the shortening of the artificial node by the use of the Fourier transform. It was revealed that the recorded force can be regarded as roughly representing the isotonic shortening of the node.

Figure 5(A1) and (A2) show action potential (V) and twitch contraction (T) when a short current pulse (I) was applied to the "artificial node" of a *Xenopus* single muscle fiber under the constant-current condition. Several of these control action potentials were stored in an FM tape recorder. After this control period, tetrodotoxin was applied to the node. Then the voltage clamp was applied, and the wave form of the action potential stored in the tape was imposed to the nodal membrane. This "simulated action potential" is shown in Fig. 5(B1) and (B2). The records show that the height of twitch

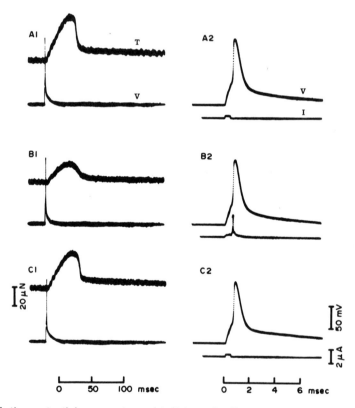

FIG. 5. Action potentials, currents, and twitches of a *Xenopus* single muscle fiber recorded with the sucrose-gap technique. **A1, A2:** real action potential (V), current, (I), and twitch (T) recorded in normal Ringer. **B1, B2:** simulated action potential and the resultant current and twitch in a solution with tetrodotoxin (2.5×10^{-8} g/ml). **C1, C2:** recovery of normal action potential 17 min after starting the wash of tetrodotoxin with normal Ringer. Fiber diameter 96 μm. Nodal length 246–261 μm. Bath temperature 23.5°C. (From Bastian and Nakajima, 1974.)

produced by the simulated action potential is far smaller than the normal control twitch. The average twitch height by the simulated action potential was 33.5% of the control twitch. The effect of tetrodotoxin was reversible, as shown in C1 and C2. Essentially the same results were obtained when a Na-free solution was used instead of tetrodotoxin to abolish the action potential.

These results indicate that there is a Na-dependent action potential in the T system. If the T system were not excitable, the real action potential and the simulated action potential should have produced the same mechanical output, since in both cases the potential changes of the surface would have conducted decrementally along the T system, and the potential and current distribution along the T system should have been the same. Thus, our results indicate that under normal conditions when an action potential occurs in the surface, an action potential is triggered in the T system, and consequently the T system is depolarized more than it would be depolarized by a decremental conduction. Since the ratio of the height of twitch resulting from the simulated action potential to that resulting from the real action potential was 33.5%, we can conclude that the action potential of the T system contributes to roughly 70% of the mechanical output of normal isotonic twitches.

The above results were obtained at room temperature. When the same kind of experiments were conducted at a lower temperature (about 12°C), the results were totally different. As shown in Fig. 6, the twitch produced by simulated action potential was not much (86%) different from the control twitch. The result indicates that at low temperature, the action potential in the T system becomes less necessary for the activation of normal twitches, although there is no reason to doubt the occurrence of action potential in the T system at low temperature.

In summary the conclusions of our experiments are: (1) The action potential is triggered in the T system when an action potential occurs in the surface membrane. (2) The action potential of the T-system is necessary to produce a quick contraction near room temperature, but becomes less necessary as temperature is lowered. (3) The action potential of the T system constitutes roughly 70% of the mechanical output of normal twitches at room temperature.

There are in addition, several reports pertaining the excitability of the T system:

(a) Gonzalez-Serratos (1966, 1971) reported that Q_{10} of the inward spread of contraction was high.

(b) Bezanilla et al. (1972) found that when single muscle fibers were stimulated at a high frequency in a Na-deficient solution, tetanic tension was not maintained, but declined. They regarded this decline of tension as reflecting a gradual decrease of Na concentration inside the tubules, leading to a decrease in the size of the T-system potential.

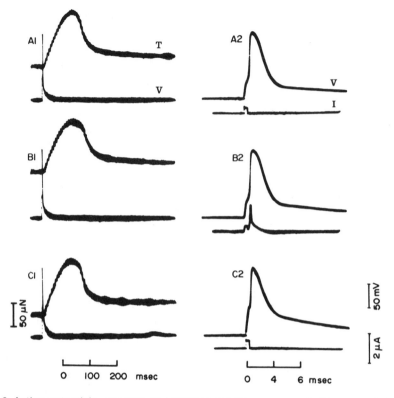

FIG. 6. Action potentials, currents, and twitches of a *Xenopus* muscle fiber recorded with the sucrose gap technique at a low temperature (12.5°C). See the legend of Fig. 5 for explanation of the symbols. **A1, A2:** real action potential in normal Ringer. **B1, B2:** simulated action potential in tetrodotoxin. **C1, C2:** real action potential in normal Ringer again. Fiber diameter 125 μm. Nodal length 347 μm. (From Bastian and Nakajima, 1974.)

(c) When normal Ringer was suddenly introduced into the bathing solution of single muscle fibers, which had been immersed in a Na-free solution, the time course of the twitch recovery is frequently very quick (Fig. 3A). Caputo and DiPolo (1973) found that the time course of the recovery was delayed by adding dextran, which increased the viscosity of the solution, and thus presumably slowed down the diffusion process of Na in the T system.

(d) As described above in (c), the recovery of twitch in single muscle fibers when normal Ringer is suddenly introduced is frequently very quick. At first sight, this quick recovery is difficult to reconcile with the idea that the T system produces a Na spike, since other phenomena which reflect a diffusion of ions in the tubules (like the slow K repolarization; Hodgkin and Horowicz, 1960a) have a half-time of a few seconds. However, Nakajima et al. (1975) have solved this somewhat puzzling problem. We found that the time course of twitch recovery was quite variable from fiber to fiber (see Fig. 3) and this variability depended on fiber size as well as on a variability of the relation between $[Na]_0$ and twitch height. We calculated the apparent diffusion constants of Na and K in the T system from the time course of twitch recovery and that of K repolarization. The calculation revealed that if we accept a value for the apparent diffusion constant of Na and K ions of about 1.5×10^{-6} cm²/sec, both twitch recovery as well as the slow K repolarization will be explained by the diffusion process in the T system. Thus, the quick recovery of twitch does not conflict with the idea of the presence of a Na spike in the T system.

(e) Adrian and Peachey's (1973) computer modeling has revealed that the hump at the beginning of early after potential (Fig. 4) can be explained, if the T system is excitable and if there is an access resistance in the T system.

(f) Rougier et al. (*personal communication*) applied tetrodotoxin to single muscle fibers. When the external solution was again replaced by normal Ringer, action potential started to recover slowly. At first, the action potential (presumably only the surface membrane is excitable at this time) did not have the hump at the beginning of the after-potential. Later the hump started to appear. This finding supports the idea described above in (e).

(g) Caillé et al. (1975) recorded the inward sodium current under the voltage clamp using the sucrose gap method. When they applied a low concentration of tetrodotoxin, the peak of inward current was initially reduced without affecting contraction (presumably only the surface was affected by tetrodotoxin); later the second slower phase of the initial current was reduced together with the reduction of contraction (presumably tetrodotoxin now abolished the action potential of the T system).

Each of the above studies alone cannot perhaps be regarded as definite evidence for the idea of the presence of the T-system action potential. Nevertheless, the idea is strengthened by these facts. Finally, it should be mentioned that Sugi (1974) has recently repeated a local stimulation experiment similar to that of Huxley and Taylor (1958) by using a larger capillary electrode. He has recorded a phasic contraction with a definite threshold propagating from the surface toward the center.

He also observed that this phasic contraction was sometimes insensitive to tetrodotoxin or to the removal of $[Na]_0$. Therefore, he suggested that some mechanism other than a Na spike operates for the active propagation in the T system.

The next question about the T system excitability is to know the density of Na channels in the T system in comparison with that in the surface. Recently Jaimovich et al. (1975) have reported that the glycerol treatment reduces the tetrodotoxin binding by about half, implying that the density of Na channels in the T system is lower than that in the surface membrane.

K Conductance Change

In many excitable tissues, sudden depolarizations produce a decrease of membrane resistance with a certain time delay. This is called delayed rectification, and is thought to represent an increase of K conductance (Hodgkin and Huxley, 1952), which is responsible for the quick repolarization of action potential. However, in 1949 Katz found a peculiar rectification in frog muscle. Depolarizing currents applied to a muscle that had already been depolarized by a high-potassium solution produced an increase of resistance rather than a decrease. This was called "anomalous rectification." The anomalous rectifying property of skeletal muscle has been confirmed by many investigators (Hodgkin and Horowicz, 1959; Hutter and Noble, 1960; Adrian, 1960; Adrian and Freygang, 1962a,b; Nakajima et al., 1962; Horowicz et al., 1968).

The relation between "delayed rectification" and "anomalous rectification" was investigated by Nakajima et al. (1962). It was revealed that when a muscle fiber that had had a conditioning membrane potential of about −90 mV was suddenly depolarized, delayed rectification showed up, but when the depolarization was maintained for a few seconds, the delayed rectification was completely inactivated [K inactivation (Grundfest, 1961; Lüttgau, 1960)] and was converted into anomalous rectification (Fig. 7A). Thus, the remarkable anomalous rectification that Katz (1949) observed is explained by the fact that delayed rectification had already been inactivated by the depolarization produced by the high K solution. This study (Nakajima et al., 1962) was conducted with two microelectrodes inserted near the center of muscle fiber. Adrian et al. (1970a,b), however, achieved voltage- and space-clamping conditions using three microelectrodes inserted near the end of muscle fibers. Using this method they analyzed the properties of Na and K permeabilities quantitatively, and determined the exact time course of K inactivation in skeletal muscle (Fig. 7B). From these studies it seems established that there are two main potassium channels in muscle membrane: (1) the delayed rectification channel, which is activated by depolarization, and is subsequently inactivated completely by maintained depolarization; and (2) the anomalous rectification channel (also called the inward rectification channel). Adrian et al.'s (1970b) experiments suggested the existence of a third kind of potassium channel, which underwent small and very slow changes in permeability.

Problem: Are Anomalous Rectification Channels Located in the T System?

Since the inward rectification is so conspicuous a phenomenon in skeletal muscle, Adrian and Freygang (1962a) thought that it might represent a property of the T system, which is again a remarkable ultrastructural entity of muscle. They proposed a model in which the T-system membrane was assumed to be permeable only to potassium ions, and this K per-

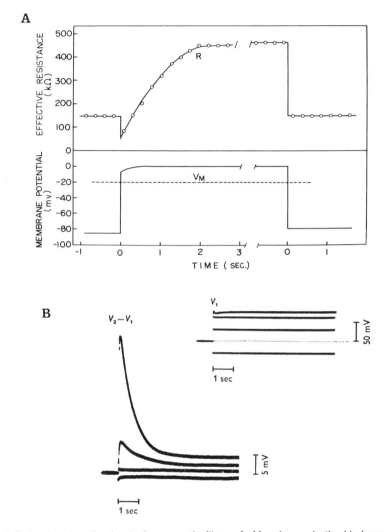

FIG. 7. Potassium inactivation in frog muscle fibers. **A:** Muscle was bathed in hypertonic 80 mM K solution. The effective resistance of a fiber was plotted (R). The membrane was hyperpolarized to −85 mV by a conditioning current, and at zero time an outward DC was passed bringing the membrane potential to about 0 mV (V_M). The effective resistance was first decreased (delayed rectification), and then increased (anomalous rectification). After a few minutes, the outward DC was turned off, bringing the potential to −80 mV. The dashed line is the resting potential. Temperature 27°C. **B:** The time courses of potassium currents (V_2-V_1), when the membrane potential (V_1) was suddenly depolarized to various levels from a holding potential of −100 mV. Hypertonic Ringer solution with tetrodotoxin. Three-electrode voltage clamping was employed. Temperature 19°C. (**A:** from Nakajima et al., 1962; **B:** from Adrian et al., 1970a.)

meability was assumed to have the inwardly rectifying property (anomalous rectification). This model or a modification of it has been shown to explain the creep phenomenon — a slow increase of membrane resistance during a hyperpolarizing current of long duration — quite well (Adrian and Freygang, 1962*a;* Almers, 1972; Barry and Adrian, 1973). On the other hand, Eisenberg and Gage (1969), by working on glycerol-treated fibers, showed that the surface membrane had an inward rectifying property. However this conclusion did not eliminate the possibility that the inward rectification channels are also located in the T-system membrane.

Existence of the inward rectifying channels in the T-system membrane has been suggested by experiments using rubidium ions (Nakajima, *unpublished*). It has been known that replacement of external K ions by Rb ions results in a complete abolishment of the inward rectification (Adrian, 1964), suggesting that K ions pass through the inward rectifier easily whereas Rb ions cannot. Nakajima has conducted experiments to see how quickly rubidium ions eliminate the anomalous rectification using the rapid solution exchanges. Changes of input resistance when Rb ions were suddenly applied were recorded under the voltage-clamp condition. The data were analyzed to give the time course of changes of membrane resistance. The time course of the elimination of the inward rectifier by rubidium was found to have a half-time of a few seconds. The time course was quicker in smaller fibers. In the glycerol-treated fibers the time course became very rapid. These results suggest that the time course is mainly determined by the diffusion of rubidium ions in the T system, and thus are indicative of the presence of the inward rectifier in the T system. Together with the result of Eisenberg and Gage (1969), it may tentatively be concluded that the inward rectification is a property of both the surface and the T-system membrane.

Problem: Do Delayed Rectification Channels Exist in the T System?

Since there is a Na-dependent action potential in the T system, it would be reasonable to suppose that the delayed rectification channels (or K activation channels, Grundfest, 1966) also exist in the T system. Yet, there is no direct evidence to support this idea. Even if the K activation mechanism does not exist in the T system, the charge stored in the T-system membrane at the peak of the T-system action potential would be discharged easily through the increased K conductance in the surface. Therefore, the T system would produce an action potential that differs little in shape from the surface action potential. In other words, there is no particular necessity for the T system to have the K activation channels in order to produce a quick repolarization.

In 1964, Freygang et al. put forward an idea that the late afterpotential (a long-lasting depolarization phase after repetitive stimulation) in skeletal muscle was a consequence of an accumulation of K ions in the T system (the K accumulation hypothesis). A corollary of this idea is that the delayed rectifying channels exist in the T system, because without an increase in K conductance it is impossible to expect a large enough accumulation of K ions to account for the magnitude of the later afterpotential.

Gage and Eisenberg (1969b) found that when the T system was disconnected from the surface by the "glycerol-treatment," the late afterpotential disappeared. This observation does suggest that the T system plays a critical role in the generation of the afterpotential, but does not necessarily indicate that the K accumulation hypothesis is correct. Recently, Adrian et al. (1970b) have presented a finding which appears to contradict the K accumulation hypothesis. They observed that the late afterpotential changed sign by changing membrane potential (i.e., there was a reversal potential). From this finding they suggested a possibility that the late afterpotential reflected a slow change in K permeability rather than a K accumulation. Because of the lack of definite evidence, it seems necessary to carry out experiments to decide whether Freygang et al.'s idea is correct.

Kirsch et al. are now carrying out experiments to answer this question. It is known that the slow K repolarization upon sudden reduction of $[K]_0$ represents the diffusion of K ions from the T system into the outside (Hodgkin and Horowicz, 1960a; Nakajima et al., 1973). Thus, if the K accumulation hypothesis of late afterpotential is correct, the time course of the late afterpotential and that of the slow K repolarization ought to be identical for each single fiber. Thus we have compared the time courses of both the phenomena for each single fiber. The data so far obtained seem to indicate that the time course of the late afterpotential coincides fairly well (not exactly though) with that of the K repolarization. The results, therefore, suggest that the K accumulation hypothesis of Freygang et al. is correct, and consequently the delayed rectifier seems to exist in the T system.

Calcium Conductance Change and the Coupling Mechanisms Between T system and SR

We now know that depolarization of the T system causes a release of calcium ions from the SR into the sarcoplasm resulting in the activation of the contractile elements. However, we don't know how the information is transmitted from the T system into the SR. There are three ways of explaining the coupling: (a) electrical hypothesis, (b) calcium-current hypothesis, and (c) macromolecular bridge hypothesis.

Electrical Hypothesis

The inside of the SR and the T-system lumen are connected by a low resistance pathway, like the one in the gap junction; thus electric currents flow directly through the two systems, and the SR is depolarized. This possibility was described clearly by Ebashi and Endo (1968) and Ebashi, Endo, and Ohtsuki (1969). Investigations on the passive electrical properties of muscle (described in the section on "Passive Electric Properties of the T system") have revealed electrical components probably corresponding to the T-system membrane, but did not reveal any substantial amount of current flowing through an electrical network that could be attributed to the SR. One might argue that this can be taken as evidence that currents do not flow directly through the SR. However, if the SR, with large capacity and low resistance, are attached in series with part of the T system, then impedance measurements could be overshadowed by the T system, even if a substantial amount of currents flow through the SR.

One of the difficulties of the electrical hypothesis is that, as calculated by Ebashi and Endo (1968), the magnitude of depolarization expected in the SR by the current flow during action potential is only of the order of a few millivolts. Assuming that some regenerative processes in the SR are initiated by this small depolarization, it would be a rather unreliable system to transmit information (noises could trigger contractions). Another difficulty of the electrical hypothesis is that the studies by Franzini-Armstrong revealed that the junctional region between the T and the SR membrane has important structural differences from the gap junction. Thus, a foot-like structure exists between the SR and the T membranes. These feet, however, seem to belong to the SR, and do not quite reach the T membrane (Franzini-Armstrong, 1970). In the freeze-fractured materials of a muscle from the spider, particles and pits that exist in the junctional SR membrane do not correspond to particles seen in the T-system membrane (Franzini-Armstrong, 1974).

Calcium-Current Hypothesis

This possibility was stated by Ford and Podolsky (1972) in a most explicit way. According to this hypothesis, when the T membrane is depolarized, Ca permeability of the T membrane increases and calcium ions flow from the T-system lumen into the sarcoplasm. This will result in an increase of calcium ion concentration in the sarcoplasm near the SR, and this increase will trigger a release of Ca from the SR (Ca-induced calcium release, see below). (In order to avoid confusion, we would like to emphasize that this hypothesis assigns a special role of calcium, as an information messenger in the form of calcium flow, and it does not merely state that calcium is somehow important.) Experimental facts supporting this calcium hypothesis are: (1) Endo et al. (1970) and Ford and Podolsky (1970) found that a calcium release from SR occurs when the sarcoplasmic calcium ion concentration was elevated in skinned muscle fibers (Ca-induced calcium release). (2) Oota et al. (1972), and Chiarandini and Stefani (1973) have shown that manganese, a competitive inhibitor of the voltage-dependent increase of Ca permeability

(Hagiwara and Nakajima, 1966; Hagiwara and Takahashi, 1967), inhibited twitch and K contracture, whereas the action potential was not highly affected. (3) Stefani and Chiarandini (1973) have found that if external calcium was reduced to zero, in the presence of 4 mM Mg, K contracture was almost abolished. This effect of the calcium free solution took place very rapidly (within 40 sec).

There are findings that are in contradiction with the calcium hypothesis. These are: (4) Armstrong et al. (1972) observed that single muscle fibers continued to produce twitch in a medium in which the free calcium ion concentration was reduced below 10^{-8} M by EGTA. (5) Endo (*in preparation*) and Thorens and Endo (*in preparation*) have studied properties of the calcium-induced calcium release in skinned muscle fibers and compared with the depolarization induced Ca release (Endo and Nakajima, 1973). They found that under the physiological concentration of magnesium ions in the sarcoplasm and the physiological degree of calcium loading in the SR, the calcium-induced calcium release occurred only at a very high myoplasmic calcium ion concentration ($>10^{-4}$ M). This calcium concentration is too high to enable one to accept the hypothesis that calcium ions are the primary transmitter of the information from the T system to SR.

Given these findings, it is difficult to reach a clear-cut conclusion about the role of calcium current in the excitation-contraction coupling. The physiological role of Ca-induced Ca release seems to be weakened by fact (5). The finding (2) could be interpreted as merely reflecting that Mn has a stabilizing effect (Shanes, 1958); namely manganese, like calcium ions, will simply shift the threshold for activation to a more depolarizing direction. In fact, Caputo and Gimenez (1967), and Frankenhaeuser and Lännergren (1967) showed that calcium itself near physiologic range produced an inhibitory effect on twitch. It seems to us that the fact (4) is a very strong argument against the calcium-current theory in the sense described here. However, the fact (3) also seems convincing by showing that calcium in the T system is very critical in producing K contracture (not twitch), although this fact itself does not necessarily prove that Ca-current theory is correct. It could be that the external calcium plays an entirely different role than described here. We hope this somewhat unsatisfactory situation is resolved in the near future.

Macromolecular Bridge Hypothesis

Franzini-Armstrong (1970, 1974) has observed that a foot-like structure exists in the SR membrane that apposes the T system. These SR feet extend to the T system, but do not quite reach it. Chandler et al. (1976b) have hypothesized that this structure could serve to transmit information from the T system to the SR. They have further suggested that the nonlinear capacity that they observed could reflect a process of this information transmission (Schneider and Chandler, 1973; Adrian et al., 1976; Chandler et al., 1976a,b). However, the causal relationship between the nonlinear capacity and the contraction activation is not yet established beyond any doubt. Calcium could play an important role in some steps of the information transmission through the feet; and thus, some of the facts mentioned under the previous heading could be interpreted in the light of this hypothesis.

COMMENTS

This review has been confined to the topics of the T system of amphibian twitch muscles. The situation in other kinds of muscle is different, but no less important. The physiological role of the T system in cardiac muscle is not clear. In muscles of the invertebrates, notably those of *Crustacea,* the T system has different properties. For example, chloride permeability seems to be high (Girardier et al., 1963; Orentlicher and Reuben, 1971), and calcium current could play a more important role in the excitation-contraction coupling (Reuben et al., 1967; Zacharová and Zachar, 1967). The readers should refer to Atwood (1972) about these topics.

ACKNOWLEDGMENTS

We are grateful to Drs. Richard H. Adrian, Robert S. Eisenberg, Makoto Endo, Sir Alan Hodgkin, and Yasuko Nakajima for reading the manuscript. Our thanks to Ms. Frances Mather for editorial help. Supported in part by grant from NIH (NS-08601).

REFERENCES

Adrian, R. H. (1960): Potassium chloride movement and the membrane potential of frog muscle. *J. Physiol. (Lond.),* 151:154–185.

Adrian, R. H. (1964): The rubidium and potassium permeability of frog muscle membrane. *J. Physiol. (Lond.),* 175:134–159.

Adrian, R. H., and Almers, W. (1974): Membrane capacity measurements of frog skeletal muscle in media of low ion content. *J. Physiol. (Lond.),* 237:573–605.

Adrian, R. H., Chandler, W. K., and Hodgkin, A. L. (1969): The kinetics of mechanical activation in frog muscle. *J. Physiol. (Lond.),* 204:207–230.

Adrian, R. H., Chandler, W. K., and Hodgkin, A. L. (1970a): Voltage clamp experiments in striated muscle fibres. *J. Physiol. (Lond.),* 208:607–644.

Adrian, R. H., Chandler, W. K., and Hodgkin, A. L. (1970b): Slow changes in potassium permeability in skeletal muscle. *J. Physiol. (Lond.),* 208:645–668.

Adrian, R. H., Chandler, W. K., and Rakowski, R. F. (1976): Charge movement and mechanical repriming in skeletal muscle (*in press*).

Adrian, R. H., Costantin, L. L., and Peachey, L. D. (1969): Radial spread of contraction in frog muscle fibres. *J. Physiol. (Lond.),* 204:231–257.

Adrian, R. H., and Freygang, W. H. (1962a): The potassium and chloride conductance of frog muscle membrane. *J. Physiol. (Lond.),* 163:61–103.

Adrian, R. H., and Freygang, W. H. (1962b): Potassium conductance of frog muscle membrane under controlled voltage. *J. Physiol. (Lond.),* 163:104–114.

Adrian, R. H., and Peachey, L. D. (1973): Reconstruction of the action potential of frog sartorius muscle. *J. Physiol. (Lond.),* 235:103–131.

Almers, W. (1972): Potassium conductance changes in skeletal muscle and the potassium concentration in the transverse tubules. *J. Physiol. (Lond.)*, 225:33–56.

Armstrong, C. M., Bezanilla, F. M., and Horowicz, P. (1972): Twitches in the presence of ethylene glycol bis (β-amino-ethylether)-N, N'-tetraacetic acid. *Biochim. Biophys. Acta*, 267:605–608.

Atwood, H. L. (1972): Crustacean muscle. In: *The Structure and Function of Muscle*, edited by G. H. Bourne, pp. 421–489. Academic Press, New York.

Barry, P. H., and Adrian, R. H. (1973): Slow conductance changes due to potassium depletion in the transverse tubules of frog muscle fibers during hyperpolarizing pulses. *J. Membr. Biol.*, 14:243–292.

Bastian, J., and Nakajima, S. (1972): A Na dependent excitation in the transverse tubular system. *Fed. Proc.*, 31:323 Abs.

Bastian, J., and Nakajima, S. (1974): Action potential in the transverse tubules and its role in the activation of skeletal muscle. *J. Gen. Physiol.*, 63:257–278.

Bezanilla, F., Caputo, C., Gonzalez-Serratos, H., and Venosa, R. A. (1972): Sodium dependence of the inward spread of activation in isolated twitch muscle fibres of the frog. *J. Physiol. (Lond.)*, 223:507–523.

Caillé, J., Ildefonse, M., and Rougier, O. (1975): Relation between membrane potential, sodium currents and contraction in frog twitch muscle fibres. *Proc. Physiol. Soc., J. Physiol. (in press)*.

Caputo, C., and DiPolo, R. (1973): Ionic diffusion delays in the transverse tubules of frog twitch muscle fibres. *J. Physiol. (Lond.)*, 229:547–557.

Caputo, C., and Gimenez, M. (1967): Effects of external calcium deprivation on single muscle fibers. *J. Gen. Physiol.*, 50:2177–2195.

Chandler, W. K., Rakowski, R. F., and Schneider, M. F. (1976a): A non linear voltage dependent charge movement in frog skeletal muscle *(in press)*.

Chandler, W. K., Rakowski, R. F., and Schneider, M. F. (1976b): Effects of glycerol treatment and maintained depolarization on charge movement in skeletal muscle *(in press)*.

Chiarandini, D. J., and Stefani, E. (1973): Effects of manganese on the electrical and mechanical properties of frog skeletal muscle fibres. *J. Physiol. (Lond.)*, 232:129–147.

Cole, K. S. (1968): *Membranes, Ions and Impulses*. University of California Press, Berkeley.

Costantin, L. L. (1970): The role of sodium current in the radial spread of contraction in frog muscle fibers. *J. Gen. Physiol.*, 55:703–715.

Costantin, L. L., and Podolsky, R. J. (1967): Depolarization of the internal membrane system in the activation of frog skeletal muscle. *J. Gen. Physiol.* 50:1101–1124.

Costantin, L. L., and Taylor, S. R. (1971): Active and passive shortening in voltage-clamped frog muscle fibres. *J. Physiol. (Lond.)*, 218:13P.

Dulhunty, A., and Franzini-Armstrong, C. (1975): Variations in internal resistivity with sarcomere length in frog semitendinosus fibers. *Biophys. J.*, 15:130a.

Dulhunty, A. F., and Gage, P. W. (1973): Differential effects of glycerol treatment on membrane capacity and excitation-contraction coupling in toad sartorius fibres. *J. Physiol.*, 234:373–408.

Ebashi, S., and Endo, M. (1968): Calcium and muscle contraction. *Progr. Biophys. Mol. Biol.*, 18:123–183.

Ebashi, S., Endo, M., and Ohtsuki, I. (1969): Control of muscle contraction. *Q. Rev. Biophys.*, 2:351–384.

Eisenberg, R. S., and Gage, P. W. (1969): Ionic conductances of the surface and transverse tubular membranes of frog sartorius fibers. *J. Gen. Physiol.*, 53:279–297.

Endo, M. (1966): Entry of fluorescent dyes into the sarcotubular system of the frog muscle. *J. Physiol. (Lond.)*, 185:224–238.

Endo, M., and Nakajima, Y. (1973): Release of calcium induced by 'depolarization' of the sarcoplasmic reticulum membrane. *Nature New Biol.*, 246:216–218.

Endo, M., Tanaka, M., and Ogawa, Y. (1970): Calcium induced release of calcium from the sarcoplasmic reticulum of skinned skeletal muscle fibres. *Nature*, 228:34–36.

Falk, G., and Fatt, P. (1964): Linear electrical properties of striated muscle fibres observed with intracellular electrodes. *Proc. Roy. Soc. Lond. B*, 160:69–123.

Ford, L. E., and Podolsky, R. J. (1970): Regenerative calcium release within muscle cells. *Science*, 167:58–59.

Ford, L. E., and Podolsky, R. J. (1972): Intracellular calcium movements in skinned muscle fibres. *J. Physiol. (Lond.)*, 223:21–33.

Frankenhaeuser, B., and Lännergren, J. (1967): The effect of calcium on the mechanical response of single twitch muscle fibres of *Xenopus laevis*. *Acta Physiol. Scand.*, 69:242–254.

Franzini-Armstrong, C. (1970): Studies of the triad. I. Structure of the junction in frog twitch fibers. *J. Cell Biol.*, 47:488–499.

Franzini-Armstrong, C. (1974): Freeze fracture of skeletal muscle from the tarantula spider. *J. Cell Biol.*, 61:501–513.

Franzini-Armstrong, C., and Dulhunty, A. F. (1974): Contribution of folds and caveolae to the surface area of frog muscle fibers: A freeze-fracture study. *J. Cell Biol.*, 63:104a.

Franzini-Armstrong, C., Landmesser, L., and Pilar, G. (1975): Size and shape of transverse tubule openings in frog twitch muscle fibers. *J. Cell Biol.*, 64:493–497.

Freygang, W. H., Goldstein, D. A., and Hellam, D. G. (1964): The after-potential that follows trains of impulses in frog muscle fibres. *J. Gen. Physiol.*, 47:929–952.

Freygang, W. H., Jr., Rapoport, S. I., and Peachey, L. D. (1967): Some relations between changes in the linear electrical properties of striated muscle fibers and changes in ultrastructure. *J. Gen. Physiol.*, 50:2437–2458.

Fujino, M., Yamaguchi, T., and Suzuki, K. (1961): 'Glycerol effect' and the mechanism linking excitation of the plasma membrane with contraction. *Nature*, 192:1159–1161.

Gage, P. E., and Eisenberg, R. S. (1969a): Capacitance of the surface and transverse tubular membrane of frog sartorius muscle fibers. *J. Gen. Physiol.*, 53:265–278.

Gage, P. W., and Eisenberg, R. S. (1969b): Action potentials, after potentials, and excitation-contraction coupling in frog sartorius fibres without transverse tubules. *J. Gen. Physiol.*, 53:298–310.

Gilai, A. (1975): Alternating current analysis in scorpion muscle fibres. *Biophys. J.*, 15:256a.

Girardier, L., Reuben, J. P., Brandt, P. W., and Grundfest, H. (1963): Evidence for anion permselective membrane in crayfish muscle fibers and its role in excitation-contraction coupling. *J. Gen. Physiol.*, 47:189–214.

Gonzalez-Serratos, H. (1966): Inward spread of contraction during a twitch. *J. Physiol. (Lond.)*, 185:20P.

Gonzalez-Serratos, H. (1971): Inward spread of activation in vertebrate muscle fibres. *J. Physiol. (Lond.)*, 212:777–799.

Grundfest, H. (1961): Ionic mechanisms in electrogenesis. *Ann. N.Y. Acad. Sci.*, 94:405–457.

Grundfest, H. (1966): Heterogeneity of excitable membrane: electrophysiological and pharmacological evidence and some consequences. *Ann. N.Y. Acad. Sci.*, 137:901–949.

Hagiwara, S., and Nakajima, S. (1966): Differences in Na and Ca spikes as examined by application of tetrodotoxin, procaine, and manganese ions. *J. Gen. Physiol.*, 49:793–806.

Hagiwara, S., and Takahashi, K. (1967): Surface density of calcium ions and calcium spikes in the barnacle muscle fiber-membrane. *J. Gen. Physiol.*, 50:583–601.

Hodgkin, A. L., and Horowicz, P. (1959): The influence of potassium and chloride ions on the membrane potential of single muscle fibres. *J. Physiol. (Lond.)*, 148:127–160.

Hodgkin, A. L., and Horowicz, P. (1960a): The effect of sudden change in ionic concentration on the membrane potential of single fibres. *J. Physiol. (Lond.)*, 153:370–395.

Hodgkin, A. L., and Horowicz, P. (1960b): The effect of nitrate and other anions on the mechanical response of single muscle fibres. *J. Physiol. (Lond.)*, 153:404–412.

Hodgkin, A. L., and Huxley, A. F. (1952): A quantitative description of membrane currents and its application to conduction and excitation in nerve. *J. Physiol. (Lond.)*, 117:500–544.

Hodgkin, A. L., and Nakajima, S. (1972a): The effect of diameter on the electrical constant of frog skeletal muscle fibres. *J. Physiol. (Lond.)*, 221:105–120.

Hodgkin, A. L., and Nakajima, S. (1972b): Analysis of membrane capacity in frog muscle. *J. Physiol. (Lond.)*, 221:121–136.

Horowicz, P., Gage, P. W., and Eisenberg, R. S. (1968): The role of the electrochemical gradient in determining potassium fluxes in frog striated muscle. *J. Gen. Physiol.*, 51:193S–203S.

Howell, J. N., and Jenden, D. J. (1967): T-tubules of skeletal muscle; morphological alterations which interrupt excitation-contraction coupling. *Fed. Proc.*, 26:553.

Hutter, O. F., and Noble, D. (1960): The chloride conductance of frog skeletal muscle. *J. Physiol. (Lond.)*, 151:89–102.

Huxley, A. F. (1971): The activation of striated muscle and its mechanical response. *Proc. Roy. Soc. Lond. B*, 178:1–27.

Huxley, A. F., and Taylor, R. E. (1958): Local activation of striated muscle fibres. *J. Physiol. (Lond.)*, 144:426–441.

Jaimovich, E., Venosa, R. A., Shrager, P., and Horowicz, P. (1975): Tetrodotoxin (TTX) binding in normal and 'detubulated' frog sartorius muscle. *Biophys. J.*, 15:255a.

Julian, F. J., Moore, J. W., and Goldman, D. E. (1962): Membrane potentials of the lobster giant axon obtained by use of the sucrose-gap technique. *J. Gen. Physiol.*, 45:1195–1216.

Katz, B. (1948): The electrical properties of the muscle fibre membrane. *Proc. Roy. Soc. Lond. B*, 135:506–534.

Katz, B. (1949): Les constantes electriques de la membrane du muscle. *Arch. Sci. Physiol.*, 3:285–300.

Krolenko, S. A. (1969): Changes in the T-system of muscle fibres under the influence of influx and efflux of glycerol. *Nature*, 221:966–968.

Lüttgau, H. C. (1960): Das Kalium-Transportsystem am Ranvier-Knoten isolierter markhaltiger Nervenfasern. *Pflügers Arch. Ges. Physiol.*, 271:613–633.

Mobley, B. A., and Eisenberg, B. R. (1975): Quantitative morphological analysis of frog skeletal muscle using method of stereology. *Biophys. J.*, 15:254a.

Nakajima, S., and Bastian, J. (1974): Double sucrose-gap method applied to single muscle fiber of *Xenopus laevis*. *J. Gen. Physiol.*, 63:235–256.

Nakajima, S., Iwasaki, S., and Obata, K. (1962): Delayed rectification and anomalous rectification in frog's skeletal muscle membrane. *J. Gen. Physiol.*, 46:97–115.

Nakajima, S., Nakajima, Y., and Bastian, J. (1975): Effects of sudden changes in external sodium concentration on twitch tension in isolated muscle fibers. *J. Gen. Physiol.*, 65:459–482.

Nakajima, S., Nakajima, Y., and Peachey, L. D. (1973): Speed of repolarization and morphology of glycerol-treated frog muscle fibres. *J. Physiol. (Lond.)*, 234:465–480.

Natori, R. (1954): The property and contraction process of isolated myofibrils. *Jikei Med. J.*, 1:119–126.

Natori, R. (1955): Repeated contraction and conductive contraction observed in isolated myofibrils. *Jikeikai Med. J.*, 2:1–5.

Oota, I., Takauji, M., and Nagai, T. (1972): Effect of manganese ions on excitation-contraction coupling in frog sartorius muscle. *Jap. J. Physiol.*, 22:379–392.

Orentlicher, M., and Reuben, J. P. (1971): Localization of ionic conductances in crayfish muscle fibers. *J. Membr. Biol.*, 4:209–226.

Peachey, L. D. (1965): The sarcoplasmic reticulum and transverse tubules of the frog's sartorius. *J. Cell Biol.*, 25:209–231.

Reuben, J. P., Brandt, P. W., Garcia, H., and Grundfest, H. (1967): Excitation-contraction coupling in crayfish. *Am. Zoologist*, 7:623–645.

Schneider, M. F. (1970): Linear electrical properties of the transverse tubules and surface membrane of skeletal muscle fibers. *J. Gen. Physiol.*, 56:640–671.

Schneider, M. F., and Chandler, W. K. (1973): Voltage dependent charge movement in skeletal muscle: a possible step in excitation-contraction coupling. *Nature*, 242:244–246.

Shanes, A. M. (1958): Electrochemical aspects of physiological and pharmacological action in excitable cells. Part II. The action potential and excitation. *Pharmacol. Rev.*, 10:165–273.

Stefani, E., and Chiarandini, D. J. (1973): Skeletal muscle: Dependence of potassium contractures on extracellular calcium. *Pflügers Arch.*, 343:143–150.

Strickholm, A. (1966): Local sarcomere contraction in fast muscle fibres. *Nature*, 212:835–836.

Sugi, H. (1974): Inward spread of activation in frog muscle fibres investigated by means of high-speed microcinematography. *J. Physiol. (Lond.)*, 242:219–235.

Sugi, H., and Ochi, R. (1967): The mode of transverse spread of contraction initiated by local activation in single frog muscle fibres. *J. Gen. Physiol.*, 50:2167–2176.

Valdiosera, R., Clausen, C., and Eisenberg, R. S. (1974a): Measurement of the impedance of frog skeletal muscle fibers. *Biophys. J.* 14:295–315.

Valdiosera, R., Clausen, C., and Eisenberg, R. S. (1974b): Circuit models of the passive electrical properties of frog skeletal muscle fibers. *J. Gen. Physiol.*, 63:432–459.

Valdiosera, R., Clausen, C., and Eisenberg, R. S. (1974c): Impedance of frog skeletal muscle fibers in various solutions. *J. Gen. Physiol.*, 63:460–491.

Zacharová, D., and Zachar, J. (1967): The effect of external calcium ions on the excitation-contraction coupling in single muscle fibres of the crayfish. *Physiol. Bohemoslov.*, 16:191–207.

Electrobiology of Nerve, Synapse, and Muscle,
edited by J. P. Reuben, D. P. Purpura, M. V. L. Bennett,
and E. R. Kandel. Raven Press, New York © 1976

Mechanism of Inward Spread of Activation in the Transverse Tubular System of Frog Skeletal Muscle Fibers

Haruo Sugi

*Department of Physiology, Teikyo University, School of Medicine,
Itabashi-ku, Tokyo, Japan*

Although it is now generally accepted that, in striated muscle, the influence of surface membrane depolarization spreads inwards along the transverse tubular system (T system) to bring myofibrils into activity, the mechanism of the inward spread of activation within the T system has not been firmly established. In 1958, Huxley and Taylor observed only a graded type of local contraction in response to a highly localized membrane depolarization, suggesting that the inward spread of contraction is due to a passive electrotonic spread of depolarization along the T tubules. On the other hand, however, evidence has been accumulating that, in addition to the electrotonic spread of depolarization, the T tubules have a kind of regenerative mechanism which may contribute to the inward spread of activation. With a local activation technique similar to that of Huxley and Taylor (1958) but stimulating many sarcomeres, Sugi and Ochi (1965*a,b*, 1967*a,b*) found that, in both crayfish and frog muscle fibers, a strong negative current caused a local contraction spreading around the whole fiber perimeter, whereas moderate depolarizations produced graded contractions. Using the same method, Strickholm (1966) reported a local contraction spreading directly across a frog muscle fiber. These findings strongly suggested some kind of regenerative mechanism in the T system.

More recently, Costantin (1970) and Costantin and Taylor (1971) showed that the radial spread of contraction in voltage-clamped frog muscle fibers was influenced by tetrodotoxin and the external Na ion concentration. Bezanilla et al., (1972) and Caputo and Dipolo (1973) reported that the contractile response in a twitch was reduced when the Na ion concentration in the tubular lumen was lowered in various ways. Bastian and Nakajima (1972, 1974) demonstrated that the twitch height of the artificial node of frog fibers decreased markedly when the node was made inexcitable by tetrodotoxin or removal of external Na ions at 20°C. These results indicate the possibility that the tubular membrane has a regenerative Na conductance mechanism similar to that of the surface membrane. For establishing the functional role of the T system, however, more experimental work is needed on the mode of inward spread of activation.

According to Strickholm (1966), a complicated seasonal variation in both electrical and mechanical responses to local membrane depolarization occurs between winter and summer frog fibers. Since the local activation experiments of Sugi and Ochi (1965*b*, 1967*b*) were made only on winter frogs, it seems desirable to repeat similar experiments on summer frogs with a much improved recording apparatus to examine whether any type of local contraction other than the graded one can be produced by moderate depolarizations.

PHASIC AND TONIC COMPONENTS OF LOCAL CONTRACTION IN RESPONSE TO MODERATE DEPOLARIZATIONS

Single fast muscle fibers showing the all-or-none twitch were isolated from the semitendinous muscles of the frog (*Rana nigromaculata* or *Rana japonica*), and mounted horizontally in a glass trough for microscopic observation. A limited area of the surface membrane was depolarized by applying rectangular current pulses to a pipette whose tip (external diameter, 50–120 μm) was in contact with the fiber surface, the approximate magni-

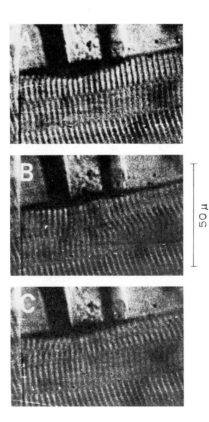

FIG. 1. Selected frames from a ciné-film (3,000 frames/sec) of the phasic response elicited by a 500 msec current pulse producing depolarization of 25 mV. **A:** resting fiber; **B,C:** frames taken at 50 and 150 msec after the onset of current pulse, respectively. The pipette for local activation is in contact with the upper edge of the fiber. (From Sugi, 1974, by permission of *J. Physiol.*)

tude of membrane depolarization being calculated by multiplying the contact resistance of the pipette, i.e., the increase of pipette resistance when the tip was brought into contact with the fiber surface, by the applied current. Further details of the method have been described elsewhere (Sugi and Ochi, 1967*a;* Sugi, 1974). The resulting local contractions were recorded with a 16-mm high-speed cinecamera (Hicam, Redlake Corp.) at 1,000 to 3,000 frames/sec, and analyzed with a film motion analyzer (Vanguard) by constructing contraction curves of the same sarcomeres at various distances from the depolarized area of the fiber surface.

The experiments were first made on fibers from *Rana nigromaculata* obtained in summer (from June to September), using pipettes of 20 to 40 μm diameter. In some of the fibers examined, moderate membrane depolarizations (20–30 mV) initiated a phasic type of local contractions as shown in Figs. 1 and 2. This type of local contraction differed from the graded local contractions in the following respects: (1) the response had a definite

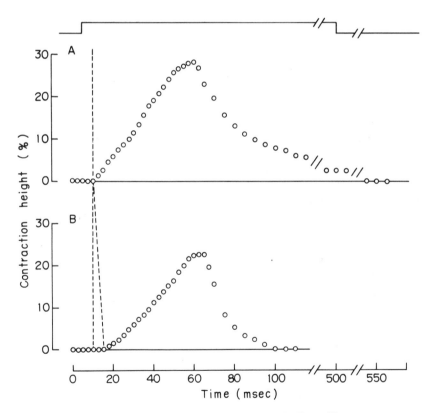

FIG. 2. Contraction curves of the phasic response shown in Fig. 1. The curves were constructed by measuring the length of five sarcomeres at the depolarized fiber surface **(A)** and at the inner part 14 μm distant from the fiber surface. Time course of the current pulse is shown at the top of the figure. (From Sugi, 1974, by permission of *J. Physiol.*)

threshold; and (2) the contraction started to relax spontaneously while the current pulse producing depolarization still continued. In Fig. 2, it can be seen that the contraction is first initiated at the depolarized fiber surface and then spreads inwards with a velocity of 0.7–2 cm/sec at 18°–26°C, and that the phasic contraction at the fiber surface is followed by a much smaller tonic contraction maintained as long as the current pulse goes on. The latter tonic component of the response was regarded to be identical with the graded contraction observed in the rest of fibers used, since the graded response was usually just barely perceptible with depolarizations of 20 to 30 mV, and its magnitude was increased in a graded manner with increasing depolarizations.

When the fiber was locally depolarized with pipettes of more than 50 to 60 μm diameter, the resulting response showed a conspicuous feature. A typical response initiated by a depolarization of nearly the threshold value is shown in Figs. 3 and 4. It can be seen in Fig. 3 that the contraction is first initiated at the inner part of the sarcomeres opposite the pipette, and the extent of contraction is greater at this part than at the depolarized fiber

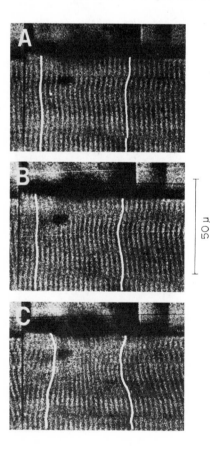

FIG. 3. Selected frames from a ciné-film (2,000 frames/sec) of a muscle fiber at rest **(A)** and during the phasic response **(B,C)** elicited by a 500 msec current pulse producing depolarization of 20 mV. Frames **B** and **C** were taken at 15 and 40 msec after the onset of current pulse, respectively. White lines in each frame mark 18 sarcomeres. The ciné-records in Figs. 1 and 3 were obtained on one and the same fiber. (From Sugi, 1974, by permission of *J. Physiol.*)

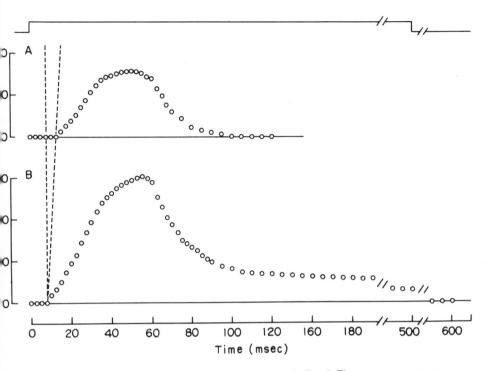

FIG. 4. Contraction curves of the phasic response shown in Fig. 3. The curves were constructed by measuring the length of 10 sarcomeres at the depolarized fiber surface **(A)** and at the inner part 15 μm distance from the fiber surface **(B)**. (From Sugi, 1974, by permission of *J. Physiol.*)

surface. In addition, the phasic contraction at the inner part was followed by the tonic contraction which relaxed only after the termination of the current pulse.

PRESENCE OF THE REGENERATIVE MECHANISM WITHIN THE T SYSTEM AND ITS POSSIBLE ROLE IN NORMAL CONTRACTION

The phasic type of local contraction with a definite threshold may be taken to indicate that, at least in fibers with the phasic response, the T system has some kind of regenerating mechanism which contributes to the inward spread of activation along the T tubules in addition to the passive electrotonic depolarization. Then, the phasic nature of the response may well be accounted for by assuming that a brief, transient potential change analogous to the action potential at the surface membrane is set up in the T tubules by a moderate depolarization to cause a rapid phasic contraction.

The duration of the phasic contraction was about 100 msec at room temperature, being comparable with the duration of isotonic twitches in frog fast muscle fibers (Buchthal and Kaiser, 1951). This suggests that the regenerative process is actually involved in normal twitches. In fibers with the initial sarcomere length of 2.5 to 3 μm, the shortening occurred almost linearly with time for the first three quarters of the change in length or more (Figs. 2 and 4). The shortening velocity at this phase of the phasic response ranged from 15 to 25 μm/sec per sarcomere, being comparable to the shortening velocity of frog fibers at a load of 0.05 P_0 (9.1 length/sec or about 20 μm/sec per sarcomere, Buchthal and Kaiser, 1951). This indicates that the locally activated sarcomeres contracted against a very small load.

On the other hand, in fibers which showed only the graded contractions, the shortening velocity of the locally activated sarcomeres in response to depolarizations of 50 to 80 mV was always less than 10 μm/sec per sarcomere, being much smaller than the shortening velocity in the phasic response though the extent of contraction finally attained was as large as that of the phasic response. This difference of shortening velocity between the phasic and the graded responses seems to indicate that the myofibrils can be activated much more rapidly by the regenerative mechanism than by the passive electrotonic spread of depolarization in the T system. This implies that the abrupt development of active state in frog muscle (Hill, 1949) may be related to the regenerative mechanism. Though it is not at present possible to exclude the possibility that the dissection procedures may impair the regenerative mechanism which exists in all the fibers examined, it is of interest that there is a large variation in the twitch-tetanus ratio in both single fibers (Ramsey and Street, 1941) and whole muscles (Close, 1972). If the large twitch is associated with the regenerative mechanism, then the twitch-tetanus ratio of whole muscles should reflect the percentage of fibers having the regenerative mechanism.

NATURE OF THE REGENERATIVE MECHANISM

In most cases, the phasic type of local contraction spread inwards only to a certain extent, even when a large area of surface membrane was depolarized. In some cases the phasic response was observed to spread right across the fiber, though the number of sarcomeres involved in the response decreased progressively with distance from the depolarized fiber surface as shown in Fig. 5. These features of the phasic response indicate that the regenerative process may propagate along the T tubules with a considerable decrement. A possible explanation for this decrement may be a low safety factor for propagation especially when the regenerative process is set up at a limited part of the T tubule network, since the T tubules branch more and more as the distance from the site of initiation of the regenerative process increases.

The effect of tetrodotoxin (TTX, 10^{-7} g/ml) or removal of external Na ions on the phasic response was somewhat variable. In two fibers of about 50 μm diameter, the phasic response was reversibly inhibited within 5 min

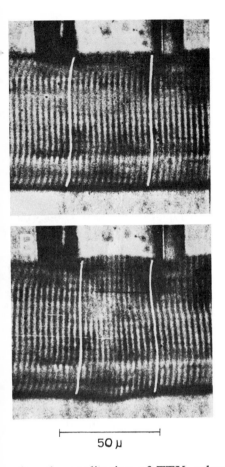

FIG. 5. Frames from a ciné-film (2,000 frames/sec) of a resting fiber **(A)** and local contraction spreading directly across the fiber **(B)**. White lines mark 15 sarcomeres. (From Sugi, 1974, by permission of *J. Physiol.*)

50 μ

after the application of TTX, whereas in three fibers of 100 to 120 μm diameter, the phasic response could be seen for more than 30 min in the presence of TTX or in the absence of external Na ions. The variability of the results suggests that, in addition to the Na conductance mechanism, the T system has some other mechanism for active propagation. The local contraction spreading around the whole perimeter of crayfish and frog muscle fibers observed by Sugi and Ochi was also not sensitive to TTX or removal of external Na.

POSSIBLE CAUSE OF THE APPARENT REVERSAL OF POTENTIAL GRADIENT ALONG THE T TUBULES

When a large area of surface membrane was depolarized, the phasic contraction was first initiated at the inner sarcomeres, and the extent of contraction was maximum at this location during the course of the response (Figs. 3 and 4). These observations suggest that the magnitude of depolarization across the T-tubule membrane is larger in the deep tubules than in the superficial tubules. This apparent reversal of potential gradient along the T tubules in the radial direction has been observed in voltage-clamped frog muscle fibers (Costantin, 1970; Costantin and Taylor, 1971). Costantin (1970) explained this phenomenon as being due to a net inward current throughout the entire T system caused by a regenerative increase in Na conductance. It seems, however, difficult to explain the presence of the tonic component of local contraction at the inner part of sarcomeres during a prolonged depolarization (Fig. 4), since the inward Na current similar to that of muscle fiber action potential decays rapidly due to inactivation during a maintained depolarization (Adrian et al., 1970).

At present, there seems to be no simple explanation for the apparent reversal of radial potential gradient along the T tubules. Some possibilities that might account for this phenomenon are as follows: (1) the regenerative mechanism(s) responsible for the net inward current throughout the entire T system has a much slower inactivation process than that of an action potential, (2) the threshold depolarization of the T tubules for activating the neighboring myofibrils is not uniform in the entire T system, being much lower in the deep tubules than in the superficial tubules, and (3) the organization of the T-tubule network is such that, during the passage of a current through a large pipette for local activation, the electrotonic depolarization is maximum at the deep tubules. The last possibility rests on the assumption that the conductivity of the network formed by the tubular lumen is not uniform in all directions; if the tubular lumen has a much higher conductivity in the radial direction than in other directions, then, with an appropriately large pipette for local activation, the current density across the tubular membrane would be expected to be larger in the deep tubules than in the superficial tubules as a consequence of the radial convergence of the T tubules. Experiments are presently being done to examine this possibility.

REFERENCES

Adrian, R. H., Chandler, W. K., and Hodgkin, A. L. (1970). Voltage clamp experiments in striated muscle fibres. *J. Physiol.*, 208:607–644.

Bastian, J., and Nakajima, S. (1972). A sodium dependent excitation in the transverse tubular system. *Fed. Proc.*, 31:323A.

Bastian, J., and Nakajima, S. (1974). Action potential in the transverse tubules and its role in the activation of skeletal muscle. *J. Gen. Physiol.*, 63:257–278.

Bezanilla, F., Caputo, C., Gonzalez-Serratos, H., and Venosa, A. (1972). Sodium dependence of the inward spread of activation in isolated twitch muscle fibres of the frog. *J. Physiol.*, 223:507–523.

Buchthal, F., and Kaiser, E. (1951). The rheology of the cross striated muscle fibre with special reference to isotonic conditions. *Dann. Biol. Medd.*, 21:7.

Caputo, C., and Dipolo, R. (1973). Ionic diffusion delays in the transverse tubules of frog twitch muscle fibres. *J. Physiol.*, 229:547–557.

Close, R. I. (1972). The relations between sarcomere length and characteristics of isometric twitch contractions of frog sartorius muscle. *J. Physiol.*, 220:745–762.

Costantin, L. L. (1970). The role of sodium current in the radial spread of contraction in frog muscle fibers. *J. Gen. Physiol.*, 55:703–715.

Costantin, L. L., and Taylor, S. R. (1971). Active and passive shortening in voltage-clamped frog muscle fibres. *J. Physiol.*, 218:13–15P.

Hill, A. V. (1949). The abrupt transition from rest to activity in muscle. *Proc. Roy. Soc. B*, 136:399–420.

Huxley, A. F., and Taylor, R. E. (1958). Local activation of striated muscle fibres. *J. Physiol.*, 144:426–441.

Ramsey, R. W., and Street, S. F. (1941). Muscle function as studied in single muscle fibres. *Biol. Symp.*, 3:9–34.

Strickholm, A. (1966). Local sarcomere contraction in fast muscle fibres. *Nature (Lond.)*, 212:835–836.

Sugi, H. (1974). Inward spread of activation in frog muscle fibres investigated by means of high-speed microcinematography. *J. Physiol.*, 242:219–235.

Sugi, H., and Ochi, R. (1965a). The mode of transverse spread of contraction initiated by local membrane depolarization in crayfish muscle fibres. *Proc. Jap. Acad. Sci.*, 41:423–427.

Sugi, H., and Ochi, R. (1965b). The mode of transverse spread of contraction initiated by local membrane depolarization in frog muscle fibres. *Proc. Jap. Acad. Sci.*, 41:864–868.

Sugi, H., and Ochi, R. (1967a). The mode of transverse spread of contraction initiated by local activation in single crayfish muscle fibers. *J. Gen. Physiol.*, 50:2145–2166.

Sugi, H., and Ochi, R. (1967b). The mode of transverse spread of contraction initiated by local activation in single frog muscle fibers. *J. Gen. Physiol.*, 50:2167–2176.

Electrobiology of Nerve, Synapse, and Muscle,
edited by J. P. Reuben, D. P. Purpura, M. V. L. Bennett,
and E. R. Kandel. Raven Press, New York © 1976

Quinidine-Induced Spikes in Lobster Muscle Fibers

Nobufumi Kawai

*Department of Neurobiology, Tokyo Metropolitan Institute for Neurosciences,
2-6 Fuchu City, Tokyo, Japan*

In crustacean muscle fibers, spike electrogenesis occurs due to an increase in membrane conductance towards Ca ions (see Fatt and Katz, 1953; Werman and Grundfest, 1961). A number of agents induce "Ca spikes" in crustacean muscle fibers by apparently either enhancing Ca conductance, e.g., caffeine (Reuben et al., 1967; Chiarandini et al., 1970) or by blocking K channels, e.g., TEA and procaine (Fatt and Katz, 1953; Reuben and Grundfest, 1960; Takeda, 1967). Quinidine was found to produce Ca spikes with characteristics significantly different from those induced by modification of the Ca and/or K conductances by agents like caffeine or procaine. A preliminary account has been published elsewhere (Kawai and Grundfest, 1972).

METHODS

The experiments to be discussed were done on the stretcher muscle of the walking leg of lobster, *Hormarus americanus*. The exoskeleton over the stretcher muscle was removed and the meropodite and propodite were clamped in order to prevent shortening of the muscle. The experiments were performed at room temperature (20°–25°C). The standard solution contained 468 mM NaCl, 15 mM KCl, and 22 mM CaCl$_2$ and the pH was adjusted with Tris buffer, 7.5). The Ca concentration was varied by stoichiometric substitution of Mg or Ba for Ca. Quinidine was used in concentrations ranging from 0.1 to 1 mM, caffeine at 10 mM, and procaine hydrochloride ranged from 10^{-4} to 10^{-3} wt/vol.

The recording microelectrode contained 3 M KCl and the resistance varied from 3 to 5 Mohms. Intracellular stimulating microelectrodes were filled with 2 M K-citrate. The distance between stimulating and recording electrodes was between 200 and 400 μm. In most of the experiments, floating electrodes were used for both stimulating and recording to minimize the muscle movement which accompanied the action potentials. The floating electrodes were made by inserting fine silver wires (100 μm) into the glass capillaries which were cut at 5–7 mm from the tip and suspended by the wire. The volume of the solution bathing the preparation was approximately 5 ml. Solutions were replaced by aspiration.

RESULTS

Characteristics of Action Potentials Induced by Quinidine

After a period of soaking (15 to 30 min) in a solution containing quinidine, the normally graded responses of the stretcher muscle were covered into all-or-none action potentials (Fig. 1A,B). A fast rising phase was followed by a plateau phase which lasted for several hundred milliseconds and terminated with a slow falling phase. Direct stimulation was applied at intervals of a few minutes. At shorter intervals, the successive responses declined and became graded. Quinidine-treated fibers continued to generate spikes for a couple of hours even after removal of quinidine from the bathing saline. However, the amplitude and duration of the spikes was dependent on the amount of quinidine applied (Fig. 1C). Because of the long induction time (15 to 30 min) it was not possible to determine the relationship between the spike overshoot and the dose of quinidine (see Chiarandini et al., 1970). The graph in Fig. 1 is an I-V curve obtained from a muscle before (open circles) and after (filled circles) treatment with quinidine. The fact that one curve describes both sets of data indicates that the resting conductance channels are not modified by quinidine.

Conductance Change During Quinidine Spike

In order to determine the conductance change during the action potential, brief hyperpolarizing currents were applied. Either single hyperpolarizing pulses were applied at a series of intervals after the onset of the action potential or trains of pulses were used (insert, Fig. 2). The relative conductance change was measured by estimating the ratio of effective resistance between the resting and active states. In Fig. 2, the dotted line, superimposed on the spike, is the time course of the relative change of effective resistance during the action potential. The value was averaged from eight muscles. A measurement of the effective resistance during the rising phase of the action potential by the use of this procedure was not possible. At the beginning of the plateau phase the relative conductance was less than one-third of the resting state and it declined rapidly in 70 to 80 msec even though the plateau persisted for about 200 msec.

Effects of Ca

The data in Fig. 3 denote that spike electrogenesis induced by quinidine is dependent upon the concentration of Ca in the medium and independent of the Na. The action potential persisted in preparations treated with tetrodotoxin (TTX) (10^{-6} g/ml) (Fig. 3B), and with solutions in which NaCl was replaced with osmotically equivalent amounts of sucrose. After soaking the

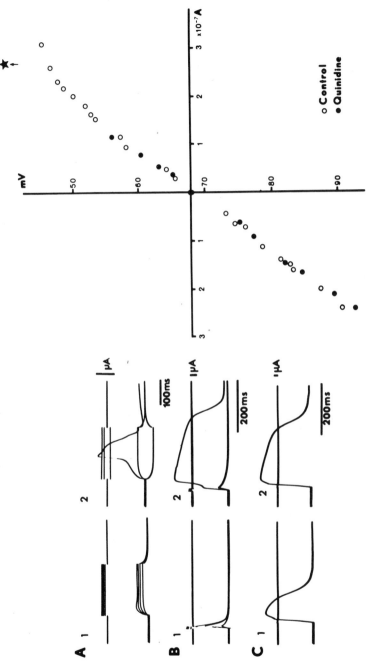

FIG. 1. Spike generation induced by quinidine. **A:1**—Graded response in normal saline. Lower tracings are records of membrane potential and upper tracings are current. In this and following figures the zero trace is the zero reference for the membrane potential of the lower trace. **A:2**—Same muscle as **A:1** but after treatment with 0.1 mM quinidine sulfate for 15 min. **B:1**—Response to short duration pulse in normal saline. **B:2**—After soaking in 1 mM quinidine. **C:1**—Spike in 0.1 mM quinidine. **C:2**—In 1 mM quinidine. Graph shows the current voltage relation before (*open circles*) and after (*filled circles*) treatment with quinidine (1 mM). *Arrow* (start) indicates threshold for spike.

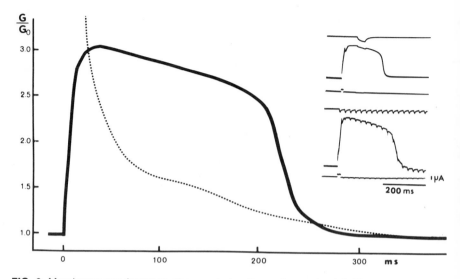

FIG. 2. Membrane conductance change during the action potential. Time course of the action potential (*solid line*) and relative conductance (*dotted line*). *Ordinate:* ratio of effective membrane resistance during action potential (G) to resting state (G$_0$). *Abscissa:* time after the onset of spike. *Inset records:* measurement of effective resistance with applied hyperpolarizing pulses. *Upper trace* is the potential displacement at rest; *middle trace*, during action potential; *bottom trace*, current recordings. (Further description is in the text.)

muscle in this Na-free solution the spike height became slightly smaller and the duration was considerably longer than that in normal saline (Fig. 3A:2). This difference may be due to the change in Cl content between the normal and NaCl-free solutions. Increasing the Ca concentration in the Na-free saline led to an enhancement of both the amplitude and duration (Fig. 3A:3). The spike overshoot in normal (open circles) and Na-free salines (filled circles) was measured for a series of increasing Ca concentrations (graph, Fig. 3). The slope is approximately 29 mV per decade Ca for Ca concentrations below 200 mM for both sets of points.

Figure 4 shows the effects of reducing the Ca concentration in external medium on the amplitude and time course of the spike. Upon reducing the Ca concentration to three-fourths of normal (16.5 mM), the amplitude of the action potential was depressed (B,C) and a further reduction to one-half abolished the spike (D). The abolition was not due to an increase in threshold since even stronger stimuli did not produce an action potential (E). The rate of rise of the action potential was also decreased upon reducing the Ca concentration. The effects of reducing Ca were reversible (G).

Effects of Ba

Quinidine spikes were markedly enhanced when a small amount (5 mM) of BaCl$_2$ was added to the bathing solution (Fig. 5B). At higher Ba concentra-

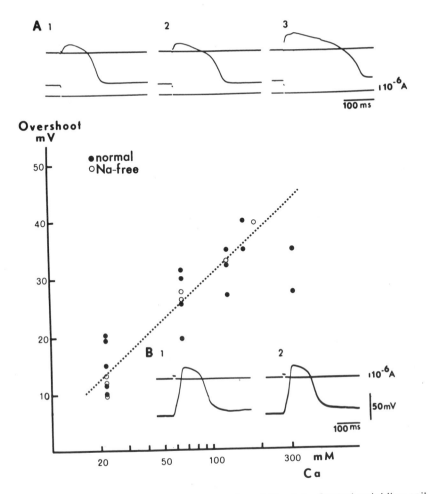

FIG. 3. Dependence of quinidine spike on external Ca. **A:1** — Control quinidine spike. **A:2** — After replacing NaCl with sucrose. **A:3** — After Ca was raised to 66 mM in the Na-free saline. **B:1** — Control. **B:2** — After addition of TTX 10⁻⁶ g/ml. The overshoot of the quinidine spike versus the log Ca concentration forms the graph. *Filled circles,* Na-saline; *open circles,* Na-free saline. The broken line indicates the slope of 29 mV for a 10-fold increase in Ca.

tions, in which the Ca and part of the Na were replaced with Ba, the action potentials were further potentiated (Fig. 4D,E). The duration of the action potentials in the presence of Ba lasted for several seconds and the refractory period was prolonged (> 30 min). In solutions containing large amounts of Ba, the resting potentials were somewhat decreased (Fig. 5D,E). This depolarization of the muscle in high Ba-containing media was previously described (Werman and Grundfest, 1961; Hagiwara and Naka, 1964; Takeda, 1967). In the graph of Fig. 4 the overshoot of the action potentials was plotted against the Ba concentration. The slope (data from four muscles)

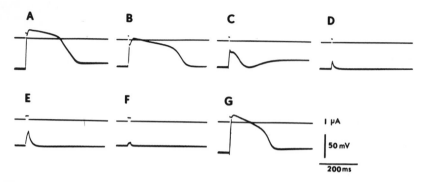

FIG. 4. Effect of reducing Ca.**A:** control; **B:** 7 min; **C:** at 10 min after reducing Ca concentration to 16.5 mM. Spikes could not be elicited at a Ca concentration of 11 mM (**D,E**) or lower (**F**). Recovery of spike after exposure to normal Ca (**G**).

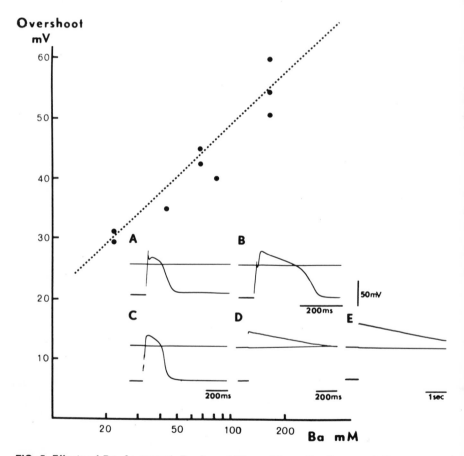

FIG. 5. Effects of Ba. **A:** control; **B:** after addition of 5 mM Ba. **C:** control; **D:** 44 mM Ba; **E:** 180 mM Ba. Overshoot of the quinidine spike is the ordinate and the log of Ba concentration is the abscissa of the graph.

is approximately 30 mV/decade Ba. It appears that Ba can replace Ca in the depolarizing electrogenesis induced by quinidine.

Effects of Mn

As described above, the action potentials induced by quinidine require a permeability increase toward divalent cations. The suppression of Ca spikes by Mn is well documented (see Fatt and Ginsborg, 1958; Hagiwara and Nakajima, 1966). When $MnCl_2$ in concentrations of more than 15 mM was applied to the muscle, the quinidine spike was blocked immediately. The data of Fig. 6 shows the effects of Mn at concentrations lower than 15 mM. After a 3 min exposure to Mn an abortive response was observed (Fig. 6B). At 5 min only a local response remained (Fig. 6C), which was essentially blocked after 7 min (Fig. 6D). The action potential reappeared after a 15-min exposure to normal saline (Fig. 6E). At a higher concentration (10 mM) the blockage was more rapid and recovery was slower (Fig. 6F–H).

Comparison with Caffeine-Induced Spikes

Caffeine induces action potentials in crayfish muscle by promoting an entry of Ca (Chiarandini et al., 1970). In the present experiment 20 mM caffeine was sufficient to generate the action potentials in the lobster muscle within a fraction of a minute. The effect of caffeine was easily removed by flushing the preparation with normal solution. The caffeine-induced action potentials do not show a prolonged plateau phase. In the scatter diagram of Fig. 7, spike overshoots induced by caffeine (open circles) and quinidine (filled circles) were plotted against their durations. Although the duration of quinidine-induced spikes increased with increasing overshoot, the duration of the caffeine spikes is not a function of the overshoot. The lower inset records of Fig. 7 show the interaction between caffeine and quinidine (A,B). Both amplitude and duration of the caffeine-spike were increased when

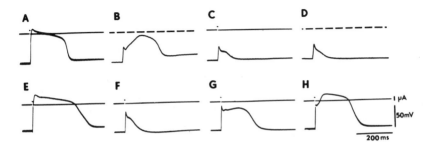

FIG. 6. Effect of Mn. **A:** control spike; **B:** 3 min after applying 5 mM Mn; **C:** 5 min; **D:** 7 min; **E:** recovery after washing out Mn; **F:** 3 min after applying 10 mM Mn; **G:** partial recovery after removal of Mn; **H:** complete recovery.

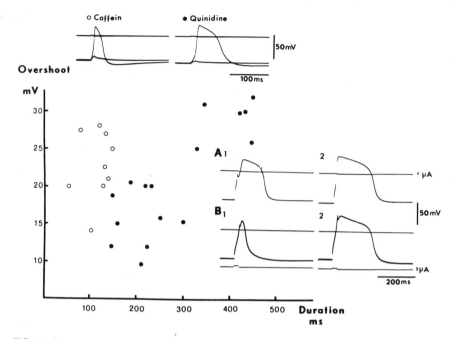

FIG. 7. Comparison between caffeine and quinidine spikes. The overshoot of caffeine (*open circles*) and quinidine (*filled circles*) spikes vs spike duration forms the scatter diagram. The upper insets are recordings of a caffeine and quinidine spike. The lower recordings are: **A:1**—spike induced by 1 mM quinidine; **A:2**—after addition of 10 mM caffeine; **B:1**—caffeine spike by 10 mM caffeine; **B:2**—after adding 1 mM quinidine. (Further description in text.)

quinidine was added (B:1,2). On the other hand, after addition of caffeine the amplitude of quinidine-evoked spikes was enhanced, but to a lesser degree (A:1,2).

Comparison with Procaine-Induced Spikes

Depolarization of procaine-treated crayfish fibers induces prolonged action potentials (Grundfest, 1961; Takeda, 1967) that are similar in duration to the quinidine spikes in lobster fibers. Prolonged action potentials were also observed in the lobster muscle fibers treated with procaine (10^{-4} to 10^{-3} wt/vol). The interaction of procaine and quinidine appears to be complicated (Fig. 8). Procaine (10^{-3} wt/vol) usually prolonged quinidine-induced spikes (7 cases out of 12 cells). In the remaining five cells the action potentials were either not affected or slightly reduced in duration. Similar results were obtained by reversing the order of exposure in which case quinidine usually prolonged the procaine-induced spikes (four out of six fibers). The amplitude and kinetics of the action potentials induced by procaine and quinidine were affected by increasing the Ca concentration of

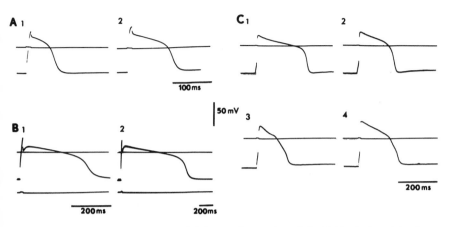

FIG. 8. A,B: Interaction between quinidine and procaine. **A:1** – Spike induced by 1 mM quinidine. **A:2** – after an addition of procaine 1 × 10⁻³ wt/vol. **B:1** – Spike induced by procaine 1 × 10⁻³ wt/vol. **B:2** – After adding 1 mM procaine-induced spike in the presence of normal Ca (22 mM) **(C:1)** and in 66 mM Ca saline **(C:2)**. Quinidine spikes in fibers bathed in normal Ca **(C:3)** and in 66 mM Ca saline **(C:4)**. (Further description in text.)

the medium. The overshoot of the procaine-induced action potential was enhanced, but the duration was shortened. This stands in marked contrast to the quinidine spike in which both overshoot and duration were increased by raising Ca (Fig. 3).

DISCUSSION

Quinidine is known as an antiarrhythmic drug for heart muscles. The drug caused prolongation of the action potential in heart muscles with therapeutic concentration (Conn, 1966) probably by prolonging the phase of elevated Ca conductance (see Reuter, 1973). In skeletal muscle, quinidine potentiates twitch tension and may induce contractures at high concentrations (Lammers and Ritchie, 1955). It has been suggested that the effects of quinidine on both skeletal and cardiac muscle are related to an increase in membrane Ca conductance (Sandow, 1965; Fuchs et al., 1968). In the present study quinidine has been shown to convert the normally graded response in lobster muscle to an all-or-none spike. The quinidine action potentials are due to Ca activation as demonstrated by their dependence on external Ca and by their persistence in the presence of TTX or absence of Na. Furthermore, Mn suppressed the action potentials.

The quinidine action potential was characterized by a long repolarizing phase. The duration of the action potential is several hundred milliseconds. In contrast, caffeine which also enhances membrane Ca conductance, induces spikes of comparatively short duration (Chiarandini et al., 1970). However, in both cases the spike overshoot increases (as predicted by the

Nernst relationship) as external Ca is elevated (Fig. 3, and Chiarandini et al., 1970).

Based on the comparative membrane pharmacology (see Sandow, 1965) and the physiology of divalent cation spikes (Reuter, 1973), it may be assumed that both caffeine and quinidine modify excitability solely by altering the membrane Ca conductance. If this is the case, the kinetics of the voltage-dependent gating of Ca must be different in fibers exposed to caffeine compared to those bathed in quinidine. That is, the durations of the quinidine spikes are long in comparison to caffeine-induced spikes. An alternative explanation for the prolonged plateau of quinidine spikes is that quinidine also has a procaine-like action and thus reduces depolarizing K activation. However, since the duration of both caffeine and quinidine spikes increases with increasing concentration of external Ca (Fig. 3, and Chiarandini et al, 1970, Fig. 11 therein), whereas the duration of procaine spikes decreases (Takeda, 1967), a blocking of K-activation by caffeine or quinidine appears unlikely. Thus, it may be concluded that agents that modify the Ca conductance–voltage relationship to allow for the development of all-or-none Ca spikes differently affect the processes that regulate the duration of Ca gating. A dependence of gating duration upon the pharmacological agents used to chemically activate the end plate of frog fibers has been demonstrated (Katz and Milledi, 1973).

REFERENCES

Chiarandini, D. J., Reuben, J. P., Brandt, P. W., and Grundfest, H. (1970): Effects of caffeine on crayfish muscle fibers. I. Activation of contraction and induction of Ca spike electrogenesis. *J. Gen. Physiol.*, 55:640–664.

Conn, H. L., Jr. (1966): Some considerations of quinidine and procaine amide action at the cellular level. In: *The Myocardial Cell*, edited by S. A. Briller and H. L. Conn, Jr., pp. 269–296. University of Pennsylvania Press, Philadelphia.

Fatt, P., and Ginsborg, B. L. (1958): The ionic requirements for the production of action potentials in crustacean muscle fibres. *J. Physiol.*, 142:516–543.

Fatt, P., and Katz, B. (1953): The electrical properties of crustacean muscle fibres. *J. Physiol.*, 120:171–204.

Fuchs, F., Gertz, E. W., and Briggs, F. N. (1968): The effect of quinidine on calcium accumulation by isolated sarcoplasmic reticulum of skeletal and cardiac muscle. *J. Gen. Physiol.*, 52:955–968.

Grundfest, H. (1961): Ionic mechanisms in electrogenesis. *Ann. NY Acad. Sci.*, 94:405–457.

Hagiwara, S., and Naka, K. (1964): The initiation of spike potential in barnacle muscle fibers under low intracellular Ca^{++}. *J. Gen. Physiol.*, 48:141–162.

Hagiwara, S., and Nakajima, S. (1966): Differences in Na and Ca spikes as examined by application of tetrodotoxin, procaine, and manganese ions. *J. Gen. Physiol.*, 49:793–818.

Katz, B., and Miledi, R. (1973): The characteristics of end-plate noise produced by different depolarizing drugs. *J. Physiol.*, 230:707–717.

Kawai, N., and Grundfest, H. (1972): Ca-spikes induced by quinidine in lobster muscle fibers. *Fed. Proc.*, 31:1039.

Lammers, W., and Ritchie, J. M. (1955): The action of quinine and quinidine on the contraction of striated muscle. *J. Physiol.*, 129:412.

Reuben, J. P., and Grundfest, H. (1960): Further analysis of the conversion of graded to all-or-none responsiveness in the electrically excitable membrane of lobster muscle fibers. *Biol. Bull.*, 119:335.

Reuben, J. P., Brandt, P. W., Garcia, H. and Grundfest, H. (1967): Excitation-contraction coupling in crayfish. *Am. Zoologist,* 7:623–645.

Reuter, H. (1973): Divalent cations as charge carriers in excitable membranes. *Progr. Biophys.,* 26:1–45.

Sandow, A. (1965): Excitation-contraction coupling in skeletal muscle. *Pharmacol. Rev.,* 17:265–320.

Takeda, K. (1967): Permeability changes associated with the action potential in procaine-treated crayfish abdominal muscle fibers. *J. Gen. Physiol.,* 50:1049–1074.

Werman, R., and Grundfest, H. (1961): Graded and all-or-none electrogenesis in arthropod muscle. II. The effects of alkali-earth and onium ions on lobster muscle fibers. *J. Gen. Physiol.,* 44:997–1027.

Electrobiology of Nerve, Synapse, and Muscle,
edited by J. P. Reuben, D. P. Purpura, M. V. L. Bennett,
and E. R. Kandel. Raven Press, New York © 1976

Voltage-Dependent Slow Conductance Changes of Frog Muscle Fiber Membranes

Kimihisa Takeda

Laboratory of Physiology, Faculty of Education, Tottori University, Tottori, Japan

It has long been recognized that frog muscle fibers exhibit both anomalous rectification (Katz, 1949) and delayed rectification (e.g., Grundfest, 1966). Anomalous rectification is also found in nerve cells (Kandel and Tauc, 1966; Nelson and Frank, 1967). In muscle fibers the analysis of rectification may be complicated with their complex membrane structures as revealed by the electron microscopy (see Peachey, 1965). The glycerol treatment which disrupts selectively the transverse tubular system (TTS) (Fujino et al., 1961; Eisenberg and Eisenberg, 1968; Howell, 1969) has provided a means to separate the electrical event of the sarcotubular system (Sandow, 1970) from that of the sarcolemma.

The idea that the tubular system may be responsible for the anomalous rectification of frog muscle fibers has been proposed prior to the use of glycerol treatment (Hodgkin and Horowicz, 1960; Adrian and Freygang, 1962). Since the Cl permeability is regarded to reside in the sarcolemma (Eisenberg and Gage, 1969) and to be voltage independent (Hodgkin and Horowicz, 1959; Hutter and Noble, 1960; but see Hutter and Warner, 1972; Warner, 1972), changes in the K conductance probably cause the rectifications. Voltage clamp analysis allows for the division of K current behavior into three components: delayed, inward (anomalous) rectification, and a depolarization-activated slow component (Adrian et al., 1970*b*). The latter two have been suggested to be in the tubular system. An analysis of the Q_{10} has shown that the inward rectifier involves a permeability change at membrane potentials more negative than -120 mV (Almers, 1972*a,b*). At smaller levels of hyperpolarization it is regarded to be caused by a depletion of K within the TTS as proposed by Adrian and Freygang (1962).

The slow hyperpolarization during an applied inward current pulse in intact fibers (Adrian and Freygang, 1962) is absent in glycerol-treated fibers (Gage and Eisenberg, 1969). However, after glycerol treatment of fibers bathed in 100 mM K, anomalous rectification still occurs and must under this condition be due to a property of the sarcolemma (Eisenberg and Gage, 1969). Thus, further analysis is required to clarify the relationship between structure and rectification.

In this article the voltage-dependent slow conductance change at the level of the sarcolemmal and sarcotubular membranes of sartorius muscle fibers from the frog (*Rana catesbiana*) are analyzed. Previous publications dealing with some aspects of the present analysis have appeared (Takeda and Oomura, 1968*a,b*, 1969, 1970*a,b*, 1971*a,b*, 1972; Takeda, 1975*a,b,c*, 1976*a,b*).

CONDUCTANCE CHANGES OF THE SARCOLEMMA

I-V Relationship in Ringer Solution

Figure 1 shows the current-voltage (*I-V*) relations of a glycerol-treated fiber in normal Ringer solution at pH 5.6 containing 1 μg/ml tetrodotoxin. Since the contribution of the sarcotubular system should be small, in glycerol-treated fibers (Eisenberg and Eisenberg, 1968), the *I-V* relations predominantly represent the properties of the sarcolemma. The Cl conductance is reduced in acidic solutions (Hutter and Warner, 1967), and the Na conductance is blocked in the presence of tetrodotoxin (e.g., Grundfest, 1966). The *I-V* plot (Fig. 1) obtained by using both 0.1 and 1 sec pulses is linear for moderate depolarization (−90 to −50 mV). Depolarizations exceeding −50 mV caused delayed rectification with a maximum at tens of milliseconds. The time course and other characteristics of the delayed rectification are comparable to those of fibers in which the sarcotubular system is intact (Adrian et al., 1970*b*). These results provide evidence for the localization of delayed rectification at the sarcolemma (Takeda, 1975*b*). The *I-V* relations for potentials less negative than about −30 mV, where delayed rectification is fully developed, are linear at both 100 msec and at 1 sec. At 1 sec of depolarization, inactivation of delayed rectification at the level of the sarcolemma was only partial and anomalous rectification was absent.

Hyperpolarizing pulses caused anomalous rectification which was greater at 1 sec than at 100 msec. During large inward current pulses the hyperpolarization decreased after attaining a peak at tens of milliseconds (inset record of Fig. 1). The sarcolemmal anomalous rectification was insensitive to changes in pH of the bathing solution (Takeda, 1975*c*), and developed much slower than the sarcotubular inward rectification (see "Conductance Changes of the Sarcotubular System").

I-V Relationship in Propionate-Ringer Solution

Figure 2 shows the *I-V* relations of a glycerol-treated fiber in a propionate-Ringer solution (NaCl replaced by Na propionate) at pH 6.3 containing 4 mM ethylenediaminetetraacetic acid disodium salt (EDTA). The replace-

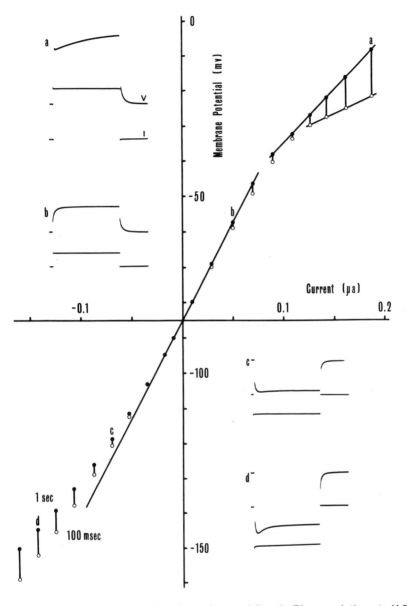

FIG. 1. Current-voltage relations of a glycerol-treated fiber in Ringer solution at pH 5.6. The solution also contained 1 μg/ml tetrodotoxin. Constant current method: *open circles,* at 100 msec; *filled circles,* at 1 sec. Open circles are omitted in this and subsequent graphs if identical with, or very close to, filled circles. Insets, current (*I*) and voltage (*V*) records (corresponding to labels on the *I-V* plot). Pulse duration, 1 sec. Resting potential, −85 mV. (Further explanation in text.)

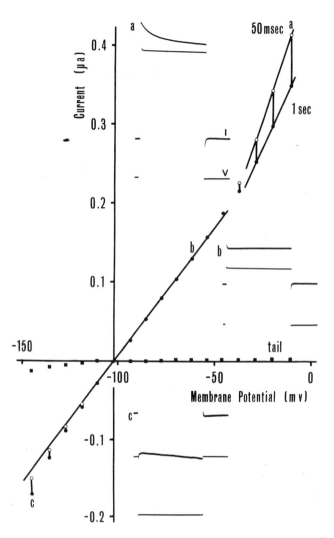

FIG. 2. Current-voltage relations of a glycerol-treated fiber in propionate-Ringer solution at pH 6.3 and containing EDTA. Point-voltage clamp method: *open circles,* at 50 msec; *filled circles,* at 1 sec; *squares,* tail current at 75 msec after voltage steps. Resting potential, −29 mV; holding potential, −102 mV.

ment of about 95% of the Cl by propionate must reduce the membrane Cl conductance.

The *I-V* relations in fiber bathed in the propionate-Ringer duplicate the features of those described for the fibers in normal Ringer solution (Fig. 1). The inset record *c* of Fig. 2 shows the inward current increasing at the end of the 1 sec hyperpolarizing voltage step. Maximum activation of this latter sarcolemmal conductance increase requires a pulse duration greater than

1 sec. The tail current following cessation of depolarizing voltage steps is very small, but an appreciable inward tail current is seen after large hyperpolarizing voltage steps.

I-V Relationship in Fibers Bathed in Fluoride-Ringer Solution

Figure 3 shows the *I-V* relations of a glycerol-treated fiber in a fluoride-Ringer solution at pH 7.8. The fluoride-Ringer solution was prepared by replacing NaCl by equimolar NaF, and $CaCl_2$ was omitted. A bicarbonate buffer was used in this solution instead of the phosphate buffer used for all other Ringer solutions.

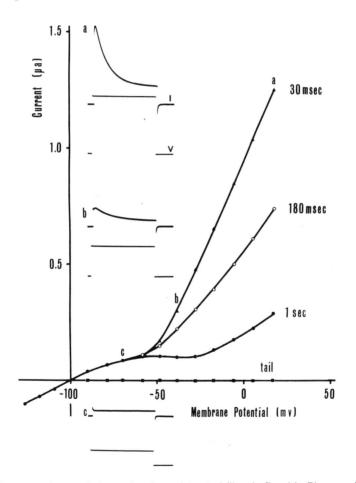

FIG. 3. Current-voltage relations of a glycerol-treated fiber in fluoride-Ringer solution at pH 7.8. Point-voltage clamp method: *triangles,* at 30 msec; *open circles,* at 180 msec; *filled circles,* at 1 sec; *squares,* at 75 msec after voltage steps. Resting potential, −45 mV; holding potential, −100 mV.

These I-V relations are not linear but anomalous rectification occurs for early and steady state depolarization of up to about -50 mV. Larger depolarization caused delayed rectification which was inactivated before 1 sec. In some fibers, the I-V relation at 1 sec showed a minor negative slope for potentials less negative than -50 mV. The tail current after depolarizing voltage steps was almost zero, which suggests that the negative slope was caused by the inactivation of the sarcolemmal conductance and not by a regenerative response as occurs in fibers with an intact tubular system (see the following section).

A depolarization-induced sarcolemmal anomalous rectification occurred only in the fluoride-Ringer solution, but not in the Cl- or propionate-Ringer solution. This anomalous rectification differs from the sarcotubular anomalous rectification observed at moderate depolarization in intact fibers (see the following section). It may be that the former represents an inactivation of the sarcolemmal conductance which is only encountered under non-physiological conditions (see Eisenberg and Gage, 1969).

CONDUCTANCE CHANGES OF THE SARCOTUBULAR SYSTEM

I-V Relationship in Ringer Solution

The data of Fig. 4, which was obtained under the same experimental conditions as those of Fig. 1 except that an intact fiber was used, shows anomalous rectification at both 100 msec and 1 sec for moderate depolarization up to about -50 mV (Adrian and Freygang, 1962; Nakajima et al., 1962). In Fig. 5A, two depolarizing potentials were produced by the same current pulses at 10 and 15 min, after returning the fiber to a normal Ringer solution at pH 7 from a 400 mM glycerol-Ringer solution. As shown by the reduction of depolarization at 15 min the I-V relations of such fibers indicated that anomalous rectification at moderate depolarization was diminished or abolished after glycerol treatment (Takeda, 1975a). Its absence in glycerol-treated fibers (Fig. 1) suggests that the anomalous rectification observed in intact fibers occurs in the sarcotubular system. This anomalous rectification appears to be almost time invariant since the outward current does not change appreciably during the depolarizing voltage step both in intact and in glycerol-treated fibers.

In Fig. 4, anomalous rectification during hyperpolarization is seen to be greater at 100 msec than at 1 sec. The slow time course of the hyperpolarization during the current pulse is shown in the inset of record b (Adrian and Freygang, 1962). For potentials more negative than about -110 mV the I-V relation is almost linear when determined by 100 msec pulses, but at 1 sec anomalous rectification is observed. The slow hyperpolarization increased and then decreased with increasing hyperpolarization. Figure 5B shows that the slow hyperpolarization is absent in glycerol-treated fibers

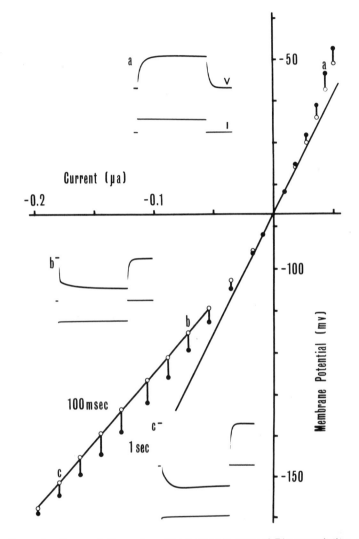

FIG. 4. Current-voltage relations of an intact fiber in normal Ringer solution at pH 5.6. Constant current method: *open circles,* at 100 msec; *filled circles,* at 1 sec. Resting potential, −87 mV.

which is apparently due to the abolition of the early conductance increase. In this figure (5B) hyperpolarizing potentials before and after disruption of the tubules can be compared. The comparison suggests that the inward rectifing component is located in the sarcotubular system. Thus, in Fig. 4 the anomalous rectification at 100 msec for large hyperpolarizing pulses is probably due to the sarcotubular inward rectifier. The anomalous rectification at 1 sec reflects the sarcolemmal slow conductance increase, which is

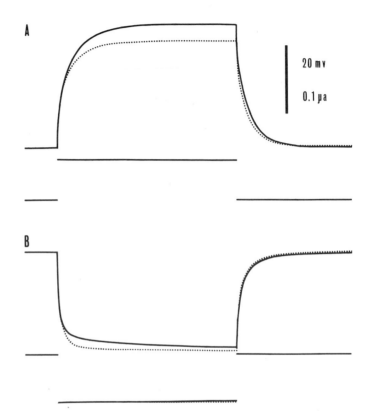

FIG. 5. Potential changes (*upper traces*) produced by 1 sec outward **(A)** and inward **(B)** constant current pulses (*lower trace*) at 10 min (*solid line*) and 15 min (*dotted line*) after return to normal Ringer from glycerol-Ringer solution.

partially masked by the slow hyperpolarization due to inactivation of the early conductance increase (Takeda and Oomura, 1968*b*; Gage and Eisenberg, 1969). An increase in conductance during hyperpolarization has also been observed in intact fibers bathed in a Rb-Ringer solution (Adrian, 1964; Hutter and Warner, 1972; Warner, 1972).

Regenerative Response of the Sarcotubular System

This section deals with a voltage- and time-dependent conductance increase within the sarcotubular system that is autogenetic (Grundfest, 1966) i.e., all-or-none prolonged depolarizing responses. Intact fibers have low resting potentials while bathed in a fluoride-Ringer solution containing bicarbonate buffer. However, if the resting potential is restored by injecting inward current, an outward current pulse induces a regenerative depolarizing response which resembles a cardiac action potential (Fig. 6A). The membrane conductance increases approximately 10 times during the regenerative response.

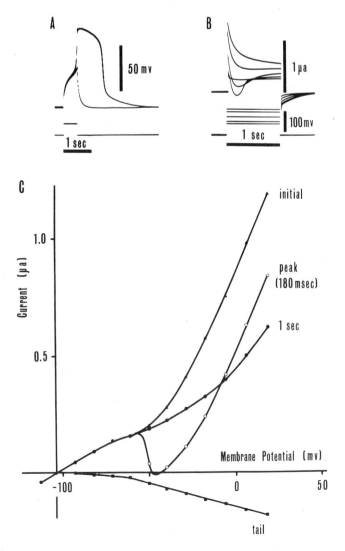

FIG. 6. Sarcotubular regenerative response in fibers in fluoride-Ringer solution. **A:** All-or-none depolarizing response (*upper trace*). Resting potential, −29 mV. Hyperpolarized to −90 mV prior to stimulating current pulse (*lower trace*). **B:** Multiple sweep record showing inward current and inward tail current (*upper trace*) produced by depolarizing voltage steps (*lower trace*). Resting potential, −56 mV; holding potential, −109 mV. **C:** Current-voltage relations. Point-voltage clamp method: *triangles,* initial (after capacitative surge); *open circles,* at 180 msec; *filled circles,* at 1 sec; *squares,* at 75 msec after voltage steps. Resting potential, −49 mV; holding potential, −104 mV.

In Fig. 6B, the inward current that gives rise to the regenerative response was obtained by using a point voltage clamp technique. The inward current reversed at large depolarizations and the equilibrium potential appears to be minus several millivolts, corresponding to the peak of the voltage response. Figure 6C shows the negative slope region (180 msec depolarizing pulses) where the inward current was maximum. Since the concurrent outward current of sarcolemmal delayed rectification was relatively large (see Fig. 3), total current at the time of maximum inward current was outward in many fibers. Since the inward current in glycerol-treated fibers was always absent (Fig. 3), the regenerative response must be generated in, and only in, the sarcotubular system.

When the phosphate buffer replaced the bicarbonate in the fluoride-Ringer solution, the regenerative response became less prominent. However, addition of 1 mM EDTA greatly enhanced the regenerative response. In the propionate-Ringer solution containing 4 mM EDTA, or 10 mM ethyleneglycoldiethyletherdiaminetetraacetic acid (EGTA), the sarcotubular regenerative response was also present.

These results may indicate that some membrane component in the sarcotubular system, i.e., the tubules or the sarcoplasmic reticulum, undergoes the permeability increase which is induced by depolarization and inactivated by maintained depolarization. These results further suggest that the sarcotubular permeability change may be responsible for the similar prolonged responses previously observed in solutions containing Ca-binding anions (see Falk and Landa, 1960; Nakajima et al., 1962). The regenerative response is also produced in normal Ringer solution containing EDTA, without a great change in the equilibrium potential (Takeda, 1976a). Therefore it is unlikely that Cl ions are responsible for the inward current, although the available data do not allow for an identification of the ion or ions that give rise to the regenerative response.

INHIBITION OF SARCOTUBULAR CONDUCTANCE CHANGES BY PICROTOXIN

Effects on *I-V* Relations in Ringer Solution

Addition of 1 mg/ml picrotoxin to normal Ringer solution caused only a slight decrease in the resting membrane conductance of intact fibers. Figure 7 shows the *I-V* relations of an intact fiber in normal Ringer solution at pH 5.6, obtained 4 hr after the addition of picrotoxin. These *I-V* relations are very similar to those of glycerol-treated fibers (Fig. 1) in every respect. Thus picrotoxin inhibits selectively the sarcotubular conductance changes, i.e., the anomalous rectification at moderate depolarization and the inward rectifier.

Effect on Sarcotubular Regenerative Response

The sarcotubular regenerative response generated in the Cl-deficient solutions was abolished with picrotoxin. Both the inward current and the inward tail current produced by depolarizing voltage steps in the propionate-

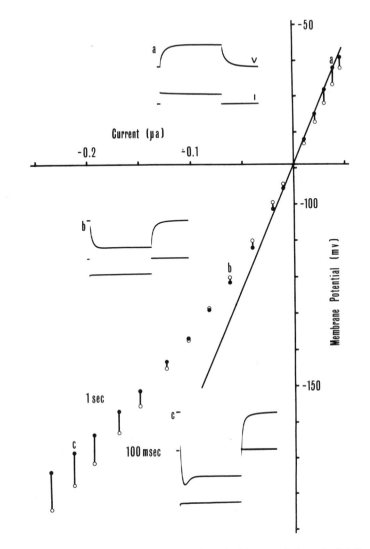

FIG. 7. Current-voltage relations of an intact fiber in Ringer solution at pH 5.6 and containing 1 mg/ml picrotoxin. Constant current method: *open circles,* at 100 msec; *filled circles,* at 1 sec. Resting potential, −89 mV.

Ringer solution containing EDTA disappeared with picrotoxin (Takeda, 1976*a*). The inhibition of the regenerative response by picrotoxin was reversible, though the recovery was incomplete.

Effects on Na-Action Potentials

Addition of 1 mg/ml picrotoxin to normal Ringer solution increased the duration of action potentials to almost twice the normal in intact fibers (Fig.

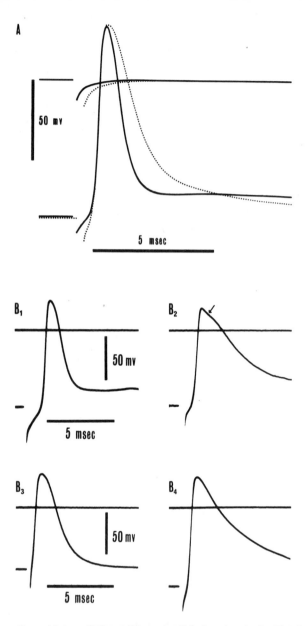

FIG. 8. Prolongation of intracellular action potentials by picrotoxin. The horizontal line registers external potential. **A:** *solid line,* before picrotoxin in intact fiber (resting potential, −85 mV); *dotted line,* 1 hr after addition of 1 mg/ml picrotoxin in another intact fiber (resting potential, −86 mV). **B:** records before (**B₁**) and 25 min after (**B₂**) 3 mg/ml picrotoxin in intact fibers; and before (**B₃**) and 32 min after (**B₄**) the picrotoxin in glycerol-treated fibers. Resting potentials (**B₁**-**B₄**), −88, −87, −75, and −95 mV. Arrow in *B₂* indicates a dip in potential. Calibrations in **B₁** also apply to **B₂**, and those in **B₃** to **B₄**.

8A). The rate of repolarization in the falling phase was diminished and the dip at the end of the spike potential (Persson, 1963) disappeared. The time course of the falling phase resembles that of action potentials computed by Adrian et al. (1970a) who assumed that responsible conductance changes are restricted to the sarcolemma. Picrotoxin (3 mg/ml) prolonged action potentials of both intact and glycerol-treated fibers (Fig. 8B). In intact fibers, however, picrotoxin induced a small plateau phase and occasionally a dip (arrow in Fig. 8B$_2$) was noticed during the plateau phase. The falling phase decays with two distinct time constants (excluding the dip) in intact fibers, in contrast to the monotonic decay in glycerol-treated fibers. Thus, it appears that the sarcotubular system is responsible for the plateau phase.

Implications of Picrotoxin's Actions

The abolition by picrotoxin of all the sarcotubular conductance changes examined, i.e., (1) the anomalous rectification at moderate depolarization, (2) the inward rectification, and (3) the regenerative response, raises the possibility that one and the same membrane component in the sarcotubular system is responsible for all these conductance changes in spite of the difference in their modes of activation. The anomalous rectification at moderate depolarization is presently regarded as a part of the inward rectification, i.e., the decrease in the K conductance with depolarization (Adrian and Freygang, 1962; Adrian et al., 1970b). If this is the case, then picrotoxin inhibits the depolarization-induced *decrease* in the K conductance, which is unlikely since it must also inhibit an *increase* in K conductance during hyperpolarization. An action of picrotoxin that both increases and decreases K conductance need not be proposed if anomalous rectification is caused by a sarcotubular permeability increase towards an ion whose equilibrium potential is inside positive. Then inhibition of the permeability by picrotoxin may abolish the anomalous rectification.

In summary, the analysis of I-V data obtained from fibers with and without an intact tubular system has provided information regarding the localization and ionic basis of slow conductance processes in frog muscle fibers. While delayed rectification appears to be due to a property of the sarcolemma, both anomalous rectification and the depolarization-activated slow component are properties of the sarcotubular system. It has also been concluded that under given conditions an autogenic response may occur within the tubular system during depolarization.

REFERENCES

Adrian, R. H. (1964): The rubidium and potassium permeability of frog muscle membrane. *J. Physiol.*, 175:134–159.

Adrian, R. H., Chandler, W. K., and Hodgkin, A. L. (1970a): Voltage clamp experiments in striated muscle fibres. *J. Physiol.*, 208:607–644.

Adrian, R. H., Chandler, W. K., and Hodgkin, A. L. (1970b): Slow changes in potassium permeability in skeletal muscle. *J. Physiol.*, 208:645–668.

Adrian, R. H., and Freygang, W. H. (1962): The potassium and chloride conductance of frog muscle membrane. *J. Physiol.*, 163:61–103.

Almers, W. (1972a): Potassium conductance changes in skeletal muscle and the potassium concentration in the transverse tubules. *J. Physiol.*, 225:33–56.

Almers, W. (1972b): The decline of potassium permeability during extreme hyperpolarization in frog skeletal muscle. *J. Physiol.*, 225:57–83.

Eisenberg, B., and Eisenberg, R. S. (1968): Selective disruption of the sarcotubular system in frog sartorius muscle. *J. Cell Biol.*, 39:451–467.

Eisenberg, R. S., and Gage, P. W. (1969): Ionic conductances of the surface and transverse tubular membranes of frog sartorius fibers. *J. Gen. Physiol.*, 53:279–297.

Falk, G., and Landa, J. F. (1960): Prolonged response of skeletal muscle in the absence of penetrating anions. *Am. J. Physiol.*, 198:289–299.

Fujino, M., Yamaguchi, T., and Suzuki, K. (1961): 'Glycerol effect' and the mechanism linking excitation of the plasma membrane with contraction. *Nature*, 192:1159–1161.

Gage, P. W., and Eisenberg, R. S. (1969): Action potentials, afterpotentials, and excitation-contraction coupling in frog sartorius fibers without transverse tubules. *J. Gen. Physiol.*, 53:298–310.

Grundfest, H. (1966): Comparative Electrobiology of Excitable Membranes. In: *Advances in Comparative Physiology and Biochemistry*, Vol. 2, edited by O. Lowenstein, pp. 1–116. Academic Press, New York.

Hodgkin, A. L., and Horowicz, P. (1959): The influence of potassium and chloride ions on the membrane potential of single muscle fibres. *J. Physiol.*, 148:127–160.

Hodgkin, A. L., and Horowicz, P. (1960): The effect of sudden changes in ionic concentrations on the membrane potential of single muscle fibres. *J. Physiol.*, 153:370–385.

Howell, J. N. (1969): A lesion of the transverse tubules of skeletal muscle. *J. Physiol.*, 201:515–533.

Hutter, O. F., and Noble, D. (1960): The chloride conductance of frog skeletal muscle. *J. Physiol.*, 151:89–102.

Hutter, O. F., and Warner, A. E. (1967): The pH sensitivity of the chloride conductance of frog skeletal muscle. *J. Physiol.*, 189:403–425.

Hutter, O. F., and Warner, A. E. (1972): The voltage dependence of the chloride conductance of frog muscle. *J. Physiol.*, 227:275–290.

Kandel, E. R., and Tauc, L. (1966): Anomalous rectification in the metacerebral giant cells and its consequences for synaptic transmission. *J. Physiol.*, 183:287–304.

Katz, B. (1949): Les constantes électriques de la membrane du muscle. *Arch. Sci. Physiol.*, 3:285–300.

Nakajima, S., Iwasaki, S., and Obata, K. (1962): Delayed rectification and anomalous rectification in frog's skeletal muscle membrane. *J. Gen. Physiol.*, 46:97–115.

Nelson, P. G., and Frank, K. (1967): Anomalous rectification in cat spinal motoneurons and effect of polarizing currents on excitatory postsynaptic potential. *J. Neurophysiol.*, 30:1097–1113.

Peachey, L. D. (1965): The sarcoplasmic reticulum and transverse tubules of the frog's sartorius. *J. Cell Biol.*, 25:209–231.

Persson, A. (1963): The negative after-potential of frog skeletal muscle fibres. *Acta Physiol. Scand.*, 58 (Suppl. 205):1–32.

Sandow, A. (1970): Skeletal muscle. *Ann. Rev. Physiol.*, 32:87–138.

Takeda, K. (1975a): Sarcotubular anomalous rectification of frog sartorius muscle. *Jap. J. Physiol.*, 25:495–506.

Takeda, K. (1975b): Properties of sarcolemmal delayed rectification in glycerol-treated fibers of frog sartorius muscle. *Jap. J. Physiol.*, 25:507–513.

Takeda, K. (1975c): Sarcolemmal slow conductance increase of frog sartorius fibers during hyperpolarization. *Jap. J. Physiol.*, 25:515–524.

Takeda, K. (1976a): Prolonged sarcotubular regenerative response in frog sartorius muscle (*in preparation*).

Takeda, K. (1976b): Potentiation of contraction by picrotoxin in frog sartorius muscle (*in preparation*).

Takeda, K., and Oomura, Y. (1968a): Conductance increase causing anomalous rectification in frog muscle in fluoride-rich solution. *Proc. Jap. Acad.*, 44:285–289.

Takeda, K., and Oomura, Y. (1968b): Dual hyperpolarizing conductance increases in frog muscle fibers. *Proc. Jap. Acad.*, 44:1072–1077.

Takeda, K., and Oomura, Y. (1969): Two component anomalous rectification in frog muscle fibers. *Proc. Jap. Acad.*, 45:814–819.

Takeda, K., and Oomura, Y. (1970a): Regenerative response in sarcotubular system of frog muscle fibers in F-rich solution. *Proc. Jap. Acad.*, 46:1046–1050.

Takeda, K., and Oomura, Y. (1970b): Picrotoxin: a potentiator of muscle contraction. *Proc. Jap. Acad.*, 46:1051–1055.

Takeda, K., and Oomura, Y. (1971a): Potentiation of muscle contraction by high concentration of picrotoxin. *J. Physiol. Soc. Japan,* 33:593–594.

Takeda, K., and Oomura, Y. (1971b): Enhancement by EDTA of sarcotubular regenerative response produced in F-rich solution. *Proc. Jap. Acad.*, 47:732–735.

Takeda, K., and Oomura, Y. (1972): Sarcotubular regenerative response induced by EDTA in propionate solution. *Proc. Jap. Acad.*, 48:753–757.

Warner, A. E. (1972): Kinetic properties of the chloride conductance of frog muscle. *J. Physiol.,* 227:291–312.

Electrobiology of Nerve, Synapse, and Muscle,
edited by J. P. Reuben, D. P. Purpura, M. V. L. Bennett,
and E. R. Kandel. Raven Press, New York © 1976

Permeability Characteristics of the Transverse Tubular System: Determinants of the Signal for Contractile Activation in Crayfish

John P. Reuben, Abraham B. Eastwood, Jenny R. Zollman, Morton Orentlicher, and Philip W. Brandt

Laboratory of Neurophysiology, Departments of Neurology and Anatomy, College of Physicians and Surgeons, Columbia University, New York, New York 10032

The earliest suggestion that events associated with the transverse tubular membranes would have to be understood before construction of a comprehensive excitation scheme for muscle was made by Bennett (1955) based on his electron microscopic observations of vertebrate muscle. Subsequent morphological studies have provided considerable information about the components which form the transverse tubular system (TTS) in a wide variety of muscles. The localization, dimensions, and continuity of the tubules with the surface and invagination membranes have been described. The complex structure referred to as triads or diads and formed in part by a portion of the tubules and the cisternae of the sarcoplasmic reticulum (SR), has also been defined in detail by the electron microscopists (Franzini-Armstrong, 1973).

Physiological studies paralleling in time the morphological ones have demonstrated the existence of localized electrically sensitive sites for inducing contraction at the fiber surface (Huxley and Taylor, 1958). These sensitive sites were shown in muscles from a number of different animals to correspond with the openings of the tubules at the fiber surface which are either located at the level of the Z-bands or the A-I junction (Huxley and Straub, 1958). This initial physiological description of the TTS was followed by a series of studies directed towards understanding the mode by which depolarization of the surface membembrane (i.e., action potentials, synaptic potentials, applied currents, and elevation of potassium) affect the tubular membranes within the fiber depths (see Sandow, 1970; Nakajima and Bastian, *this volume*). On the basis of these studies three mechanisms have been proposed to explain the inward spread of an electrical signal via the TTS. (1) A passive decay of the surface potential signal along the tubules as determined by their cable-like properties (Huxley and Taylor, 1958). (2) Propagation of an action potential along the tubular membrane network (see Nakajima and Bastian, *this volume*). (3) A flow of current between the surface membrane and high conductance sites (triads or diads) throughout the tubular network (Girardier et al., 1963; Reuben et al., 1967*a*). In vertebrate muscle there is now strong evidence that a regenerative increase in Na conductance occurs within the TTS and it may give rise to a propagated action potential (see Nakajima and Bastian, *this volume*). A propagated response is less likely to occur within the TTS of the crustacean fibers used in the studies to be described, since they are incapable of generating propagated responses under physiological conditions (see Suarez-Kurtz et al., 1972).

The second step in the excitation process, the conveyance of a signal to the intracellular systems across the diads or triads, may occur by the same mechanism in different muscles despite the above mentioned dissimilarity. Two hypotheses have been given to explain the mode of involvement of the tubules in the second step. (1) Depolarization of the diads or triads per se, whether brought about by current flow between membranes of different ionic selectivity or by a tubular action potential, signals the intracellular processes (see Schneider and Chandler, 1973). (2) The transport of current by specific ions across the diads or triads serves as the signal for mobilization of SR-bound Ca to initiate contractile activation (see Atwood, 1972). The development of and support for the latter hypothesis which we have called the channeled current model (Girardier et al., 1963; Brandt et al., 1965; Reuben et al., 1967*a;* and Brandt et al., 1968) is particularly dependent upon a thorough characterization of the resting and active ionic permability of the tubular membranes.

In this chapter we will review the previous findings, describe our recent data on the ionic permeabilities of the TTS of crayfish fibers, and extend the channeled current hypothesis to encompass the new data.

MORPHOMETRIC DETERMINATION OF TUBULAR PROPERTIES

In the course of investigating the processes involved in the regulation of the distribution of KCl in crayfish fibers (Reuben et al., 1964) we noted a dramatic change in their appearance when viewed under the light microscope (see Fig. 1 in Girardier et al., 1963). The fibers became grainy and opaque whenever they were exposed to solutions that induced an efflux of KCl. Electron micrographs of the darkened fibers (Brandt et al., 1968) revealed a swelling of the TTS which was predominantly localized at the diadic portion of the tubules. The swollen tubules maintain their connections with the surface and invagination membranes and unlike vertebrate fibers subjected to similar conditions (Howell and Jenden, 1967) the openings are not constricted ("detubulate"). The tubular swelling evoked by KCl efflux was initially thought to be due to an osmotic imbalance caused by KCl effluxing from the fibers into the extracellular space formed by the TTS. The darkening of fibers was in turn ascribed to the modification of transmitted light pathways. The latter would occur if the index of refraction of the saline within the swollen tubules is different from that of the myoplasm.

Localization of Cl Permeability at the Diads

Since the tubular swelling was also shown to be induced by an inward current applied through an intracellular microelectrode (see Fig. 4, Girardier et al., 1963 therein), the initial explanation suggesting an accumulation of KCl within the tubules had to be modified. During the application of an inward current only Cl ions move outward and K ions are transported into the fiber. Thus, the swelling under this condition must be related to a translocation of Cl from the myoplasmic to the tubular space. We concluded that the current-mediated movement of Cl could only account for the swelling of the diadic portion of the TTS if the latter were predominantly permeable to Cl. Thus, during an applied current Cl transports most of the transtubular membrane current into the tubules whereas only about one-half of the current leaving the tubules via their core is transported by Cl. The other fraction of the core current is transported by Na ions (saline is approximately 200 mM NaCl and $t_{Na} \cong t_{Cl}$) entering the tubules from the medium. An accumulation of NaCl at the diads must occur and the resulting osmotic gradient will swell the tubules. To our knowledge this is the only demonstration which indicates that the ionic properties of one region within the TTS (diads) is distinct from the other portions.[1]

Other Evidence Supporting the Separation of K and Cl Permeable Sites

Another technique which allows conclusions to be drawn regarding the difference in permeability of the membrane components of the TTS from those of the surface membrane was first described by Hodgkin and Horowicz (1959). The kinetics and amplitudes of membrane potential changes induced by rapidly changing bathing solutions of different ionic composition were measured in single muscle fibers. The comparatively rapid change in potential of the membrane of frog fibers to a change in Cl concentration led them to conclude that the Cl permeable sites are limited to the surface of these fibers. In contrast, increasing K caused an initial rapid depolarization followed by a slow phase of depolarization. The slow component was ascribed by Hodgkin and Horowicz to the additional time required for K ions to reach the K permeable sites within the TTS. Similar experiments with crayfish fibers indicate that Cl permeable sites are within the TTS whereas the K sites are superficial. Crayfish fibers respond slowly to Cl concentration changes and rapidly to step changes in the K concentration (Orentlicher and Reuben, 1971). The rapid depolarization of crayfish fibers exposed to elevated K, however, is limited to concentrations of K which do not exceed 20 mM. The dependence of the potential kinetics on the concentration of K is a recent finding and it will be dealt with in a subsequent section. Let it

---

[1] Krolenko and Schwinka (1974) have recently reported swelling of the TTS in frog fiber during applied currents (10^{-8} to 10^{-7} A). The data, however, are insufficient for localizing the swellings to a given portion of the TTS.

suffice at this point to emphasize that two independent types of evidence indicate that the ion permeability of the TTS is distinct from that of the surface membranes.

CHANNELED CURRENT HYPOTHESIS

The spatial separation of membranes possessing different ionic permeabilities led us to propose a mechanism for excitation-contraction coupling which was solely based upon this described mosaic structure of the muscle membranes (Girardier et al., 1963). We suggested that the current which must flow between the diadic or junctional portions of the tubules and the other membranes of the muscle during either physiological (synaptic or action potentials) or experimentally induced activations (variation in the ionic composition of the medium and applied currents) constituted the ECC signal. Furthermore, since diads forming these portions of the tubules are sites of high Cl permeability we concluded that Cl ions were directly involved in the ECC process. The word channel was selected to distinguish this signalling process from that of a passive electronic spread of a signal along the tubular membranes. In other words, the length constant of the small (about 10 μm length) tubules must be considerably longer than the length of the tubules. Under this condition the current flow between the surface or invagination membranes of the diads would be channeled through the core of the tubules to the high conductance Cl-permeable membranes at the junctional portion of the tubules. The current transported by specific ions across the diadic complex would convey information to the intracellular organelles.

Testing of the channeled current hypothesis was sought by turning to measurements of the initiation and development of tension in single crayfish fibers (Reuben et al., 1967a).

INITIATION AND DEVELOPMENT OF TENSION

Although the channeled current hypothesis was not developed by analyses of tensional data, its predictions regarding the relationship between membrane parameters and the initiation of tension are clearly defined. The coupling factor between the membrane and the contractile system is membrane current and since a specific ion current has been postulated the coupling factor must be given by the ionic current equation

$$I_x = g_x (V - V_x)$$

The ideal conditions for testing the postulate that a specific ionic current constitutes the ECC signal are simultaneous measurements of tension and membrane current by voltage-clamp techniques. Our attempts to voltage-clamp crayfish fibers under adequate spatial control conditions have not been successful. The primary hinderance to voltage clamping with microelectrodes is the large decrease (from 1.5 to less than 0.1 mm) in length constant as the membrane potential approaches zero. Nevertheless, by using other techniques the initiation of tension has been readily shown to be correlated with an ionic current (Suarez-Kurtz et al., 1972). Furthermore, a membrane potential change independent of a specific ionic current has been shown to be an unlikely signal for inducing tension in crayfish fibers (Reuben et al., 1967a).

The initial observation that tension persists in the absence of Cl (see Fig. 21, Reuben et al., 1967a; Gainer and Grundfest, 1968) dismissed the possibility that the transport of current by Cl ions at the diadic junctions constitutes the ECC signal. Based on our measurements of tensions from crayfish fibers (Reuben et al., 1967a) and those of Chiarandini and Stefani (*this volume*) from frog, the specific ionic current carrier is most likely Ca. The initiation of tension was found to be dependent upon external Ca and upon conditions that promote an inward Ca current. Furthermore, the tensional data obtained from crayfish fibers suggested that the nature of Cl involvement in ECC was due to an interaction with Ca. That is, the membrane conductance towards Ca and the Ca distribution across the fiber boundary were found to depend upon the Cl concentration of the bathing medium. An interaction between Cl and Ca ions has also been described in other preparations. In skinned fibers of frog (Costantin and Podolsky, 1967), human (Wood et al., 1975), and crayfish (Reuben et al., 1967b; Orentlicher et al., 1974) a change in Cl concentration induces a Ca redistribution and, as a consequence, tension is elicited. Ca regulation by isolated SR preparation is also altered when the Cl content of the medium is varied (Kasai and Miyamoto, 1973).

There are also numerous nonphysiological ions and agents that have been noted to modify either Ca permeability and/or Ca fluxes in various muscle preparations (see Sandow, 1965). By comparing the effects of a number of these nonphysiological ions on the threshold for tension initiation with that of the onset of an inward Ca current, substantial support was obtained for the role of Ca as a transmembrane messenger in ECC. For crayfish fibers the onset of an inward Ca current can be monitored without voltage clamping by measuring threshold depolarization for induction of a Ca spike. Since Ca spikes can be induced in crustacean fibers by various reversible treatments (Suarez-Kurtz et al., 1972), the threshold for tension (induced by an applied current of fixed duration) can be compared before and after the treatment to the measurement of the onset of Ca electrogenesis. When the experimentally induced variation in thresholds were measured they were found to be directly related by the regression equation $\Delta t = 1.23 \ \Delta s + 2.96$ (Suarez-Kurtz et al., 1972). In the equation Δt is the change in tension threshold under a given experimental condition and Δs is the change in spike threshold for the same condition (Suarez-Kurtz et al., 1972).

FURTHER CHARACTERIZATION OF THE TTS

Our most recent work dealing with the properties of the TTS has been directed along two lines. One entails an investigation of the membrane electrical parameters and ECC in fibers before and after swelling the TTS. The volume of the TTS was increased either by using our previously described procedure for inducing a KCl efflux (Girardier et al., 1963) or by glycerol treatment which is commonly used to "detubulate" vertebrate muscle (Howell and Jenden, 1967). For crayfish, glycerol treatment changed the geometry of the TTS in exactly the same way as that brought about by KCl efflux. The membrane potential is not changed by 200 mM glycerol treatment, but concentrations near 400 mM, commonly used to "detubulate" vertebrate fibers, depolarized and irreversibly damaged crayfish fibers (Eastwood et al., 1973). Independent of the treatment for swelling the TTS, no changes in the measured electrical parameters nor in the initiation or development of tensions induced by applied currents and action potentials have been detected (Zollman et al., 1974). Although this work is still in progress the findings to date are of particular interest in light of the recent suggestion that ECC is blocked in vertebrate muscle due to swelling and not pinching-off ("detubulation") of the tubules (Dulhunty and Gage, 1973).

The second line of investigation, which is discussed below in some detail, has been concerned with the response of normal and TTS-swollen fibers to sudden changes in the ionic composition of the bathing saline. This work has provided further characterization of the ionic permeability of the TTS.

KINETICS OF ION-INDUCED DEPOLARIZATION IN CONTROL AND TTS SWOLLEN FIBERS

The rationale for comparing membrane potential changes induced by varying K and/or Cl concentrations of the bathing saline before and after swelling the TTS is straightforward. If any of the component membranes of the TTS are permeable to K and/or Cl ions or become permeable under experimental conditions, then enlargement of the extracellular space formed by the TTS should slow the rate of potential change.

Depolarization Induced by Cl Withdrawal

Since Cl-permeable sites have been shown to reside within the TTS, the membrane depolarization induced by withdrawing Cl from the medium (see Grundfest, 1962) should be slower to attain a peak value after swelling the TTS. The data of Fig. 1 fulfill this expectation. The membrane potentials were measured by repeated microelectrode penetrations following

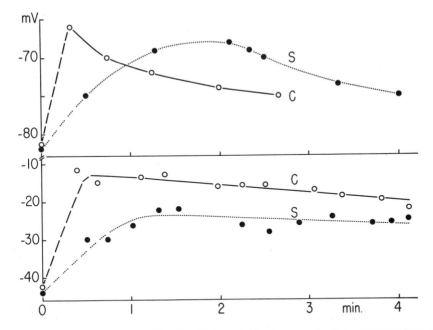

FIG. 1. Depolarization induced by Cl withdrawal. Membrane potential determinations at times following substitution of an impermeant anion (propionate) for Cl form the graphs of this figure. The potential measurements in the upper portion were obtained from a fiber bathed in normal K (5 mM) both before (C) and after swelling the TTS (S). The same procedure was used to obtain the data of the lower portion of the figure, but from a fiber bathed in high K (30 mM). Further description is given in text.

substitution of the impermeant anion propionate for Cl. The potential between the ground electrode and the microelectrode was balanced to zero before each penetration. The two experiments of Fig. 1 were similar in that potentials were recorded both before and after swelling the TTS. However, the lower recordings were obtained from a fiber continuously bathed in high K (30 mM). In both normal K (5 mM) and in elevated K the time to reach peak depolarization was prolonged after swelling the TTS. For a more complete description of the potential time course induced by Cl withdrawal the reader is referred to an earlier publication (Orentlicher and Reuben, 1971), in which the slow time course of the control Cl withdrawal responses was analyzed theoretically. The concentration of Cl within the TTS during the transient response, which determines in part the change in membrane potential, varies due to the efflux of intracellular Cl into the tubules and the diffusion of Cl from the tubules to the medium. This variation in the Cl gradient across the tubular membrane accounts for the slow rise to peak depolarization (15 to 30 sec) even before swelling the TTS. Swelling further prolongs the interval of time to as long as 3 min in some fibers.

Depolarization Induced By Elevating K < 20 mM

The step depolarizations shown in Fig. 2 were elicited by increasing the K concentration from 5 to 12 mM. The upper tracing is the control response (depolarization from 82 to 65 mV) before swelling the TTS. The fiber was then exposed to 200 mM glycerol for 30 min and returned to control saline for an additional 30 min. In the lower record of Fig. 2 the fiber was again exposed to 12 mM K and the membrane potential decreased from 82 to 65.5 mV. The large increase in the extracellular space formed by the TTS did not modify the response as it did for the Cl-withdrawal-induced potential change or those induced by higher levels of K which are described below.

Depolarization Induced by High Concentrations of K (>20 mM)

The depolarizing steps of Fig. 3 were elicited by elevating K to the indicated concentrations from an initial level of 40 mM. Exposing the fiber to 40 mM K caused a transient tension and reduced the membrane potential to 35 mV. While continuously bathed in 40 mM K saline a further elevation of K does not evoke tension and continuous recordings of potential can be obtained without the impaling microelectrode damaging the fiber. The three responses of the upper line (A, B, and C) were elicited by increasing K to 80, 120, and 180 mM, respectively. Although the changes in potential increased from 14 to about 30 mV, the shapes of the three responses were the same. After swelling the TTS by treating the fiber with 200 mM glycerol as described above, the time courses of the potential changes were greatly prolonged while the respective amplitudes were not changed from the corresponding control values (D, E, and F). In this experiment the K concentration was elevated by substituting KCl for NaCl, but similar changes were observed when K was increased in a propionate medium in the complete absence of Cl ions.

A comparison of the time course of depolarization induced by low K (Fig. 2) to that elicited by high K (Fig. 3) has led us to conclude that some

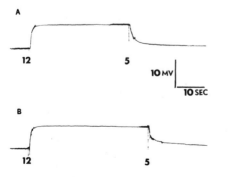

FIG. 2. Depolarization induced by elevating K from 5 to 12 mM. The depolarization and subsequent repolarization of the membrane following, respectively, the elevation of K to 12 mM and return to 5 mM are shown both before **(A)** and after swelling the TTS **(B)**. Further description in text.

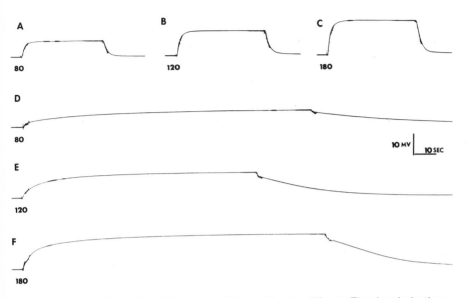

FIG. 3. Depolarization induced by varying K from 40 up to 180 mM. The depolarizations elicited by increasing K from 40 to 80, 120, and 180 mM were recorded before (**A, B,** and **C**) and after swelling the TTS (**D, E,** and **F**). Further description in text.

membrane component within the TTS became permeable to K upon exposing the fiber to high K. Before swelling the TTS the time interval between elevating K and attainment of a steady level of depolarization is measured in tenths of seconds in fibers exposed to low K and in seconds in those bathed in high K. After swelling the TTS the interval was not changed in low K and it expanded to minutes in fibers bathed in high K. These differences can be ascribed to the additional period of time for K to equilibrate with membrane sites within the TTS that become permeable to K in depolarized fibers bathed in high K. If the volume of the TTS increases the time required for K to equilibrate between the bath and the swollen TTS increases.

The results obtained with crayfish fibers after glycerol treatment stand in marked contrast with those obtained from frog fibers treated in a similar manner. The latter respond more rapidly to a challenge with K after glycerol treatment than before the treatment (Nakajima et al., 1973).

K-INDUCED TENSION IN TTS SWOLLEN FIBERS

After swelling the TTS, the K tensions are slower to develop and they are not maintained for as long a period as those induced before swelling the TTS (Fig. 4). The tensions induced by increasing K from 5 to 100 mM in the control state (C) and after swelling the TTS (S) are shown in the upper line of Fig. 4. The difference in the time course of the tensions is

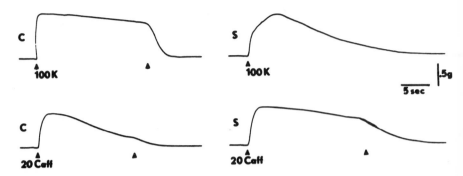

FIG. 4. Modification of K- and caffeine-induced tension following swelling of the TTS. The tensions evoked by high K and 20 mM caffeine before swelling the TTS are the tracings on the left **(C)**. The corresponding responses after swelling the TTS **(S)** are shown in right-hand portion of the figure. Description of the procedure is given in the text.

predicted on the basis of the potential measurements of Fig. 3. The amount of intracellular Ca that is mobilized and becomes available for activating the contractile system depends upon both the amplitude and time of membrane depolarization (Reuben et al., 1967a; Sugi, 1968; Edwards et al., 1964; Adrian et al., 1969). This dependence is consistent with the channeled current hypothesis because the degree of membrane Ca activation is also dependent upon both time and potential. Due to membrane accommodation processes a slow rate of depolarization is generally less effective than a rapid depolarization for eliciting an increase in ionic conductance.

To demonstrate that the contractile system is not modified after swelling the TTS, tensions were induced by exposing fibers to caffeine both before and after swelling the TTS (lower line Fig. 4). The rate of rise and amplitude of the caffeine tension were not changed after swelling the TTS. The slower rate of relaxation in TTS-swollen fibers has been described previously (Chiarandini et al., 1970) and may be related to an action of caffeine at the level of the tubules (Lüttgau and Oetliker, 1968).

POSSIBLE ROLES OF K-ACTIVATION WITHIN THE TTS

The development of a membrane conductance towards K ions within the TTS of depolarized fibers may serve as a means for regulating the diadic signal for ECC. The regulation may occur in the following possible ways: (1) K-activation would rapidly repolarize the junctional membranes within the TTS and consequently reduce Ca conductance that is voltage dependent and necessary for ECC. (2) A reduction in the length constant of the tubules would occur due to an increase in K-conductance of the tubular membranes. Such a change would oppose both the channeling of current between the surface and diadic membranes as well as an inward electrotonic spread of potential.

The refractory period following contractile activation (Caputo, 1972; Suarez-Kurtz and Sorenson, *this volume*) may also be regulated by K activation within the TTS. The persistence of an increase in membrane conductance following complete repolarization of the membrane (see Suarez-Kurtz and Sorenson, *this volume*) would antagonize a subsequent excitatory signal. We prefer this explanation for the refractory period to that of a temporary depletion of the Ca source, because of the responsiveness of fibers under experimental conditions to caffeine. That is, fibers in high K or during the refractory period immediately following removal of excess K, respond with maximal tensions to the application of caffeine (Chiarandini et al., 1970). This demonstrates that the Ca load of the SR is not depleted under conditions in which tension cannot be elicited by membrane depolarization.

Although the regulation of the ECC signal by tubular K activation is speculative, the localization of K sites within the TTS of depolarized crayfish fibers has been demonstrated.

ACKNOWLEDGMENTS

Work in the laboratory is supported in part by grants from the Muscular Dystrophy Associations of America, Inc.; by Public Health Service Research Grants (HL 16082, NS 05920, GM 18640); Training Grant (NS 05328) and NS 11766 from the National Institute of Neurological Diseases and Stroke, and the H. Houston Merritt Clinical Research Center for Muscular Dystrophy and Related Diseases. Dr. Zollman held a Research Fellowship from the MDAA and Dr. Orentlicher held a Research Fellowship from the MDAA.

REFERENCES

Adrian, R. H., Chandler, W. M. and Hodgkin, A. L. (1969): The kinetics of mechanical activation in frog muscle. *J. Physiol.*, 204:204–230.

Atwood, H. L. (1972): Crustacean muscle. In: *The Structure and Function of Muscle,* edited by G. H. Bourne, pp. 421–489. Academic Press, New York.

Bennett, H. S. (1955): Modern concepts of structure of striated muscle. *Am. J. Phys. Med.*, 34:46.

Brandt, P. W., Reuben, J. P., Girardier, L. and Grundfest, H. (1965): Correlated morphological and physiological studies on isolated single muscle fibers. I. Fine structure of the crayfish muscle fiber. *J. Cell Biol.*, 25:233–261.

Brandt, P. W., Reuben, J. P. and Grundfest, H. (1968): Correlated morphological and physiological studies on isolated single muscle fibers. II. The properties of the crayfish transverse tubular system: localization of the sites of reversible swelling. *J. Cell Biol.*, 38:115–129.

Caputo, C. (1972): The effect of low temperature on the excitation-contraction coupling phenomena of frog single muscle fibers. *J. Physiol.*, 223:461.

Chiarandini, D. J., Reuben, J. P., Brandt, P. W. and Grundfest, H. (1970): Effects of caffeine on crayfish muscle fibers. I. Activation of contraction and induction of Ca-spike electrogenesis. *J. Gen. Physiol.,* 55:640–664.

Chiarandini, D. J., and Stefani, E. (1976): Ca and excitation-contraction coupling in frog skeletal muscle fibers. In: *Electrobiology of Nerve, Synapse, and Muscle,* edited by J. P. Reuben, D. P. Purpura, M. V. L. Bennett, and E. Kandel. Raven Press, New York.

Costantin, L. L., and Podolsky, R. J. (1967): Depolarization of the internal membrane system in the activation of frog skeletal muscle. *J. Gen. Physiol.,* 50:1110–1124.

Dulhunty, A. F., and Gage, P. W. (1973): Differential effects of glycerol treatment on membrane capacity and excitation-contraction coupling in toad sartorius fibers. *J. Physiol.,* 234:373–408.

Eastwood, A. B., Zollman, J. R., Katz, G. M., and Reuben, J. P. (1973): Disruption of the TTS in crayfish muscle fibers. *Fed. Proc.,* 32:373 (Abst. No. 880).

Edwards, C., Chichibu, S., and Hagiwara, S. (1964): Relation between membrane potential changes and tension in barnacle muscle fibers. *J. Gen. Physiol.,* 48:225–234.

Franzini-Armstrong, C. (1973): Membraneous Systems in Muscle Fibers. In: *Structure and Function of Muscle,* edited by G. H. Bourne, pp. 532–619. Academic Press, New York.

Gainer, H., and Grundfest, H. (1968): Permeability of alkali metal cations in lobster muscle. A comparison of electrophysiological and osmometric analyses. *J. Gen. Physiol.,* 51:399–425.

Girardier, L., Reuben, J. P., Brandt, P. W., and Grundfest, H. (1963): Evidence for anion permselective membranes in crayfish muscle fibers and its possible role in excitation-contraction coupling. *J. Gen. Physiol.,* 47:189–214.

Grundfest, H. (1962): Ionic transport across neural and non-neural membranes. In: *Properties of Membranes and Diseases of the Nervous System,* edited by M. D. Yahr, pp. 71–99. Springer, New York.

Hodgkin, A. L., and Horowicz, P. (1959): The influence of potassium and chloride ions on the membrane potential of single muscle fibers. *J. Physiol.,* 148:127–160.

Howell, J. N., and Jenden, D. J. (1967): T-tubules of skeletal muscle: morphological alterations which interrupt excitation-contraction coupling. *Fed. Proc.,* 26:553.

Huxley, A. F., and Straub, R. W. (1958): Local activation and interfibrillar structures in striated muscle. *J. Physiol.,* 143:40P.

Huxley, A. F. and Taylor, R. E. (1958): Local activation of striated muscle fibres. *J. Physiol.,* 144:426–441.

Kasai, M., and Miyamoto, H. (1973): Depolarization induced calcium release from sarcoplasmic reticulum membrane fragments by changing ionic environment. *FEBS Lett.,* 34:299–301.

Krolenko, S. A. and Schwinka, N. E. (1974): Vacuolation of skeletal muscle fibers. II. Formation of vacuoles at the action of direct current. *Cytology (USSR),* 16:12.

Lüttgau, H. C., and Oetliker, M. (1968): The action of caffeine on the activation of the contractile mechanism in striated muscle fibers. *J. Physiol.,* 194:51–74.

Nakajima, S., and Bastian, J. (1976): Membrane properties of the transverse tubular system of amphibian skeletal muscle. In: *Electrobiology of the Nerve, Synapse, and Muscle,* edited by J. P. Reuben, D. P. Purpura, M. V. L. Bennett, and E. Kandel. Raven Press, New York.

Nakajima, S., Nakajima, Y., and Peachey, L. D. (1973): Speed of repolarization and morphology of glygerol-treated frog muscle fibers. *J. Physiol.,* 234:465–480.

Orentlicher, M., and Reuben, J. P. (1971): Localization of ionic conductances in crayfish muscle fibers. *J. Membrane Biol.,* 4:209–226.

Orentlicher, M., Reuben, J. P., Grundfest, H., and Brandt, P. W. (1974): Calcium binding and tension development in detergent-treated muscle fibers. *J. Gen. Physiol.,* 63:168–186.

Reuben, J. P., Brandt, P. W., Garcia, H., and Grundfest, H. (1967a): Excitation-contraction coupling in crayfish. *Am. Zoologist,* 7:623–645.

Reuben, J. P., Brandt, P. W., and Grundfest, H. (1967b): Tension evoked in skinned crayfish muscle fibers by anions, pH and drugs. *J. Gen. Physiol.,* 50:2501.

Reuben J. P., Girardier, L., and Grundfest, H. (1964): Water transfer and cell structure in isolated crayfish muscle fibers. *J. Gen. Physiol.,* 47:1141–1174.

Sandow, A. (1965): Excitation-contraction coupling in skeletal muscle. *Pharmacol. Revs.,* 17:265–320.

Sandow, A. (1970): Skeletal muscle. *Ann. Rev. Physiol.,* 32:87–138.

Schneider, M. F., and Chandler, W. K. (1973): Voltage dependent charge movement in skeletal muscle: a possible step in excitation-contraction coupling. *Nature,* 242:244–246.

Suarez-Kurtz, G., Reuben, J. P., Brandt, P. W., and Grundfest, H. (1972): Membrane calcium activation in excitation-contraction coupling. *J. Gen. Physiol.,* 59:676–688.

Suarez-Kurtz, G., and Sorenson, A. L. (1976): The roles of external calcium in excitation-contraction coupling in crab muscle fibers. In: *Electrobiology of Nerve, Synapse, and Muscle,* edited by J. P. Reuben, D. P. Purpura, M. V. L. Bennett, and E. Kandel. Raven Press, New York.

Sugi, H. (1968): Local activation of frog muscle fibers with linearly rising currents. *J. Physiol.,* 199:549–567.

Wood, D. S., Zollman, J. R., Reuben, J. P., and Brandt, P. W. (1975): Human skeletal muscle: properties of the "chemically skinned" fiber. *Science,* 187:1075–1076.

Zollman, J. R., Eastwood, A. B., Reuben, J. P. and Brandt, P. W. (1974): Ionic permeabilities and equilibria in the TTS of crayfish muscle. *Fed. Proc.,* 33:1402 (Abstr. 1011).

Electrobiology of Nerve, Synapse, and Muscle,
edited by J. P. Reuben, D. P. Purpura, M. V. L. Bennett,
and E. R. Kandel. Raven Press, New York © 1976

Ca and Excitation-Contraction Coupling in Frog Skeletal Muscle Fibers

D. J. Chiarandini and E. Stefani*

*Department of Ophthalmology, New York University Medical Center, New York, New York 10016; and *Departamento de Fisiología, Centro de Investigación y Estudios Avanzados del IPN, Mexico City, Mexico*

Since the pioneering work of Ringer (1882), it has been well established that Ca ions in the external medium are essential for contraction. The possibility that extracellular Ca plays a direct role in contraction activating the contractile proteins has been raised several times in the past (Bailey, 1942; Heilbrunn and Wiercinski, 1947; Bianchi and Shanes, 1959). Lately, however, it has been disregarded because calculations have shown that the Ca influx during contraction is insufficient to account for the increase of myoplasmic Ca required for triggering the contraction (Sandow, 1965).

It is considered now that the role of extracellular Ca on contraction is indirect, as a factor necessary to maintain the electrical excitability of the muscle membrane (Jenden and Reger, 1963; Edman and Grieve, 1964). This view is based on the fact that incubating muscles in salines considered to be "Ca free" has no inhibitory effect on contraction provided that the depolarization that follows this treatment is prevented by the addition of other divalet cations or by the intracellular injection of current (Frank, 1962; Jenden and Reger, 1963; Lüttgau, 1963).

In our opinion, however, this evidence does not rule out completely a direct role of extracellular Ca in tension development. In the above-mentioned studies no special care was taken to determine and control the Ca contamination that most likely existed in the "Ca-free" salines. The contamination Ca present in an analytical grade NaCl might be enough to produce a Ca concentration of 8 μM in frog saline (Frankenhaeuser, 1957), and very recently, Ca contaminations between 10 and 25 μM have been reported in "Ca-free" salines under conditions close to those of the experiments mentioned above (Milligan, 1965; Hurlbut et al., 1971; Miledi and Thies, 1971).

Calcium contaminations of these magnitudes cannot be ignored when it is considered that, at rest, the Ca concentration in the myoplasm may be as low as 10^{-7} M (Ebashi and Endo, 1968). It is evident that under these conditions the Ca contamination in the external solution may set up a force

---

* A. Rosenblueth Visiting Professor, supported by the Grass Foundation.

that will drive Ca into the muscle. Therefore, tensions recorded when muscles were bathed with salines assumed to be "Ca free," can be due to an influx of Ca from the external medium.

In the past years we have explored the possibility that a Ca influx can be the triggering signal for contraction. We have studied the effects of very low Ca concentrations and the action of Mn, an inhibitor of cell membrane permeability to Ca, on tension development. Two previous papers dealing with this matter have been published (Chiarandini and Stefani, 1973; Stefani and Chiarandini, 1973).

RESULTS

Effects of Very Low External Ca Concentrations

The object of these series of experiments was to analyze the effects of extremely low (Ca) in the external medium on the electrical properties and tension development in the frog muscle.

The control saline was made from stock solutions and contained (mM) 114.5 NaCl, 2.5 KCl, 1.8 $CaCl_2$, 4.0 $MgSO_4$, and 2.0 Tris-Cl, with a pH of 7.3. A "Ca-free" saline was prepared by omitting the $CaCl_2$ from the control fluid and adding 1 mM EGTA (ethylene glycol-bis-(β-aminoethylether) N,N'-tetraacetic acid) previously neutralized to pH 7.0. The main sources of Ca contamination were the chemicals and the Ca leak from the muscle. To minimize the (Ca) in the "Ca-free" salines we selected reagents with low levels of Ca content and used repeated or continuous exchange of the bathing fluid. The (Ca) was determined by atomic absorption spectrophotometry in the stock solutions and was found to be detectable (i.e., more than 1 ppm) only in the $MgSO_4$ and the KCl solutions. Thus, the (Ca) in the "Ca-free" salines with 2.5 mM KCl was 2.7×10^{-7} M and 1.4×10^{-6} M in the "Ca-free" saline with 117 mM KCl, used to induce contractures. Assuming an apparent binding constant for the Ca-EGTA complex of 7.6×10^6 M^{-1} (Portzehl et al., 1964), the addition of 1 mM EGTA reduced the ionized Ca in these two salines to 0.6×10^{-10} M and 0.3×10^{-9} M, respectively.

A first series of experiments was performed to study the effects of the "Ca-free" salines on the resting potential, action potential and K-induced depolarizations. The electrical measurements were performed in superficial fibers of pairs of sartorius muscles of frogs *Leptodactylus ocellatus* with conventional intracellular technique. One muscle was bathed with control saline while the other was soaked in the "Ca-free" saline for 25 to 35 min. Table 1 shows that in the five pairs of sartorii, there was no difference between the resting potential of the control muscles and of the muscles exposed to extremely low (Ca).

To test the effect of Ca deprivation on the K-induced depolarizations, the

TABLE 1. Effect of "Ca-free" saline on the resting potential and K-induced depolarizations[a]

$(Ca)_0 = 1.8$ mM			$(Ca)_0 = <3 \times 10^{-9}$ M		
2.5 mM K	40 mM K	80 mM K	2.5 mM K	40 mM K	80 mM K
-88.1 ± 0.4	-46.9 ± 0.9		-89.0 ± 0.8	-47.1 ± 0.7	
-91.9 ± 0.9	-44.2 ± 1.3		-89.3 ± 1.1	-44.5 ± 0.9	
-92.2 ± 1.3		-19.7 ± 0.8	-93.0 ± 0.8		-22.9 ± 0.6
-94.2 ± 0.6		-15.3 ± 0.4	-94.9 ± 0.7		-16.5 ± 0.5
-90.3 ± 1.0		-26.7 ± 1.8	-90.2 ± 1.1		-24.7 ± 0.8

[a] Each value is the mean $\pm$ SE of 8 to 12 fibers of one muscle.

muscles were exposed thereafter to 40 or 80 mM KCl and the resting potential was recorded between 5 and 8 min after increasing $(K)_0$. In these solutions KCl was substituted for NaCl in equivalent amounts. Table 1 shows that the virtual absence of extracellular Ca does not affect the K-induced depolarizations.

Action potentials were elicited by brief intracellular depolarizing pulses. The exposure to the "Ca-free" saline for about 20 min. reduced the overshoot from 34.7 ± 0.9 mV (28) (mean $\pm$ SE; number of fibers) to 26.4 ± 0.9 mV (24) and the action potential duration, measured at a membrane potential of 0 mV, from 1.06 ± 0.08 msec (28) to 0.72 ± 0.02 msec (20). These changes are statistically significant ($p < 0.01$).

These measurements showed that the fibers had normal resting potential and excitability, but that the action potential was somewhat smaller and briefer. Since the twitch amplitude depends on the action potential duration and overshoot height (Taylor et al., 1969), and these parameters were modified, we had to limit our analysis to K contractures.

In these experiments we used single muscle fibers dissected from the muscle tibialis anticus longus. Tension was recorded isometrically and tetrodotoxin (10^{-7} g/ml) was used throughout to prevent twitches during the K depolarization.

The application of a solution with a 117 mM KCl to the fibers produced a sudden tension that developed and subsided in about 7 sec (Fig. 1, left traces). These contractures were biphasic with a peak and a slow component as has been reported (Costantin, 1971). Fifteen minutes after the control contractures, a "Ca-free" saline [(Ca) $= 0.6 \times 10^{-10}$ M] with a normal K concentration was flushed through the chamber at a rate of 0.5 ml/sec for 40 sec. Preliminary measurements showed that 98% of the solution in the chamber was replaced after flowing 5 ml of the new solution. Immediately after, a "Ca-free" saline with 117 mM KCl was applied for 2 to 3 sec at a very fast flow. The presoaking for 40 sec in the virtual absence of Ca markedly reduced the K-induced contractures (Fig. 1, middle traces).

In the six fibers studied, the main inhibitory effect was on the slow

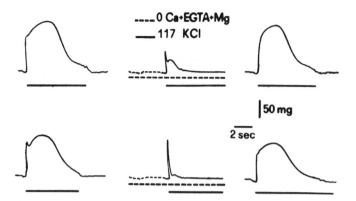

FIG. 1. Effects of "Ca-free" saline on K contractures in two single muscle fibers. **Left records:** control K contractures induced with 117 mM KCl saline. **Middle records:** the fibers were exposed to "Ca-free" saline for 40 sec (*broken line*) before inducing tension with the 117 mM KCl "Ca-free" saline. **Right records:** control K contractures. The interval between contractures was 15 min.

component of the tension, which was briefer and reduced to 39 ± 16.5% (mean ± SE) of the control value (mean: 105 mg). The peak phase was affected to a lesser degree, its amplitude was 78 ± 10.5% of the control (mean: 100 mg). In preliminary experiments we observed that if the fibers were exposed to the "Ca-free" saline without continuous flow of the solution, the inhibitory effect was less obvious, even if the presoaking time was extended to several minutes. This could be explained by the existence of unstirred layers and a Ca accumulation in the saline adjacent to the fiber surface.

After allowing 15 min, the 117 mM KCl was applied again to test the reversibility of the low Ca treatment. The tension thus evoked was consistently similar to the first control. Usually, the sequence shown in Fig. 1 was repeated for a second time, in some cases using 60 mM KCl with similar results.

Effects of Manganese on the Mechanical Responses

Twitch and Tetanus

A concentration of Mn of 5 mM or above produced a reduction in the twitch amplitude. In 12 single muscle fibers 10 mM Mn decreased the twitch amplitude by 45.0 ± 6.7% (mean ± SE). Control tests showed that this effect was not related to the slight increase in the osmolarity of the saline that resulted from the addition of $MnCl_2$.

Figure 2 shows the effect and velocity of action of 7.5 and 10 mM Mn in the same single muscle fiber. In both experiments the reduction of the twitch

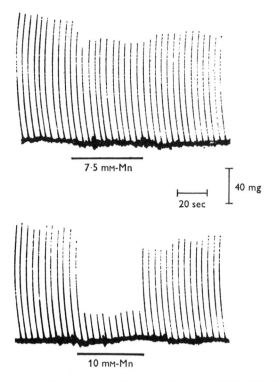

FIG. 2. Action of Mn on twitches in a single muscle fiber. Twitches evoked by extracellular stimulation at a frequency of 1 every 4 sec. **Upper record:** the application of a saline with 7.5 mM Mn (*continuous line*) somewhat reduced the amplitude of the twitch. **Bottom record:** same fiber with 10 mM Mn (*continuous line*); the twitch was markedly reduced in about 8 sec. Upon returning the fiber to control saline the twitch recovered the amplitude.

amplitude was maximal within less than 8 sec after the application of Mn. The inhibitory action was reversed quickly after returning the preparation to normal saline.

Simultaneous records of the extracellular action potential and twitch showed that under Mn the extracellular action potential was broader and had somewhat reduced positive and negative deflections. The twitch response was diminished without appreciable change in its time course.

The depressant action of Mn on the twitch cannot be accounted for by changes in the electrical properties of the muscle fibers. The resting potential of 13 fibers was slightly increased from a control value of -82.6 ± 0.8 mV to 90.0 ± 0.7 mV after equilibrating the muscle in a saline containing 10 mM Mn. The action potential overshoot was unchanged by Mn whereas its duration was increased. Measured at 0 mV level, the action potential duration was 0.95 ± 0.02 msec (10) in control saline and 1.10 ± 0.03 msec (8) under Mn.

The effect of 10 mM Mn on tetanus amplitude was studied in six single fibers. The cells were stimulated at frequencies of 50, 75, and 100 Hz for 0.5 sec. Whereas in all the fibers the twitch was reduced by Mn, the effect on tetanus was variable. In two fibers no change was detected and in the others a reduction of 10,16,16, and 42% was recorded.

K-Induced Contractures

The effects of Mn on K contractures was studied in 10 single fibers. To induce tension, salines with a constant (K) × (Cl) product with (K) ranging from 30 to 75 mM and isotonic K_2SO_4 saline (190 mM K) were used (Hodgkin and Horowicz, 1959). Submaximal contractures, elicited with 75 mM K or less, were consistently reduced or blocked by 10 mM (Fig. 3). In five single fibers, 10 mM Mn reduced by 73 ± 4% the K contractures induced with 75 mM K. Maximal K contractures elicited with 190 mM K, on the other hand, showed only relatively minor changes in their amplitude.

Mn consistently prolonged the K contractures, this action being more evident in the case of maximal contractures.

The observed diminution of the tension output could be due to a reduction of the ability of K to depolarize the fibers since in the case of submaximal K contractures, the amplitude of the tension depends on the magnitude of the triggering depolarization (Hodgkin and Horowicz, 1960a). This possibility, however, was ruled out since it was found in several fibers that 10 mM

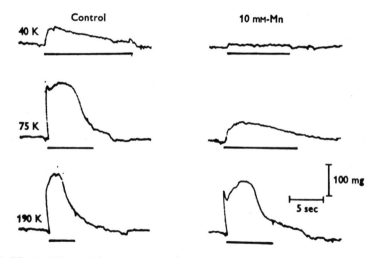

FIG. 3. Effect of Mn on K contractures in a single muscle fiber (diameter 89 μm). K contractures were induced with solutions having a constant (K) · (Cl) product. A saline with 10 mM Mn was flushed 1 min before eliciting tension. The fiber was alternately exposed for 10 to 15 sec (*continuous lines*) to the different K salines without and with 10 mM Mn. The interval between contractures was 10 to 15 min. Mn reduces 40 and 75 mM K tensions and slows down the contractures induced with 190 mM K. The effect was reversible.

Mn did not change the depolarizations induced by salines with (K) × (Cl) product constant and (K) of 10, 20, 30, and 75 mM.

The relationship between tension amplitude and different $(K)_0$ was studied in three single fibers in the absence and presence of 10 mM Mn. Figure 4 illustrates the results obtained in two fibers. Mn shifted the curve relating tension versus log $(K)_0$ to the right changing the minimal $(K)_0$ necessary to produce a detectable tension from 20 to 35 mM. According to our previous measurements this represents a change in the mechanical threshold from −48 to −33 mV.

Caffeine-Induced Contractures

The inhibition of the contractile responses induced by electrical stimulation by Mn could be due to different effects. For example, it could be due to a reduction of the efficiency of the coupling between membrane depolarization and the increase in myoplasmic Ca responsible for tension, to a diminution of the amount of Ca released from the sarcoplasmic reticulum (SR) or to a decrease in the sensitivity of the contractile proteins towards

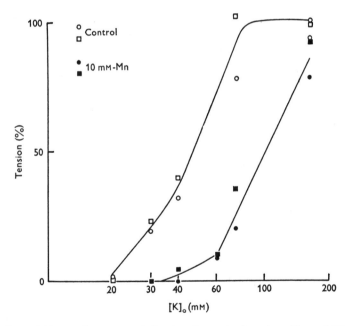

FIG. 4. Effect of Mn on the curve relating tension output vs. logarithm of $(K)_0$. Results from two fibers. Tensions were induced with solutions having a constant $(K) \cdot (Cl)$ product. The fiber was alternately exposed to solutions with different K concentrations and without or with 10 mM Mn. Mn was added one minute before each contracture. *Open symbols:* control contractures. *Filled symbols:* effect of 10 mM Mn. Mn shifts the curve towards the right increasing the mechanical threshold. Control 190 mM K tensions were about 2.5 kg/cm² in both fibers.

Ca. To distinguish between these possibilities, the effect of Mn on caffeine contractures was examined since this alkaloid induces tension by a movement of Ca from the SR to the myoplasm (Weber and Herz, 1968), without involving the excitation-contraction coupling step (Axelsson and Thesleff, 1958).

In the three fibers studied, 10 mM Mn did not affect submaximal caffeine contractures induced with 3 to 4 mM caffeine even after presoaking the fibers in a solution with Mn for 17 min. These results are in keeping with previous data obtained in crayfish muscle fibers (Zachar and Zacharova, 1968; Chiarandini et al., 1970).

DISCUSSION

Measurements with radioactive calcium have shown that during muscle depolarization and contraction there is an increased Ca influx into the muscle (Bianchi and Shanes, 1959; Winegrad, 1970). The present results show that treatments that decrease Ca movements across the muscle membrane, either by reducing the driving force for the ion or by decreasing the muscle membrane permeability, result in a partial inhibition of tension output. These findings suggest that this Ca influx may be involved in the triggering of contraction.

The reduction of $(Ca)_0$ to a value of about 0.3×10^{-9} M consistently produced a reversible inhibition of the K contractures. This effect is not due to a loss of membrane potential, which was kept normal by the presence of Mg in the saline, or a consequence of a depletion of the Ca content of the SR. The exposure to "Ca-free" saline was very brief as compared to 200 min, the half-time of the Ca efflux from the compartment thought to represent the SR (Curtis, 1970).

The marked reduction of the tension output found when muscle were exposed to extremely low $(Ca)_0$ can be explained assuming that the virtual removal of the external Ca reduces the driving force for this cation and, therefore, its influx during the muscle contraction.

The driving force for Ca is given by $(E_{Ca} - E_m)$, with $E_{Ca} = (RT/zF) \ln (Ca)_0/(Ca)_i$, and E_m the membrane potential. An exact determination of the value of the driving force when the muscle is bathed with control or "Ca-free" saline is not possible at the present time. The value of $(Ca)_i$ at rest can only be estimated to be between 10^{-8} and 10^{-7} M considering that a $(Ca)_i$ of 0.3 to 1.2×10^{-7} M induces threshold tension in frog skinned fibers (Ebashi and Endo, 1968; Hellam and Podolsky, 1969). The value of $(Ca)_0$ in the "Ca-free" saline can be calculated to be between 0.2 and 3.0×10^{-9} M, using the two extreme values given in the literature for the apparent binding constant of the Ca-EGTA complex (Portzehl et al., 1964; Ebashi and Endo, 1968). Considering this range of values it can be estimated that E_{Ca} in control saline is at least 120 mV and in "Ca-free" medium, some value between

−16 and −80 mV. Thus, in the "Ca-free" condition a drastic change in the driving force for Ca takes place and the Ca entrance into the muscle has to be severely limited. If the triggering of contraction is related to a Ca influx, it is expected that the tension output should be reduced under this condition.

The possible relationship between Ca influx and triggering of contraction was further explored by the study of the action of Mn on the twitch and K contractures.

Manganese is a well-known blocker of the membrane permeability to Ca in a large variety of excitable cells. It reduces or blocks the inward Ca current in barnacle muscle and frog atrial muscle (Hagiwara, 1966; Rougier et al., 1969) and the overshoot of the Ca-dependent spikes in barnacle and crayfish muscle and in snail neurons (Hagiwara and Nakajima, 1966; Takeda, 1967; Meves, 1968). Furthermore, the Ca-dependent depolarizing response in the presynaptic terminal of the giant synapse of the squid and the Ca entry associated with K depolarization in squid axon are also blocked by Mn (Katz and Miledi, 1969; Baker et al., 1971).

The foregoing data suggest that Mn may also be a blocker of Ca permeability in the case of frog muscle and indicates that the observed reduction of the K contractures and twitches, as well as the shift of the mechanical threshold, could be due to this pharmacological action.

The inhibitory action of Mn on tensions induced by depolarization, reported previously in crustacean muscle (Orkand, 1962; Zachar and Zacharova, 1968), is not due to changes in the electrical properties or in the contractile elements of the fibers. The action potential mechanism and the response of the cell membrane to the depolarizing effect of high $(K)_0$ were found to be essentially normal. Similarly, as shown by the integrity of the responses to 190 mM K and to caffeine and by the minimal effect observed on the tetanus, the release of Ca from the SR and the subsequent response of the contractile proteins appear to be unaffected.

These findings and the observed change in the mechanical threshold to a more depolarized level, suggest that Mn may be acting at the coupling step between the electrical events and the release of Ca from the SR. The fact that the reduction of tension takes place within less than 8 sec after adding Mn suggests that the site of action may be the surface and transverse tubular surfaces.

Twitches were less reduced by Mn than were K contractures. This difference can be attributed to the observed prolongation of the action potential which should increase the mechanical output (Taylor et al., 1969) and thus, counteract the blocking action of Mn.

As has been mentioned before, the Ca influx during muscle activation has been considered too small to have a significant role in tension development. There is, however, recent evidence that suggests the existence of a mechanism capable of amplifying this Ca influx to a sarcoplasmic Ca concentration adequate to activate the contractile proteins.

Some years ago Bianchi and Bolton (1967) suggested that during muscle activation a Ca release from the transverse tubules could induce a secondary release of Ca from the SR, which in turn could trigger the contraction. This possibility is now supported by experimental data. In frog skinned fibers it has been suggested that an increase in the free myoplasmic Ca induces a release of Ca from the SR (Endo et al., 1970; Ford and Podolsky, 1970; 1972). A similar mechanism appears to exist in crayfish muscle fibers in which intracellular injections of Ca produce local contractures that, under certain treatments, propagate (Reuben et al., 1974).

If this mechanism operates in physiological conditions, it is possible that the process that couples the excitation (depolarization) of the muscle with the contraction is a transient Ca influx that would be determined by the magnitude of the driving force for Ca and by a brief increase of a voltage-dependent Ca permeability. The present results, which show a reduction in the tension output when either the driving force for Ca or the Ca membrane permeability were reduced, support this hypothesis. This hypothesis has also been offered as an explanation for excitation in crayfish muscle fibers (Suarez-Kurtz et al., 1972).

If the coupling signal between excitation and contraction is a Ca influx, it is expected that within certain limits, the tension output would depend on the ability of Ca to cross the cell membrane and that there will be a close correlation between mechanical threshold and Ca influx. Indeed, several reports in the literature show that such a relationship may exist. Nitrate, caffeine at low doses, and low external ionic strength enhance ^{45}Ca uptake in muscle and, at the same time, reduce the mechanical threshold and potentiate the tension (Bianchi and Shanes, 1959; Hodgkin and Horowicz, 1960b; Bianchi, 1961; Sandow et al., 1964; Lorković, 1967). On the other hand, tetracaine and Mn, which reduce ^{45}Ca uptake, decrease tension and increase the mechanical threshold (Feinstein, 1963; Lüttgau and Oetliker, 1968; Sabatini-Smith and Holland, 1969; Chiarandini and Stefani, 1973).

Recent studies on the possible role of a Ca entry in excitation-contraction coupling (Armstrong et al., 1972; Sandow et al., 1974) have found that frog muscle fibers are capable of twitching with a $(Ca)_0$ of 2×10^{-9} M for relatively long periods, before inexcitability appears. The discrepancy between these results and our findings may be due to several factors. It is possible that the (Ca) at the level of the sarcolemma, $(Ca)_s$, was much larger in the experiments of Armstrong et al. and Sandow et al. than in ours, since there was 4 mM Mg in our saline whereas the authors mentioned had no divalent cations in the salines they studied.

It is presently thought that negative fixed charges in the plasma membrane give rise to a surface potential: ψ. The existence of ψ will determine a $(Ca)_s$ according to the Boltzmann equation:

$$(Ca)_s = (Ca)_b \, \exp^{-2F\psi/RT}$$

in which $(Ca)_b$ is the (Ca) in the bulk solution. If ψ has a value of -100 mV (McLaughlin et al., 1971), $(Ca)_s$ would be about 5×10^{-6} M when $(Ca)_b$ is 2×10^{-9} M. Such a $(Ca)_s$ would, most likely, favor a Ca entry. In our case the initial $(Ca)_b$ was 0.3×10^{-9} M, that is lower than in the experiments of the authors mentioned and, which is more important, 4 mM Mg was added to the saline. Divalent cations have a marked screening action on fixed charges (McLaughlin et al., 1971) and should reduce ψ. Consequently, $(Ca)_s$ should have been lower than in the experiments of Armstrong et al. and Sandow et al. and close to $(Ca)_b$.

The apparent lack of stirring of the bathing solution in the experiments performed by both groups of investigators could be another contributing factor to the difference in the results. As was mentioned before, we found that constant mixing of the solution bathing the preparation was essential to fully evidence the depressant action of the "Ca-free" saline.

Finally, it should be considered the possibility that twitches and K contractures respond differently to the low Ca treatment. This possibility, however, seems rather unlikely. Twitches and K contractures appear to be initiated by a common mechanism. They are triggered by a sudden depolarization and have similar thresholds (Hodgkin and Horowicz, 1960a; Reuben et al., 1967; Adrian et al., 1969).

ACKNOWLEDGMENTS

This work was supported by the Consejo Nacional de Investigaciones Cientificas y Tecnicas, Argentina and, partially, by grant EY01297 from the USPHS.

REFERENCES

Armstrong, C. M., Bezanilla, F. M., and Horowicz, P. (1972): Twitches in the presence of ethylene glycol bis (β-amino-ethyl ether)N, N'-tetraacetic acid. Biochim. Biophys. Acta, 267:605–608.

Axelsson, J., and Thesleff, S. (1958): Activation of the contractile mechanism in striated muscle. Acta Physiol. Scand., 44:55–66.

Bailey, K. (1942): Myosin and adenosine triphosphatase. Biochem J., 36:121–139.

Baker, P. F., Meves, H., and Ridgway, E. B. (1971): Phasic entry of calcium in response to depolarization of giant axons of Loligo forbesi. J. Physiol., 216:70–71.

Bianchi, C. P. (1961): The effect of caffeine on radiocalcium movement in frog sartorius. J. Gen. Physiol., 44:845–858.

Bianchi, C. P., and Bolton, T. C. (1967): Action of local anesthetics on coupling systems in muscle. J. Pharmacol. Exp. Ther., 157:388–405.

Bianchi, C. P., and Shanes, A. (1959): Calcium influx in skeletal muscle at rest. J. Gen. Physiol., 42:803–815.

Chiarandini, D. J., Reuben, J. P., Girardier, L., Katz, G. M., and Grundfest, H. (1970): Effects of caffeine on crayfish muscle fibres. II. Refractoriness and factors influencing recovery (repriming) of contractile responses. *J. Gen. Physiol.,* 55:665–687.

Chiarandini, D. J., and Stefani, E. (1973): Effects of manganese on the electrical and mechanical properties of frog skeletal muscle fibres. *J. Physiol.,* 232:129–147.

Costantin, L. L. (1971): Biphasic potassium contractures in frog muscle fibers. *J. Gen. Physiol.,* 58:117–130.

Curtis, B. A. (1970): Calcium efflux from frog twitch muscle fibers. *J. Gen. Physiol.,* 55:243–253.

Ebashi, S., and Endo, M. (1968): Calcium ions and muscle contraction. *Progr. Biophys. Mol. Biol.,* 18:123–183.

Edman, K. A. P., and Grieve, D. W. (1964): On the role of calcium in the excitation-contraction process of frog sartorius muscle. *J. Physiol.,* 170:138–152.

Endo, M., Tanaka, M., and Ogawa, Y. (1970): Calcium induced release of calcium from the sarcoplasmic reticulum of skinned skeletal muscle fibres. *Nature,* 228:34–36.

Feinstein, M. B. (1963): Inhibition of caffeine rigor and radiocalcium movements by local anesthetics in frog sartorius muscle. *J. Gen. Physiol.,* 47:151–172.

Ford, L. E., and Podolsky, R. J. (1970): Regenerative calcium release within muscle cells. *Science,* 167:58–59.

Ford, L. E., and Podolsky, R. J. (1972): Intracellular calcium movements in skinned muscle fibres. *J. Physiol.,* 223:21–33.

Frank, G. B. (1962): Utilization of bound calcium in the action of caffeine and certain multivalent cations on skeletal muscle. *J. Physiol.,* 163:254–268.

Frankenhaeuser, B. (1957): The effect of calcium on the myelinated nerve fibre. *J. Physiol.,* 137:245–260.

Hagiwara, S. (1966): Membrane properties of the barnacle muscle fiber. *Ann. NY Acad. Sci.,* 137:1015–1024.

Hagiwara, S., and Nakajima, S. (1966): Differences in Na and Ca spikes as examined by application of tetrodotoxin, procaine, and manganese ions. *J. Gen. Physiol.,* 49:793–818.

Heilbrunn, L. V., and Wiercinski, F. J. L. (1947): The action of various cations on muscle protoplasm. *J. Cell. Comp. Physiol.,* 29:15–32.

Hellam, D. C., and Podolsky, R. J. (1969): Force measurements in skinned muscle fibres. *J. Physiol.,* 200:807–819.

Hodgkin, A. L., and Horowicz, P. (1959): The influence of potassium and chloride ions on the membrane permeability of single muscle fibres. *J. Physiol.,* 148:127–160.

Hodgkin, A. L., and Horowicz, P. (1960a): Potassium contractures in single muscle fibres. *J. Physiol.,* 153:386–403.

Hodgkin, A. L., and Horowicz, P. (1960b): The effect of nitrate and other anions on the mechanical response of single muscle fibres. *J. Physiol.,* 153:404–412.

Hurlbut, W. P., Longenecker, H. B., Jr., and Mauro, A. (1971): Effects of calcium and magnesium on the frequency of miniature endplate potentials during prolonged tetanization. *J. Physiol.,* 219:17–38.

Jenden, D. J., and Reger, J. F. (1963): The role of resting potential changes in the contractile failure of frog sartorius muscles during calcium deprivation. *J. Physiol.,* 169:889–901.

Katz, B., and Miledi, R. (1969): Tetrodotoxin-resistant electric activity in presynaptic terminal. *J. Physiol.,* 203:459–487.

Lorković, H. (1967): The influence of ionic strength on potassium contractures and calcium movements in frog muscle. *J. Gen. Physiol.,* 50:883–891.

Lüttgau, H. C. (1963): The action of calcium on potassium contractures of single muscle fibres. *J. Physiol.,* 168:679–697.

Lüttgau, H. C., and Oetliker, H. (1968): The action of caffeine on the activation of the contractile mechanism in striated muscle fibres. *J. Physiol.,* 194:51–74.

McLaughlin, S. G. A., Szabo, G., and Eisenman, G. (1971): Divalent ions and the surface potential of charged phospholipid membranes. *J. Gen. Physiol.,* 58:667–687.

Meves, H. (1968): The ionic requirements for the production of action potentials in *Helix pomatia* neurons. *Pflügers Arch. Ges. Physiol.,* 304:215–241.

Miledi, R., and Thies, R. (1971): Tetanic and post-tetanic rise in frequency of miniature endplate potentials in low-calcium solutions. *J. Physiol.,* 212:245–257.

Milligan, J. V. (1965): The time course of the loss and recovery of contracture ability in frog striated muscle following exposure to Ca-free solutions. *J. Gen. Physiol.,* 48:841–858.

Orkand, R. K. (1962): Chemical inhibition of contraction in directly stimulated crayfish muscle fibres. *J. Physiol.*, 164:103–115.

Portzehl, H., Caldwell, P. C., and Rüegg, J. C. (1964): The dependence of contraction and relaxation of muscle fibres from the crab *Maia squinado* on the internal concentration of free calcium ions. *Biochim. Biophys. Acta*, 79:581–591.

Reuben, J. P., Brant, P. W., García, H., and Grundfest, H. (1967): Excitation-contraction coupling in crayfish. *Am. Zool.*, 7:623–645.

Reuben, J. P., Brandt, P. W., and Grundfest, H. (1974): Regulation of myoplasmic calcium concentration in intact crayfish muscle fibers. *J. Mechanochem. Cell Motility*, 2:269–285.

Ringer, S. (1882): A further contribution regarding the influence of different constituents of the blood on the contraction of the heart. *J. Physiol.*, 4:29–42.

Rougier, O., Vassort, G., Garnier, D., Gargouil, Y. M., and Coraboeuf, E. (1969): Existence and role of a slow inward current during the frog atrial action potential. *Pflügers Arch. Ges. Physiol.*, 308:91–110.

Sabatini-Smith, S., and Holland, W. C. (1969): Influence of manganese and ouabain on the rate of action of calcium on atrial contraction. *Am. J. Physiol.*, 216:244–248.

Sandow, A. (1965): Excitation-contraction coupling in skeletal muscle. *Pharmacol. Rev.*, 17:265–320.

Sandow, A., Pagala, M. K. D., and Sphicas, E. C. (1974): "Zero" Ca effects on excitation-contraction coupling (ECC). *Fed. Proc.*, 33:1259.

Sandow, A., Taylor, S. R., Isaacson, A., and Seguin, J. J. (1964): Electrochemical coupling in potentiation of muscular contraction. *Science*, 143:577–579.

Stefani, E., and Chiarandini, D. J. (1973): Skeletal muscle: Dependence of potassium contractures on extracellular calcium. *Pflügers Arch.*, 343:143–150.

Suarez-Kurtz, G., Reuben, J. P., Brandt, P. W., and Grundfest, H. (1972): Membrane calcium activation in excitation-contraction coupling. *J. Gen. Physiol.*, 59:676–688.

Takeda, K. (1967): Permeability changes associated with the action potential in procaine-treated crayfish abdominal muscle fibers. *J. Gen. Physiol.*, 50:1049–1074.

Taylor, S. R., Preiser, H., and Sandow, A. (1969): Mechanical threshold as a factor in excitation-contraction coupling. *J. Gen. Physiol.*, 54:352–368.

Weber, A., and Herz, R. (1968): The relationship between caffeine contracture of intact muscle and the effect of caffeine on reticulum. *J. Gen. Physiol.*, 52:750–759.

Winegrad, S. (1970): The intracellular site of calcium activation of contraction in frog skeletal muscle. *J. Gen. Physiol.*, 55:77–88.

Zachar, J., and Zacharova, D. (1968): Modification of the excitation-contraction link by divalent cations in crustacean muscle fibres. *Abstr. XXIV Int. Physiol. Congr.*, p. 1435.

Electrobiology of Nerve, Synapse, and Muscle,
edited by J. P. Reuben, D. P. Purpura, M. V. L. Bennett,
and E. R. Kandel. Raven Press, New York © 1976

Role of External Calcium in Excitation-Contraction Coupling in Crab Muscle Fibers

G. Suarez-Kurtz and A. L. Sorenson

Departamento de Farmacologia, Instituto de Ciencias Biomedicas, Universidade Federal do Rio de Janeiro, Rio de Janeiro, Brazil

It has been proposed that the conveyance of electrical information from the surface membrane to the junctional membranes (diads and triads) within the transverse tubular system (TTS) of striated muscle occurs by: (1) an electrotonic spread of the surface depolarization along the tubular membranes (Huxley and Taylor, 1958); (2) propagation of an action potential along the tubular network (see Nakajima and Bastian, *this volume*); and (3) channeling of current between the surface membrane and the high-conductance junctional membranes within the depths of the TTS (Girardier et al., 1963; Reuben et al., 1967).

The junctional membranes, in turn, are believed to be involved in conveying a signal to the sarcoplasmic reticulum (SR) by: (1) membrane depolarization *per se* (Kuffler, 1946). A potential-induced molecular displacement within the junctional membranes of the tubules may convey information to the SR via molecular projections across the junctional gap (Schneider and Chandler, 1973). (2) An influx of Ca across the tubular membranes supplies the total amount of Ca required for any degree of contractile activation (Bianchi and Shanes, 1959; Zachar, 1971; Atwater et al., 1974). (3) An influx of Ca causes the release of SR-stored Ca by a positive feedback process (Frank, 1960; Bianchi and Bolton, 1967; Endo et al., 1970; Ford and Podolsky, 1972). (4) An influx of Ca signals the release of SR-stored Ca via an intermediatory process that remains to be defined (Hagiwara and Naka, 1964; Reuben et al., 1967; Suarez-Kurtz et al., 1972; Chiarandini and Stefani, 1973; *this volume*).

As a result of studies originating from Professor Grundfest's laboratory (Girardier et al., 1963; Reuben et al., 1967; Suarez-Kurtz et al., 1972), a membrane Ca activation and the subsequent influx of Ca is seen as an integral step in excitation-contraction coupling (ECC) in crayfish muscle fibers. The present experiments extend this conclusion to the fibers of the South American crab *Callinectes danae,* which, in contrast to both barnacle and crayfish muscle fibers, are fast acting (Suarez-Kurtz and Reuben, 1975). Depolarizing Ca activation in these crab fibers is more prominent than in other crustaceans and can be studied without resorting to pharmacological treatments. Furthermore, the kinetics of contraction are comparable to those of frog twitch fibers.

We will first describe the electrical properties of this new preparation and then discuss experiments which point to the participation of a membrane Ca current in excitation and tension development. Finally, we present evidence that membrane depolarization per se is not adequate for initiation of tension development and that the entry of extracellular Ca does not provide a sufficient quantity of Ca for contractile activation.

Experiments were performed on single fibers isolated from the flexor and extensor muscle of the walking legs of *Callinectes danae*. The procedures followed for isolating the fibers, mounting them in experimental chambers, and recording membrane parameters and isometric tension were previously described (Suarez-Kurtz, 1974). The normal saline employed in this study was similar to that used by Fatt and Katz (1953) with the deletion of part of the NaCl to adjust for the osmotic blood concentration of these estuarine crabs.

ELECTRICAL PROPERTIES OF THE RESTING MEMBRANE

The resting permeability of these crab fibers is determined primarily by K and Cl since the fibers depolarize readily in solutions of elevated K, or when Cl is replaced by an impermeant anion such as sulfate or propionate. The former depolarization is steady, the latter is transient, which signifies that here as in frog fibers (Hodgkin and Horowicz, 1959), K plays the dominant role. The normal resting potential is -62 mV for an external K concentration of 12.5 mM, and Na and Mg are without important effect.

The cable characteristics of the single muscle fibers of *Callinectes danae* as determined by the method of Hodgkin and Rushton (1946; Fatt and Katz,

TABLE 1. *Low-frequency electrical constants of marine crab muscle fibers[a]*

Ref.[b]	D (microns)	R_{eff} (KΩ)	τ_m (msec)	λ (mm)	R_i (Ω × cm)	R_m (Ω × cm²)	C_m μF × cm⁻²	Species
1	181	20.0	3.0	0.7	103	128	29	Callinectes
2	180	10	4.6	0.9	69	116	42	Carcinus and Portunus
3	105	115	36	2.39	53	1,170	41	Carcinus "B"
4	210	30	55	1.55	63	282	15	Carcinus "C"

[a] D is the measured fiber diameter, R_{eff} is the effective (or input) resistance, τ_m is the membrane time constant, λ is the membrane length constant, R_i is the internal resistivity, R_m is the specific membrane resistance, and C_m is the specific membrane capacitance. Average values are presented. In the case of the present study, fibers with diameters of 250 μm or less are included; the references from other sources were selected for similar fiber sizes, saline solutions, and experimental conditions.
[b] References: (1) present study, average values of 18 fibers; (2) Fatt and Katz, 1953; (3) Atwood, 1963; (4) Atwood, 1963.

1951) are shown in Table 1. It can be seen that our results agree reasonably well with those derived from muscle fibers of *Portunus* and *Carcinus*, the species studied by Fatt and Katz (1953). A few fibers with cable characteristics different from those shown in the table were occasionally encountered. The electrical properties of these fibers were similar to those designated as "tonic" by Atwood et al. (1965). We shall, however, restrict our analysis of results to the more common type of fiber shown in Table 1. An interesting point is that this type of *Callinectes* fiber and those fibers studied by Fatt and Katz (1953) have different cable properties than those of other commonly used crustaceans. The significance of these differences for the study of ECC coupling has not been analyzed.

PROPERTIES OF THE ELECTRICALLY EXCITABLE MEMBRANE

Fibers of *C. danae* present a variety of membrane responses to constant current pulses. The current–voltage relationship shown in Fig. 1 illustrates the most common pattern observed in our experiments. Weak currents in either direction evoke little electrical response other than the ohmic voltage drop across the electrically inert membrane. With stronger inward currents, hyperpolarizing activation is observed; this is a common finding in crustacean muscle fibers and seems to be due to increase in Cl conductance (Grundfest, 1966a). Increasing outward currents evoke little if any in-

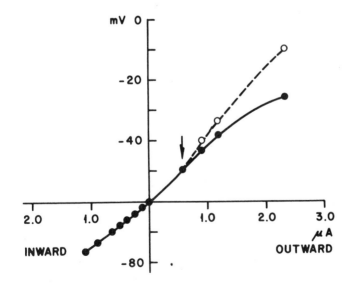

FIG. 1. The current–voltage relationship of *Callinectes danae* muscle fibers. Membrane responses are plotted both as the voltage deflection at the end of current pulses of 20-msec duration (*filled circles*) and as maximal displacement of potential during the pulses (*open circles*) versus the intensity of the current pulses.

activation before the appearance of delayed rectification. The latter is most probably due to increase in K conductance whereas the former might in fact result from an increase in Ca conductance at membrane potential levels where K activation is not obscuring the depolarization due to inward Ca currents.

In some fibers large inward stimuli cause hyperpolarizing inactivation followed by a secondary increase in conductance which persists beyond the duration of the current pulses. The return of membrane conductance to control values occurs slowly and during this period of high conductance another hyperpolarizing response cannot be elicited. Hyperpolarizing responses have been previously described for other muscle fibers and have attributed to inactivation of K conductance (Grundfest, 1966*b*).

MODULATION OF MEMBRANE CALCIUM ACTIVATION AND CONTRACTION

The fibers of *C. danae* seldom show all-or-none responses to depolarizing current pulses, but graded activations are normally prominent, as illustrated in Fig. 2. In all cases the membrane responses show a smooth time course

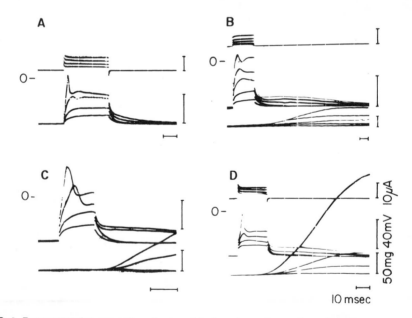

FIG. 2. Representative examples of current-induced membrane Ca activation and tension. Results from four fibers are shown: all show the presence of a fast-rising depolarization due to Ca activation. Note the afterpotentials in **B, C,** and **D**; both the degree of Ca activation and the degree of afterpotential are correlated with the development of tension. For **A, B,** and **D**, the top trace represents the current record and the bottom trace is the record of membrane potential changes. The bottom record in **B, C,** and **D** is that of tension.

for depolarizations less than 20 to 30 mV; for larger depolarizations a brief (2 to 5 msec) initial transient is observed, followed by delayed rectification. These graded membrane responses are accompanied by local contractions and are followed by depolarizing afterpotentials. It seems unlikely that this afterdepolarization is caused by movement of the fiber during contraction since it is smooth in appearance and shows none of the irregularities observed with mechanical artifacts as noted by Fatt and Katz (1953). Long pulses tend to obscure the afterpotential but when short pulses are used a hyperpolarizing dip in the record is often observed to lead the repolarizing phase; in this regard it is similar to the afterpotentials seen with frog muscle. However, unlike the case of frog fibers, the time constant of the decay of the after depolarization in crab fibers is far greater than the τ_m for the resting membrane. Since the afterpotentials are not observed in the absence of the initial transient, it seems that they are coupled with the early increase in ionic conductances which underlie the graded responses.

Through the work of many investigators, a quartet of electrophysiological criteria for the identification of Ca-dependent membrane electrogenesis has become available. The first test is that the active responses be insensitive to Na or Mg removal—yet they must disappear in the absence of Ca. Next, the rate of rise and the degree of overshoot must be sensitive to the external Ca concentration; in addition, Sr and Ba should be able to substitute for Ca. The third criterion is that the active responses be unaffected by tetrodotoxin (TTX), but be depressed by the divalent cations Mn and Co. Finally the expression of Ca activation is enhanced by agents which block or depress depolarizing K activation such as tetraethylammonium (TEA), Ba, and procaine. We have tested these points in isolated muscle fibers of *C. danae* and found no exceptions. Figure 3A–D illustrates the lack of effect of Na and Mg on the active response and, in Fig. 3E–F, the inhibition of the active response and of contraction when Ca is removed from the bathing medium. The inhibitory effect of Mn on the graded activation and tension development is shown in Fig. 4; note the marked appearance of depolarizing K activation when Ca activation is blocked. In contrast to these effects of Mn, TTX (10^{-6} g/ml) is without effect on the graded electrogenesis of these fibers (Suarez-Kurtz and Reuben, 1975).

The ability of TEA and procaine to convert the graded responses in all-or-none spikes is shown in Fig. 5. The mechanical output associated with the procaine-induced spikes increases as external Ca is augmented (Fig. 5A); the dependence of the overshoot of procaine spikes in crustacean muscle has been demonstrated by Takeda (1967). The amplitude and duration of the TEA-induced spikes as well as the time course and peak tension of the accompanying twitches are also modified by the Ca concentration of the bathing medium (Fig. 5C). When external Ca is 12.5 mM, the maximal rate of rise (V_{max}) of both procaine and TEA-induced spikes is in the range of 20 V/sec; spike duration at half-maximal amplitude is about 20 to 40 msec

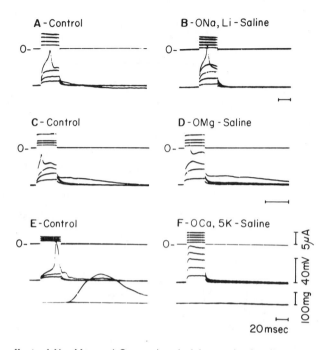

FIG. 3. The effect of Na, Mg, and Ca on depolarizing activation in response to current injection. In all cases the top two traces are records of current and membrane potential respectively; in **E** and **F** the third line is the record of tension. Results from two fibers are displayed. The first fiber **(A–D)** illustrates the lack of effect of removal of Na **(A,B)** when replaced by Li, and of Mg **(C,D)** when replaced by Na. Choline replacement of Na likewise did not abolish the activation. The second fiber **(E,F)** shows that Ca removal abolished the large overshooting spike in this fiber. The depolarization due to Ca withdrawal was counteracted by lowering K.

for both agents. However, the tension derived from the procaine spikes is much smaller that induced by TEA-action potentials. This difference might reflect the inhibitory effect of procaine on the source of the activator Ca (Bianchi and Bolton, 1967). The experiment shown in Fig. 5D further illustrates the depressing effect of procaine on contractility. The fiber was first exposed to TEA alone and then to TEA plus procaine. Procaine reduced the rate of tension development to half without any important effect on V_{max}. The increased overshoot as well as the increase in duration of the action and consequent prolongation of the time to peak tension observed in the presence of procaine could be attributed to further blockade of K activation. These results can also be taken as evidence against a "direct coupling" mechanism (Bianchi, 1969) in these fibers, a point which we will take up again in a later section.

Membrane Ca activation can be depressed by a number of treatments and it is relatively simple to show that tension is depressed at the same time. Figure 4 shows this for the case of Mn. The fact that elevated external Ca

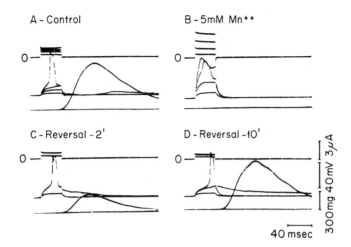

FIG. 4. The effect of Mn on membrane Ca activation and tension. Four records from a single fiber; all records display, from top to bottom: current, potential, and tension. The introduction of Mn for 2 min abolished any appreciable tension and raised the threshold for the onset of membrane Ca activation. The amount of regenerative membrane potential change is smaller in the presence of Mn. Reversal of Mn effects is also rapid, being nearly complete 2 min after the experiment.

can overcome the depression of tension and electrical response adds strength to the argument for the importance of extracellular Ca in ECC. Analogous results have been found for crayfish muscle (Suarez-Kurtz et al., 1972). Additional means of depressing membrane Ca activation and consequently inhibiting tension development are treatment with aminoglycoside antibiotics, hypertonic saline solutions and prolonged exposure to high-K salines.

Neomycin and streptomycin have been recently shown to inhibit both graded and spike electrogenesis in crab muscle fibers (Suarez-Kurtz, 1974). These effects of neomycin, similarly to those of Mn, can be partially antagonized by increasing the external Ca concentration (Fig. 5A). As a consequence of its effects on membrane Ca activation, neomycin increases the threshold for tension development and displaces the curve relating tension to depolarization towards more positive values of membrane potential (Fig. 5B). Antagonism between aminoglycoside antibiotics and Ca was first suggested by Vital-Brazil and Corrado (1957) to explain the neuromuscular blockade caused by these antibiotics. Since then, a great variety of Ca-dependent membrane phenomena have been shown to be inhibited by these compounds (Pittinger and Adamson, 1972) and in most cases, increasing extracellular Ca concentration reverses the inhibition (Corrado et al., 1975).

Another means of depressing membrane Ca activation lies in the use of hypertonic solutions (Suarez-Kurtz and Reuben, 1975). The action of

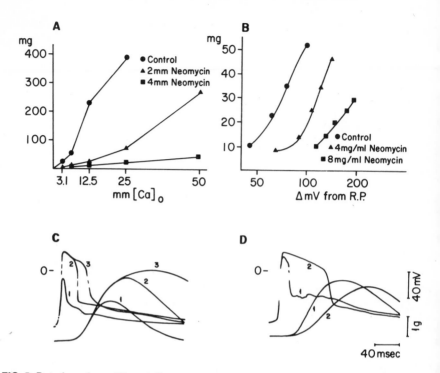

FIG. 5. Data from four different fibers are plotted. **A:** influence of Ca and neomycin on tension induced by procaine spikes. Tension is proportional to external Ca; the inhibitory effect of neomycin on peak tension is partially antagonized by raising external Ca. **B:** effect of neomycin on the amplitude of local contractions induced by graded electrogenesis. Note the displacement of the curve towards larger membrane depolarizations in the presence of neomycin. **C:** effect of external Ca on the action potentials and twitches induced in the presence of 25 mM TEA. Three concentrations of Ca are shown: 2 mM(1),12.5 mM(2), and 25 mM(3). Increase from 2 to 12.5 mM increases both amplitude and duration of the action potential whereas further increase to 25 mM increases only the duration of the action potential. The size of the tension increases as the external Ca is increased. **D:** influence of procaine on TEA spikes and tension. The fiber was first exposed to 25 mM TEA (records marked 1) and then to TEA and procaine (records marked 2). Procaine (7 mM) increases the amplitude and duration of the electrical change and depresses the peak tension and rate-of-rise of the tension (2) whereas TEA alone (1) produced faster and larger tension development even though the duration of the spike and its amplitude was smaller. In records **C** and **D**, the top traces represent the changes in membrane potential and the bottom traces represent tension records. The currents used to elicit the TEA spikes are not shown.

hypertonic solutions on muscle has received a great amount of attention in the past several years because of an apparent lack of effect on electrically excitable membranes which made it possible to use these solutions as an experimental tool to suppress contractions (Hodgkin and Horowicz, 1957). Studies on crayfish have suggested that hypertonic solutions act directly on myofibrils through an increase in ionic strength (April et al., 1968). We find that solutions made hypertonic by a variety of electrolytes and nonelectrolytes block membrane calcium activation in these crab fibers; these solutions do so at tonicities in which there is still a well-developed caffeine contracture which suggests that the Ca release mechanism and the activity of the myofibrils are both functional. Figure 6 shows the effect of hypertonic solutions under our conditions; we found this inhibition of membrane Ca activation to be overcome by extra Ca but not by extra Mg. There were several other effects on the electrical properties of the membrane, the most conspicuous being a doubling of the membrane capacitance and also an elevated internal resistivity as noted for single frog fibers by Hodgkin and Nakajima (1972). Investigation of the current–voltage relationship showed that the threshold for delayed rectification was elevated as was the threshold for hyperpolarizing activation. It is apparent that hypertonic solutions are

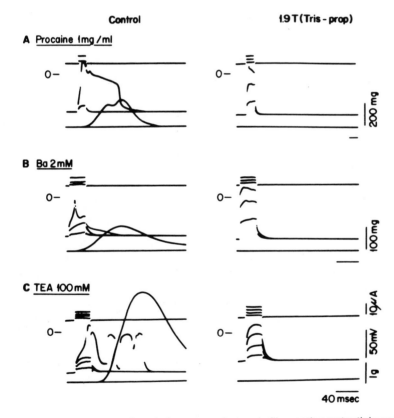

FIG. 6. The effect of hypertonic solutions on crab muscle fiber action potentials and tension development. In all sections the top lines show the current pulse, the middle lines show the membrane potential changes and the bottom lines show tension. One fiber was treated successively with procaine, Ba, and TEA, to produce spiking. Each time the fiber was tested with the hypertonic solution. Introduction of a saline solution made hypertonic (1.9 times) by the addition of tris propionate blocked the depolarizing activation in all three cases. The irregular afterpotential in **C** was the result of movement artifact.

not entirely without membrane effects in crab muscle. The action of hypertonic solutions on ECC in crab muscle, where both spike and tension are blocked, differs from the effects in frog fibers where the action potential is not affected in any important aspect although tension is inhibited (Hodgkin and Horowicz, 1957). This might be due to the different ionic mechanisms underlying the membrane electrogenic responses in frog and crab muscle; the mechanisms that give rise to Ca activation seem to be sensitive to hypertonic media whereas those generating Na spikes are not.

The use of high-K solutions (Hodgkin and Horowicz, 1960) provide further evidence for the inseparability of membrane Ca activation from the development of tension. Fibers of *C. danae* respond to elevated K with a phasic contracture; during the continued exposure to high-K salines the fibers remain depolarized and show no sign of activation of Ca conductance in response to applied current. After removal of K, repolarization for a period of time is necessary before membrane Ca activation and contraction reappear. During this period we find that the effective membrane resistance remains low; addition of TEA or procaine also fails to induce spike electro-

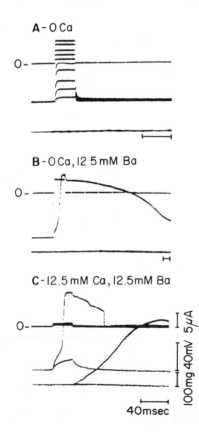

FIG. 7. The effect of Ca on tension development in the presence of Ba. A single fiber treated successively in solutions. **A:** without Ca; **B:** without Ca, but with Ba present; **C:** with both Ca and Ba present. In all three records the top trace is the current, the middle trace is the membrane potential change in response to the current, and the bottom record is the tension recording. Ca lack abolished electrical and mechanical activity. The addition of Ba to the zero-Ca solution caused the appearance of an electrical change without tension, whereas the addition of both Ba and Ca caused an increase in the amplitude of the electrical response and in addition there was development of tension.

genesis and tension development. We are currently exploring the mechanism underlying this aspect of K action.

We have already shown that Ca withdrawal blocks the graded responses of these crab muscle fibers. Another example of this effect of Ca-lack is shown in Fig. 7A. Replacement of Ca with Ba restores the ability of the fiber to generate action potentials (Fig. 7B). However, even though the temporal characteristics of these spikes are similar to those elicited by Ba in the presence of Ca (Fig. 7C), there is no contraction in the absence of external Ca. Thus it appears that Ba activation cannot substitute for membrane Ca activation where tension is concerned; this observation suggests a specific role for Ca entry in the coupling process. In connection to this experiment, we wish to mention the interesting observation of Hagiwara and Naka (1964) showing that membrane Ba conductance can be inactivated for some time after the elicitation of a Ba-spike whereas Ca activation is unaffected.

The uncoupling observed in Fig. 7B appears to occur at a different stage than that caused by either hypertonic solutions or after prolonged exposure to high-K media, where the electrotonic depolarization of the membrane fails to elicit any regenerative response. We suggest that Ca entry *per se,* apart from any electrical change, seems to be a step in the coupling process in crustacean muscle.

EXCITATION-CONTRACTION COUPLING IN CRAB MUSCLE FIBERS

The situation for crustacean muscle seems to be somewhat clearer now than it was a few years ago. A first step in ECC requires the activation of membrane Ca conductance; it results from electrotonic depolarization following current injection, or follows transmitter action in physiological conditions. Tension development is correlated with the occurrence of this membrane Ca activation.

It is of importance to determine the morphological location of the voltage-sensitive Ca conductance mechanism; there is indication from studies on crayfish muscle (see Zachar, 1971) that the Ca channels involved in the coupling process are located in the transverse tubule system. Previous studies from Grundfest's laboratory indicated the importance of Cl for tension development and showed that the Cl channels are also located in the tubule system (Girardier et al., 1963; Reuben et al., 1967; see also Selverston, 1967; Zachar, 1971). According to the "channeled current" hypothesis (Girardier et al., 1963) the current flow between the tubule system and the surface membrane would pass through tubular Cl channels and surface K channels; the resulting electrotonic depolarization in the tubules presumably would cause activation of voltage-sensitive Ca channels. The role of Cl in frog fibers would be different since much evidence (Eisenberg and Gage, 1969) suggests that Cl channels are confined to the surface membrane whereas K channels are in both tubular and surface membranes.

The second question of whether the Ca delivered by the membrane activation process activates the contractile system directly or whether it acts by means of another "triggering" action, as suggested by Bianchi and Bolton for frog muscle (1967), remains unsolved. Tracer studies by Atwater et al. (1974) suggest that enough Ca enters during depolarization to fully activate the myofibrils in TEA-treated barnacle muscle fibers. We are unable to answer this second question for crab muscle fibers. It appears though, that the entry of Ca, besides carrying inward current during membrane excitation, plays an additional role in the coupling process.

ACKNOWLEDGMENTS

The work in Dr. Suarez-Kurtz's laboratory is supported in part with grants from Conselho Nacional de Pesquisas (TC-16.272, TC-16.897) and from Conselho de Pesquisas para Graduados, U.F.R.J.; Dr. Suarez-Kurtz's attendance at the Symposium was sponsored by a grant from Secretariade Ciencia e Tecnologia do Estado da Guanabara. Dr. Sorenson is a Visiting Scientist sponsored by Conselho Nacional de Pesquisas (TC-16.841).

REFERENCES

April, E., Brandt, P. W., Reuben, J. P., and Grundfest, H. (1968): Muscle contraction: The effect of ionic strength. Nature, 220:182–184.

Atwater, I., Rojas, E., and Vergara, J. (1974): Calcium influxes and tension development in perfused single barnacle muscle fibres under membrane potential control. J. Physiol, 243:523–541.

Atwood, H. L. (1963): Differences in muscle fibre properties as a factor in "fast" and "slow" contraction in Carcinus. Comp. Biochem. Physiol., 10:17–32.

Atwood, H. L., Hoyle, G., and Smyth, T. (1965): Mechanical and electrical responses of single innervated crab muscle fibres. J. Physiol., 180:449–482.

Bianchi, C. P. (1969): Pharmacology of excitation-contraction coupling in muscle. Fed. Proc., 28:1624–1627.

Bianchi, C. P., and Bolton, T. C. (1967): Action of local anesthetics on coupling systems in muscle. J. Pharmacol. Exp. Ther., 157:388–405.

Bianchi, C. P., and Shanes, A. M. (1959): Calcium influx in skeletal muscle at rest, during activity, and during potassium contracture. J. Gen. Physiol., 42:803–815.

Chiarandini, D. J., and Stefani, E. (1973): Effects of manganese on the electrical and mechanical properties of frog skeletal muscle fibres. J. Physiol., 232:129–147.

Corrado, A. P., Prado, W. A., and Pimenta de Morais, I. (1975): Competitive antagonism between calcium and aminoglycoside antibiotics in skeletal and smooth muscles. In: Concepts of Membranes in Regulation and Excitation, edited by M. Rocha e Silva and G. Suarez-Kurtz, pp. 201–215. Raven Press, New York.

Eisenberg, R. S., and Gage, P. W. (1969): Ionic conductances of the surface and tubular membranes of frog sartorius fibers. J. Gen. Physiol., 53:279–298.

Endo, M., Tanaka, M., and Ogawa, Y. (1970): Calcium induced release of calcium from the sarcoplasmic reticulum of skinned skeletal muscle fibres. Nature, 228:34–36.

Fatt, P., and Katz, B. (1951): An analysis of the endplate potential recorded with an intracellular electrode. J. Physiol., 115:320–370.

Fatt, P., and Katz, B. (1953): The electrical properties of crustacean muscle fibers. J. Physiol., 120:171–204.

Ford, L. E., and Podolsky, R. J. (1972): Intracellular calcium movements in skinned muscle fibres. *J. Physiol.*, 223:21–23.

Frank, G. B. (1960): Effects of changes in extracellular calcium concentration on the potassium-induced contracture of frog's skeletal muscle. *J. Physiol.*, 151:518–538.

Girardier, L., Reuben, J. P., Brandt, P. W., and Grundfest, H., (1963): Evidence for anion-permselective membrane in crayfish muscle fibers and its possible role in excitation-contraction coupling. *J. Gen. Physiol.*, 47:189–214.

Grundfest, H. (1966a): Heterogeneity of excitable membranes: Electrophysiological and pharmacological evidence and some consequences. *Ann. NY Acad. Sci.*, 137:901–949.

Grundfest, H. (1966b): Comparative electrobiology of excitable membranes. *Advan. Comp. Physiol. Biochem.*, 2:1–116.

Hagiwara, S., and Naka, K. (1964): The initiation of spike potential in barnacle muscle fibers under low intracellular Ca^{2+}. *J. Gen. Physiol.*, 48:141–162.

Hodgkin, A. L., and Horowicz, P. (1957): The differential action of hypertonic solutions on the twitch and action potential of a muscle fibre. *J. Physiol.*, 136:17P–18P.

Hodgkin, A. L., and Horowicz, P. (1959): The influence of potassium and chloride ions on the membrane potential of single muscle fibres. *J. Physiol.*, 148:127–160.

Hodgkin, A. L., and Horowicz, P. (1960): Potassium contractures in single muscle fibres. *J. Physiol.*, 153:386–403.

Hodgkin, A. L., and Nakajima, S. (1972): The effect of diameter on the electrical constants of frog skeletal muscle fibres. *J. Physiol.*, 221:105–120.

Hodgkin, A. L., and Rushton, W. A. H. (1946): The electrical constants of crustacean nerve fibres. *Proc. Roy. Soc. Lond.*, 133B:444–479.

Huxley, A. F., and Taylor, R. E. (1958): Local activation of striated muscle fibres. *J. Physiol.*, 144:426–441.

Kuffler, S. W. (1946): The relation of electric potential changes to contracture in skeletal muscle. *J. Neurophysiol.*, 9:367–377.

Pittinger, C., and Adamson, R. (1972): Antibiotic blockade of neuromuscular function. *Ann. Rev. Pharmacol.*, 12:169–184.

Reuben, J. P., Brandt, P. W., Garcia, H., and Grundfest, H. (1967): Excitation-contraction coupling in crayfish. *Am. Zool.*, 7:623–645.

Schneider, M. F., and Chandler, W. K. (1973): Voltage dependent charge movement in skeletal muscle: a possible step in excitation-contraction coupling. *Nature*, 242:244–246.

Selverston, A. (1967): Structure and function of the transverse tubular system in crustacean muscle fibers. *Am. Zool.*, 7:515–525.

Suarez-Kurtz, G. (1974): Inhibition of membrane calcium activation by neomycin and streptomycin in crab muscle fibers. *Pflügers Arch.*, 349:337–349.

Suarez-Kurtz, G., and Reuben, J. P. (1975): Is a Ca current necessary for excitation-contraction coupling in skeletal muscle? In: *Concepts of Membranes in Regulation and Excitation*, edited by M. Rocha e Silva and G. Suarez-Kurtz, pp. 41–54. Raven Press, New York.

Suarez-Kurtz, G., Reuben, J. P., Brandt, P. W., and Grundfest, H. (1972): Membrane calcium activation in excitation contraction coupling. *J. Gen. Physiol.*, 59:676–688.

Takeda, K. (1967): Permeability changes associated with the action potential in procaine-treated crayfish abdominal muscle fibers. *J. Gen. Physiol.*, 50:1049–1074.

Vital-Brazil, O., and Corrado, A. P. (1957): The curariform action of streptomycin. *J. Pharmacol. Exp. Ther.*, 120:452–459.

Zachar, J. (1971): Electrogenesis and contractility in skeletal muscle. *Slovak. Acad. Sci.*, Bratislava.

Electrobiology of Nerve, Synapse, and Muscle,
edited by J. P. Reuben, D. P. Purpura, M. V. L. Bennett,
and E. R. Kandel. Raven Press, New York © 1976

Role of the Plasma Membrane in Metabolic Regulation: Brown Adipose Tissue as Experimental Model

Lucien Girardier

Département de Physiologie, Ecole de Médecine, Université de Genève,
Geneva, Switzerland

The choice of adipose tissue as the subject of a chapter on electro-physiology might understandably be questioned. In order to justify my reasons for this choice, I would like to show how the techniques and concepts of electrophysiology can contribute to the study of metabolic regulation of tissues. To do this, I will survey a study that was undertaken 6 years ago with my group in Geneva on brown adipose tissue (BAT) and will briefly describe its relation to its physiological context.

LOCALIZATION AND FUNCTION OF BAT

BAT is found in all hibernating mammals and in numerous permanently homeothermic animals including man, in whom it is particularly developed during the perinatal period. Its anatomic localization is similar in all species. An important deposit, often used for the study of this tissue, is found in the interscapular region where it forms a bilobed mass that extends laterally in two deposits surrounding the brachial and subclavial veins. In the upper cervical region, two deposits, right and left, are in contact with the vertebral veins. It can also be found surrounding the azygous vein and on the posterior side of the aorta with which it traverses the diaphragm and extends laterally to surround the renal veins; it surrounds the inferior vena cava and there are some small deposits on the iliac veins.

Smith and Roberts (1964) have stressed the importance of a functional association of BAT with the circulatory system. BAT, which functions as an endocrine gland whose product is heat, is actually a "biological furnace." Its purpose is the preferential heating of the thoracic organs and nervous system. It is interesting to note that structures of particular thermosensitivity like the cardiac pacemaker are surrounded with BAT (Cottle et al., 1971).

INNERVATION

The activation of BAT depends on the sympathetic nervous system. Morphologists have described a meshwork of fibers surrounding the adipocytes and fluorescent histochemical studies of the adult rat (Cottle et al., 1971; Derry et al., 1969) have demonstrated the adrenergic nature of these fibers. Observation by electron microscope has revealed direct contacts of nerve terminals with the invaginated cell membrane and, more frequently, loose "en passant" contacts. Norepinephrine (NE) might thus be secreted either directly in contact with the cell or in the narrow interstitial space separating the adipocytes. Such innervation would facilitate a mass response of BAT to sympathetic stimulation.

Nexus-like junctions have been observed in BAT of mouse (Revel and Sheridan, 1968), rat (Girardier and Seydoux, 1971b), and hamster (Linck et al., 1973). These junctions, the only ones connecting BAT adipocytes, are obviously responsible for the electrical coupling observed in these cells (Sheridan, 1971).

RESPONSE TO EXOGENOUS CATECHOLAMINES

In order to obtain continuous monitoring, a thermic flux differential calorimeter was designed.

The basal heat production of BAT was measured and found to be 1.6 μcal sec^{-1} (mg wet wt)$^{-1}$, almost the same as the basal metabolism of the living adult male rat. Under stimulation, however, it is characteristic of BAT to sustain very large increases in heat production without producing any external work. Figure 1 shows the calorimetric reading of the dose-response

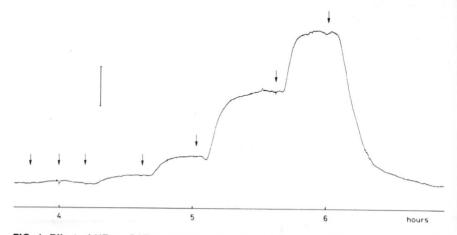

FIG. 1. Effect of NE on BAT as measured by direct calorimetry. This reading shows the response of BAT to increasing doses of NE beginning with a threshold dose (24 nmoles) at first arrow. The second arrow shows the effect of removal of this dose. The concentration of NE was then increased stepwise: 35, 60, 160, and 600 nmoles. The last arrow indicates the removal of the last dose of NE followed by rapid return to basal. Rat adapted at 22°C. It can be seen that each dose elicited a steady-state response. Vertical bar, 10 μcal sec^{-1}.

curve of NE of a piece of tissue weighing 11 mg. Each increase of the hormone concentration can be seen to be followed by a *steady-state increase in heat production*. Upon removal of NE, the tissue heat production rapidly returned to basal. Since NE is known to be bound to the surface of the plasma membrane, the steady-state response observed can only be explained by assuming that BAT heat production is continuously regulated by a membrane-bound system.

THE SOURCE OF HEAT PRODUCTION IN BROWN ADIPOCYTES

It is important for our purpose to localize the source of heat production within the cell. The primary energy-releasing reaction in biological oxidations is the oxidative breaking down of carbon–hydrogen bonds with the consequent formation of water and carbon dioxide. The general trend in phylogeny has been toward the development of systems for the conversion of chemically bound energy into physical work with the highest possible efficiency. The system that has reached the highest degree of efficiency is the mitochondrial oxidative phosphorylation in which the cell's energy requirement regulates the release of bound chemical energy by controlling the rate of phosphate acceptor formation.

Although, logically, heat production in BAT should require only a low-efficiency system, which would make mitochondrial regulation of respiration unnecessary, the fact is that there are far more mitochondria in BAT than in most other tissues. These mitochondria have a classical electron transport system and the basal respiration of BAT has been shown to be coupled with oxidative phosphorylation (Hittelman and Lindberg, 1970).

Since the breakdown of the ATP synthesized during respiration represents only about one-quarter of the amount of the total thermal energy resulting from substrate oxidation (Prusiner and Poe, 1970), it is apparent that the bulk of this energy is liberated in the form of heat in the mitochondrial respiratory chain. Thus, the enzymatic reactions that control the rate of heat production are almost certainly the same as those that regulate the mitochondrial respiratory chain when there is an optimal supply of substrate and oxygen.

The Problem: How Can a Membrane-Bound System Regulate the Mitochondrial Respiratory Chain?

It is known that NE increases the rate of lipolysis in BAT and it has been claimed (Skala et al., 1970; Beviz et al., 1971) that this increase is triggered by a membrane-bound adenylate cyclase system that is NE sensitive. Thus, the binding of the hormone to the membrane results in an increased supply of oxidizable substrate, i.e., free fatty acids, to the mitochondria.

This substrate release, however, cannot explain the *sustained* increase in respiration since a system in which the flux of electrons along the respiratory chain is coupled with phosphorylation would be automatically limited by the decreasing availability of phosphate acceptors.

It is necessary, therefore, to postulate a second effect of hormone binding that would in some way liberate the electron transport from the phosphorylation system. The need for this hypothesis was also demonstrated by the following experiment performed by J. Seydoux in Brauser's laboratory in Munich: low-noise spectra of a light beam reflected from perfused BAT were calculated by averaging 256 primary spectra recorded within 13 sec. The average spectrum was used as the control spectrum and stored in the memory system of the averaging computer. A physiological concentration of NE was then added to the perfusing fluid. Ten minutes after the addition of the hormone, 256 primary spectra were again averaged, and from this mean test spectrum, the control spectrum was subtracted. The difference spectrum thus obtained can be more easily interpreted than primary spectra

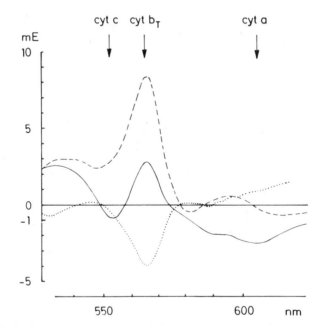

FIG. 2. Effect of NE on the redox state of cytochromes of BAT. mE, optical density expressed in milliextinction units. Positive values correspond to a reduction, negative values to an oxydation. The abcissa represents the wavelength. Each spectrum represents the difference between the mean of 256 test spectra (obtained at 6 min after injection for NE and at steady level for the other test substances) and the mean of 256 control spectra registered at time 0. (———) NE, 10 nmole (6 min); (– – –) Na-octanoate, 0.12 mM; ($\cdots$) 2.4 DNP, 13 μM. Rat adapted at 22°C. It can be seen that the change in the cytochrome redox state of BAT induced by NE includes characteristics of both the substrate and the decoupler effects.

since the difference spectrum would be perfectly flat if the redox state of the cytochromes remained constant during the test period. Figure 2 shows that this was not the case. Cytochrome b was reduced whereas cytochromes c and a were oxidized. A comparison was made of this effect of NE on cytochromes with that of the addition of substrate on the one hand, and with that of a known uncoupler, on the other. When a fatty acid [Na-octanoate (0.12 mM)] was added to the perfusion medium, cytochrome b was reduced and there was no effect on cytochromes a and c. The major effect of 13 μM of the uncoupler DNP was the oxidation of cytochrome b. Seydoux and Brauser interpret these results to mean that a physiological concentration of NE has two different effects on the respiratory chain of BAT: (1) a stimulation of the respiratory chain that would explain oxidation of cytochromes c and $a;$ and (2) an increase in the substrate supply to the respiratory chain as indicated by the reduction of cytochrome b. The resulting increased concentration of reduced equivalents would mask the oxidation expected of cytochrome b when there is only a stimulation of respiration.

THE STIMULATION OF THE RESPIRATORY CHAIN

The mechanism of this stimulation has not yet been established and the numerous hypotheses that have been advanced fall into two categories. On the one hand, it is thought that during NE stimulation the BAT mitochondria become less tightly coupled, thus enabling the respiratory chain to become independent of phosphate acceptor concentration. In contrast to this view is the concept that NE-induced thermogenesis is sustained by an increase in the energy requirements of the cell. In other words, one or several ATP-consuming systems are stimulated concomitantly with the adenylate cyclase system, which would keep the concentration of phosphate acceptors at a high level. Thus, in contrast to the uncoupling concept, there is the concept of what might be called an energy trap. These two mechanisms, however, are not necessarily mutually exclusive, and may even be complementary. The observation that BAT mitochondria are more susceptible to uncoupling by fatty acids than are those isolated from other tissues lends support to the hypothesis of the uncoupling mechanism. The increase of free fatty acid concentration caused by NE stimulation of lipase activity would set off the decoupling mechanism (Rafael et al., 1969; Lindberg et al., 1970).

On the other hand, it is very likely that the energy requirement of the cell during NE stimulation is increased even if only because ATP is required for the activation of fatty acids and for cyclic AMP formation. However, several other energy-requiring cycles could also be involved (Prusiner and Poe, 1970). Consequently, the controversial question should be seen as a quantitative one, i.e., given the theoretical amount of ATP produced in a tightly coupled BAT respiratory chain, what fraction of the total ATP could be utilized by the energy-trap systems?

THE SODIUM PUMP AND THE
REGULATION OF THERMOGENESIS

The Na-K-sensitive ATPase might be important to the entire energy-trap system for the following reasons:

(1) Brown adipocytes were found to have a transmembrane potential of about 55 mV (Girardier et al., 1968).

(2) NEs action on the adipocyte membrane causes depolarization both *in vitro* (Girardier et al., 1968) and *in vivo* (Horwitz et al., 1969) as well as a decrease in membrane resistance (Horowitz et al., 1971).

(3) NE causes an increase in the Na^+ content and a decrease in that of K^+ in BAT (Girardier and Seydoux, 1971a).

The following sequence of events, therefore, seems plausible: first, NE would cause not only an increase in adenylate cyclase activity but also in the resting permeability of Na^+ which would, in turn, cause an influx of sodium to the cell. The resulting rise in cytoplasmic sodium content would then increase the ATP requirement of the sodium pump as is the case in other tissues. This entire sequence can be seen as an energy trap that would therefore be regulated directly by the hormone at the cytomembrane level.

If this mechanism is to be considered quantitatively significant, the following would have to be demonstrated:

(1) Na^+ *turnover* in the cytoplasm of the adipocytes is increased by NE and the increase is in proportion to heat production.

(2) The calorigenic effect of NE is inhibited in low-sodium Ringer solutions.

(3) Ouabain has a strong inhibitory effect on NE heat production.

The following series of experiments were therefore performed.

The Effect of NE on Sodium Turnover

Fragments of tissue were loaded by incubation in a physiological solution containing trace amounts of ^{22}Na and ^{42}K. After the loading period (90 min), the efflux of radioisotopes was monitored at 30°C or at 2°C in continuously renewed, nonradioactive Krebs–Ringer solution. The washout curves thus obtained were analyzed by computer, using a modification of an automatic peeling technique (Mancini and Pilo, 1970).

Based on the data obtained from the computer, the most likely model to explain the shape of the washout curve would be two compartments in series, one having a significantly faster washout than the other:

$$Y(t) = A_1 e^{-\lambda_1 t} + A_2 e^{-\lambda_2 t}$$

The washout time constant λ_1 of the first compartment was found to be substantially the same for Na and K. It corresponded to a half-time value of 6.9 min at 30°C and 9.4 min at 2°C giving a Q_{10} of 1.1, which can be explained by the effect of the temperature on the diffusion coefficient of the solute. The passive behavior of compartment 1 suggests that we are dealing with extracellular space. The apparent volume of both compartments was therefore calculated by using the values obtained for A_1 and A_2 for the washout curves of both potassium and sodium. For compartment 1, a mean fractional value of 20% was obtained as compared with 21% for ^{14}C saccharose space.

For compartment 2, which must therefore consist of intracellular space, the following half-time values were obtained:

> For potassium   51 min at 30°C;
> 205 min at 2°C.
> For sodium   52 min at 30°C;
> 69 min at 2°C.

These values yielded a Q_{10} value of 2.1 for potassium suggesting that its washout is chemically controlled. For the sodium, on the other hand, the Q_{10} was found to be only 1.1. Thus, it is entirely possible that all of the sodium turned over in 90-min incubation could originate in compartments in which the sodium exchange takes place by free diffusion. The kinetics of this exchange was not modified by NE. However, under the experimental conditions of the present study, a small intracellular pool of actively turned-over Na^+ could exist but be undetectable because of the noise of our measurements.

The Effect of Low Sodium on BAT Respiration and Membrane Potential

This was studied by monitoring membrane potential, oxygen consumption, and heat flow of BAT samples throughout the transition from a normal to a low-sodium medium. It was found that a depolarization of the adipocytes takes place during this transition. The relationship between membrane potential and the logarithm of the sodium concentration varies somewhat depending on the Na^+ substitute used, but the shape of the curve is always sigmoidal (Fig. 3). Thus, the major cationic species in the extracellular fluid must be sodium if the BAT cell is to develop a resting potential above 30 mV. This can readily be explained as follows: the membrane capacity of BAT cells may be shunted by a sizable ionic leak in which case steady-state or resting potential would depend on the minute-to-minute loading of the membrane capacity by the sodium pump. Any slowing down of the pumping activity would therefore lead to a rapid loss in membrane polarization.

This explanation is compatible with the observations that the resting potential of BAT is very sensitive to ouabain, is reversibly decreased in a potassium-free solution, and has a high Q_{10} (Girardier et al., 1968). The depolarization of BAT exposed to low-Na^+ solution would thus be the re-

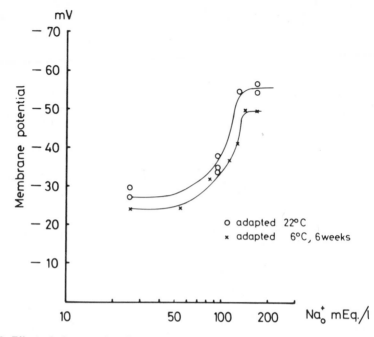

FIG. 3. Effect of change of sodium concentration on membrane potential of BAT. Each point is the mean of 10 intracellular recordings starting 10 min after the change in Na⁺ content of the medium. The experiment was performed with tissue of rats adapted at two different temperatures. It can be seen that the cell depolarized in low-Na⁺ media.

sult of the slowing down of Na⁺ pumping caused by the decrease of the inward leak of Na⁺, which would cause a drop in its cytoplasmic concentration and consequently a decrease in activation of the membrane Na-K ATPase. In the context of this hypothesis, it seemed of interest to compare oxygen consumption in low- and high-Na⁺ media and therefore a study was undertaken by Y. A. Barde.

Using a Clark electrode, a determination was made of the time required for a fragment of BAT in an air-tight, bubble-free chamber to decrease the partial pressure of oxygen (Po₂) by a given amount. The apparatus was so designed that when this amount was reached, the medium was automatically renewed with fresh oxygenated and sterile solution and a new measurement started. This allowed for measurements over a long period of time and for the Po₂ in the medium to be kept within a narrow range. With this set-up it was established that decreasing the external Na⁺ concentration from the normal 140 mEq to 25 mEq causes an *increase rather than a decrease* in respiration, which was found to be as high as 50%.

Measurements of oxygen consumption in BAT samples submitted to a K-free solution (Fig. 4) or ouabain also revealed an increase in respiration.

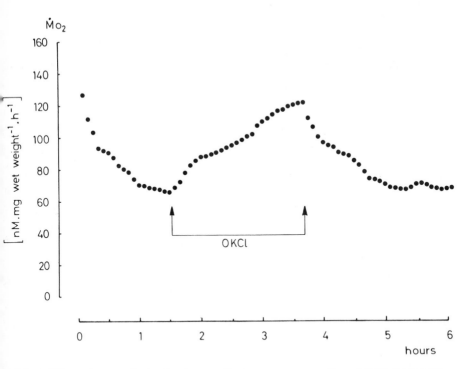

FIG. 4. Effect of removal of potassium on the oxygen consumption of BAT. During the first 2 hr after the introduction of the tissue into the metabolic chamber, its respiration slowly drifts from a high level toward a steady state. This effect was due to a massive discharge of NE caused by dissection of the tissue that cut off the nerve supply. When the tissue entered the steady-state respiration period, the K^+ was removed from the medium by rinsing with potassium-free solution. This caused a very large increase in the respiration rate which was found to be reversible. Rat adapted at 22°C.

It is surprising that steps known to cause a decrease in the active pumping of Na^+ would result in an increase in respiration. This increase develops slowly, however, and could therefore be due to a progressive modification of the ionic content of the cytoplasm consequent to the blocking of the sodium pump. A modification of this kind has actually been shown in heart, for instance, where the internal Ca^{2+} concentration has been found to be inversely related to the sodium gradient across the cell membrane (Glitsch et al., 1970).

Considering the possibility of an ionic modification of this kind, it is necessary to record the evolution of the basal metabolism of the tissue *immediately* after the change in composition of the Krebs–Ringer solution in order to determine the energy consumption of the sodium pump itself. Since continuous recording was not possible with the apparatus described above, direct calorimetry was used by A. Chinet to study the ouabain effect.

The Effect of Ouabain on Membrane Potential and on Heat Flow of BAT as Measured by Direct Calorimetry

Continuous recording of heat flow revealed that the addition of ouabain is immediately and invariably followed by a *decrease in heat production* (Fig. 5). This decrease is small, amounting to about 5% of the basal heat production, and is followed by a gradual increase that can reach a steady state at 160% of basal. It was found that this increase could be considerably delayed by replacing the calcium in the bathing solution with magnesium, and that this delay did not increase the amplitude of the initial response. Thus, the sodium pump activity in the resting state must represent only about 5% of the total energy consumption of the resting cell. In NE-stimulated tissue, however, the contribution of the sodium pump must be much greater since it was found that ouabain cut down the extra heat production by 25%.

One of the most interesting conclusions that can be drawn from the results of the present investigation is a quite unexpected one, i.e., that the basal metabolism of BAT cannot be represented by a fixed value since

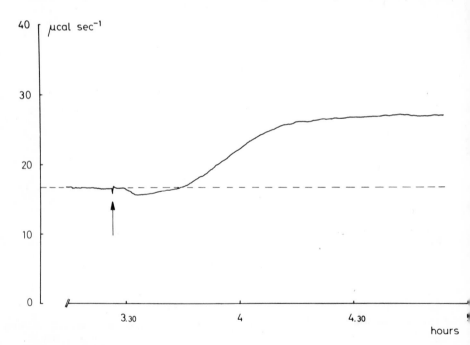

FIG. 5. Effect of 10^{-4} M ouabain on the heat production of BAT. *Arrow,* the point at which the drug was added. The 3-min latency period is due to the dead space represented by the heat exchanger in the calorimeter. *Abscissa,* the time of introduction of the BAT into the apparatus. Rat adapted at 22°C. It can be seen that at first ouabain elicited a decrease in metabolic rate followed by a gradual increase reaching a steady state considerably above basal.

variations of the ionic content of its bathing medium were found to considerably affect its steady-state heat production.

A second conclusion is that the basal metabolism of BAT in Krebs–Ringer solution is minimal when the Na pumping proceeds freely but that any inhibition of this pumping results in higher steady-state heat production.

Finally, it was found that when the Na pump is operating freely, its contribution to the total energy consumption of the cell at rest is low but increases when the cell is NE stimulated. It can therefore be concluded that although the Na-K-sensitive ATPase can hardly be considered the major controlling factor of heat production in BAT, it represents a substantial contribution to the total energy-trap system. Unfortunately, measurement of the sodium turnover, which would allow a quantification of this contribution, proved to be much less simple than was hoped (see section on "The Effect of NE on Sodium Turnover").

The finding that BAT metabolism cannot be represented by a fixed value but rather is dependent on the ionic environment of the cell, prompted us to further investigation of this problem. Since low-sodium, low-potassium medium or ouabain caused depolarization concomitantly with an increase in respiration in BAT, it seemed likely that membrane depolarization might be a signal for the respiratory regulation system. The obvious question to be asked then is discussed in the following section.

IS THERE A CORRELATION BETWEEN DEPOLARIZATION AND HEAT PRODUCTION IN BAT?

It is known that nonsteroidal hormones modify the membrane potential of their target cells (Rassmussen, 1970; Peterson, 1974). Rassmussen has proposed a general scheme of the activation of these cells. According to his theory, the hormone, as primary signal, would induce both membrane depolarization and activation of adenylate cyclase. The depolarization would cause a dissociation of the membrane-bound calcium which would in turn affect the permeability to Na^+, K^+, and Ca^{2+}. The resulting change in ionic content of the cell is thus seen as a prerequisite to the cell's response to the hormone.

In order to test Rassmussen's hypothesis, the effect of depolarization of BAT samples on respiration was studied. This depolarization was achieved by submitting the tissue to one of the following:

(1) K^+-free medium
(2) ouabain-containing medium
(3) low-Na^+ medium
(4) high-K^+ medium
(5) glucose-free medium
(6) medium containing glycolysis inhibitors

It has already been shown in this chapter that the first four of these media cause depolarization. The choice of the last two media requires some explanation. In the present study, it was shown by B. Lasserre that glucose was an adequate substrate for the energy-requiring system that generates membrane potential. Figure 6 shows that hypoxia causes depolarization in a substrate-free medium but not in one containing glucose. Moreover, glucose appears to be the only possible energy source. As shown in Fig. 7, when pyruvate was used as substrate instead of glucose, the cells depolarized. This depolarization cannot be attributed to a lack of energy source, since it was verified that exogenous pyruvate was being effectively utilized by BAT cells in the metabolic chamber.

The results showed that regardless of which method was used to bring about depolarization, all six of them resulted in an increase in cell metabolism (three cases are illustrated in Figs. 4, 5, and 8). It was therefore concluded at this stage that membrane potential does have some regulatory effect on BAT heat production. Bearing in mind the fact that BAT is a richly innervated tissue, a further verification of this conclusion was attempted by testing whether the depolarization induced by the various methods was actually the result of a direct effect on the adipocytes or rather an indirect effect caused by the release of NE by the cut nerve endings.

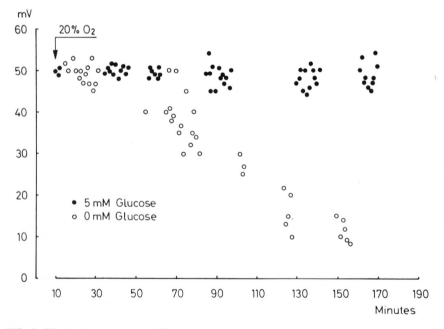

FIG. 6. Effect of hypoxia on BAT membrane potential in the presence and absence of glucose. Arrow shows the moment in which hypoxia was induced by modification of the gas phase, from 95% O_2 + 5% CO_2 to 20% O_2 + 5% CO_2 + 75% N_2. Rat adapted at 22°C. It can be seen that in the absence of glucose, hypoxia induced depolarization.

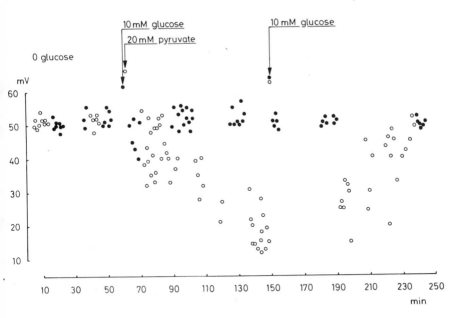

FIG. 7. Effect of prolonged glucose deprivation on BAT membrane potential. The tissues were well supplied with oxygen throughout the experiment. After 60 min in glucose-free solution, during which time the glycogen store of the cell was largely depleted, glucose or pyruvate was introduced as substrate. Rat adapted at 22°C. It can be seen that prolonged glucose deprivation caused a loss of membrane potential, reversible with the reintroduction of glucose.

All six experiments were therefore repeated with propranolol, a blocker of the β effect of catecholamines, added to the bathing medium. Results showed that for experiments with glucose-free media, glycolysis inhibitors, and high K^+, propranolol completely blocked the increase in respiration. For those using low K^+, low Na^+, and ouabain, however, the original results were unmodified.

This result, pointing to an indirect effect of high K^+ on BAT respiration, was thoroughly checked by Y. A. Barde who found that the increase in BAT respiration induced by K^+ could be blocked not only by the addition of propranolol to the bathing medium, but also in the following ways: by a chemical denervation with 6-OH dopamine [a drug known to selectively destroy sympathetic nerve endings (Thoenen and Tranzer, 1968)]; by lowering the Ca^{2+} and increasing the Mg^{2+} concentrations in the medium (which has been found to block synaptic transmission in many tissues); and, as illustrated in Fig. 9, by pretreatment of the animal with reserpine (a drug known to deplete the nerve endings of their catecholamine content).

In a concurrent series of experiments performed by J. Seydoux in order to check the effect of high K^+ on resting potential, it was found that neither

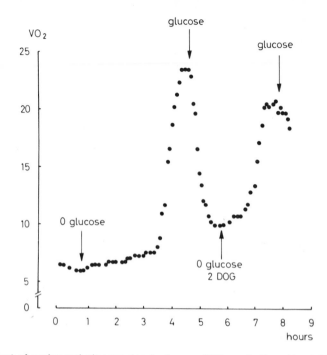

FIG. 8. Effect of prolonged glucose deprivation on BAT respiration. About 1 hr after the introduction of the tissue into the metabolic chamber, the bathing medium was replaced with one that was glucose-free. A large increase in respiration occurred after 2.5 hr which could be largely reversed by reintroducing glucose into the medium. In a second run, when an inhibitor of glycolysis – deoxyglucose (2 DOG) – was added to the glucose-free medium, the increase in respiration occurred after only 0.5 hr. Rat adapted at 22°C.

propranolol nor reserpine pretreatment had any effect on the depolarizing action of potassium (Fig. 10). Comparison of Figs. 9 and 10 shows that: (a) depolarization alone did not trigger heat production (KCl on BAT of reserpinized rat, Figs. 9 and 10); (b) depolarization prior to the addition of NE did not modify the heat production triggered by the hormone (NE after KCl on BAT of reserpinized rat, Fig. 9).

It can thus be concluded that depolarization of the adipocytes *cannot be a signal for the system regulation BAT respiration.*

Based on the above results of Barde, Lasserre and Seydoux, it can also be concluded that the increase in BAT respiration observed when glucose utilization is blocked and when external potassium concentration is increased, is due to a release of NE by the nerve endings rather than to a direct effect on the adipocyte. On the other hand, since β blockers were found to have no effect on the depolarization or on the increase in heat production in BAT induced by low K+, low Na+, and ouabain, it must be concluded that these agents act by direct effect on the adipocytes and it is almost

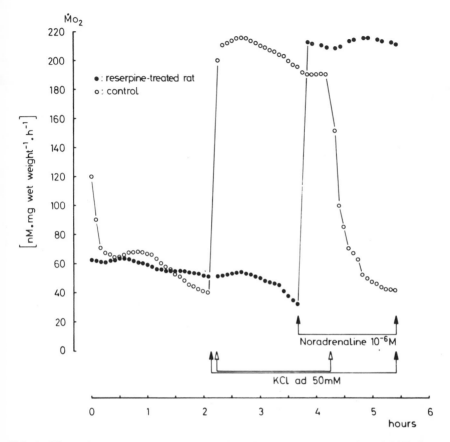

FIG. 9. Effect of reserpine on potassium-induced increase in respiration of BAT. *Open symbols,* sample taken from control animal; *filled symbols,* sample taken from reserpine-treated animal. Both animals were adapted at 22°C. The control shows the normal, reversible response to KCl medium. The reserpine-treated rat shows no response upon exposure to KCl medium but an increase in oxygen consumption upon the addition of NE.

certain that the mechanism of this effect must be related to changes in ionic transmembrane distribution. Now, since all three of these agents cause a decrease in transmembrane sodium gradient, either by inducing an increase in internal concentration (ouabain, low K⁺), or by decreasing the external concentration (low Na⁺), it is entirely possible that a high-Na⁺ gradient is required for optimal basal metabolism, i.e., one that is maintained by the least possible energy consumption. Conceivably, the potential energy stored in the Na⁺ gradient, which is thermodynamically similar to that inherent in a chemical bond, could function as a direct energy source for membrane-bound structures such as carriers, as is the case for the active extrusion of calcium by exchange with sodium.

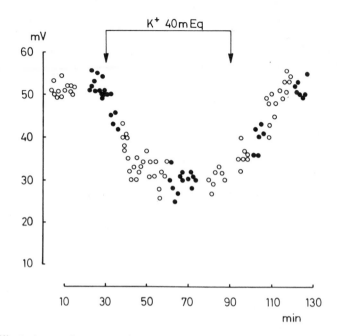

FIG. 10. Effect of reserpine on potassium-induced depolarization in BAT. *Open symbols,* sample taken from control animal; *filled symbols,* sample taken from reserpine-treated animal. Both animals were adapted at 22°C. The control shows the normal, reversible response to KCl medium. The reserpine-treated rat gave the same response.

SUMMARY AND CONCLUSIONS

In examining the role of the plasma membrane in metabolic regulation of BAT, emphasis has been placed on the sodium pump rather than on the well-known adenylate cyclase system.

The sodium pump activity in the resting state was found to represent 5% of the total energy consumption of the resting cell. In NE-stimulated tissue, however, the contribution of the sodium pump to the total heat production was much greater.

The sodium gradient generated by the pump appears to be a regulatory factor of the cell's heat production. The energy requirement for basal metabolism increases when the sodium gradient is either diminished or destroyed. There is strong evidence that this is true for striated muscle as well as for BAT (Chinet, Clausen, and Girardier, *in preparation*).

Depolarization, even prolonged, caused by high external K⁺ does not induce an increase in heat production of BAT if the NE release by the nerve endings is prevented.

Since the conductance of BAT membrane is increased by the hormone but not by changes in potential it must be concluded that brown adipocytes have a nonelectroexcitable membrane (Grundfest, 1957, 1959). In this context, the functional role of the gap junctions existing between brown adipocytes and the resulting electrical coupling remains to be determined. In studying metabolic regulation in organ samples, the role of the still-functioning cut nerve endings must not be underestimated. In the present study, for example, the results, which at first seemed to indicate that the glucose required for the cell to maintain its resting potential was utilized by the adipocytes, later revealed that it is the nerve endings that require glucose to maintain the resting release of catecholamines at a subliminal level. Thus, exposing BAT to a glucose-free medium was found to be tantamount to exposing adipocytes to NE.

ACKNOWLEDGMENTS

I am deeply indebted to Mrs. Judith Noebels for her uncompromising and patient collaboration in the editing and translating of this paper. This research was supported by the Swiss National Foundation for Scientific Research.

REFERENCES

Beviz, A., Lundholm, L., and Mohme-Lundholm, E. (1971): Cyclic AMP as a mediator of hormonal metabolic effects in brown adipose tissue. *Acta Physiol. Scand.*, 81:145–156.

Cottle, M. K., Cottle, W. H., Nash, C. W., and Bickman, S. (1971): Cardiac brown fat. In: *International Symposium on Environmental Physiology. Bioenergetics*, edited by R. E. Smith, pp. 122–126. Federation of American Societies for Experimental Biology, Bethesda, Maryland.

Derry, D. M., Schönbaum, E., and Steiner, G. (1969): Two sympathetic nerve supplies to brown adipose tissue of the rat. *Can. J. Physiol. Pharmacol.*, 47:57–63.

Girardier, L., Seydoux, J., and Clausen, T. (1968): Membrane potential of brown adipose tissue. *J. Gen. Physiol.*, 52:925.

Girardier, L., and Seydoux, J. (1971a): Cytomembrane phenomenon during stimulation of brown fat thermogenesis by norepinephrine. In: *Nonshivering Thermogenesis*, edited by L. Jansky, pp. 255–270. Academia, Prague.

Girardier, L., and Seydoux, J. (1971b): Le contrôle de la thermogénèse du tissu adipeux brun. *J. Physiol. (Paris)*, 63:147–186.

Glitsch, H. G., Reuter, H., and Scholz, H. (1970): The effect of the internal sodium concentration on calcium fluxes in isolated guinea-pig auricles. *J. Physiol. (Lond.)*, 209:25–43.

Grundfest, H. (1957): Electrical inexcitability of synapses and some of its consequences in the central nervous system. *Phys. Rev.*, 37:337–361.

Grundfest, H. (1959): Synaptic and ephatic transmission. In: *Handbook of Physiology, Section I, Neurophysiology I*, edited by J. Field, pp. 147–197. American Physiological Society, Washington, D.C.

Hittelman, K. J., and Lindberg, O. (1970): Fatty acid uncoupling in brown fat mitochondria. In: *Brown Adipose Tissue*, edited by O. Lindberg, pp. 245–262. Elsevier, New York.

Horowitz, J. M., Horowitz, B. A., and Smith, R. E. (1971): Effect *in vivo* of norepinephrine on the membrane resistance of brown fat cells. *Experientia*, 27:1419.

Horwitz, B. A., Horowitz, J. M., and Smith, R. E. (1969): Norepinephrine-induced depolarization of brown fat cells. *Proc. Natl. Acad. Sci. USA*, 64:113.

Linck, G., Stoeckel, M. E., Porte, A., and Petrovic, A. (1973): An electron microscope study of the specialized contacts and innervation of adipocytes in the brown fat of the European hamster (*Cricetus cricetus*). *Cytobiologie*, 7:431–436.

Lindberg, O., Prusiner, S., Ching, T. M., Cannon, B., and Eisenhardt, R. H. (1970): Metabolic control in isolated brown fat cells. *Lipids*, 5:204.

Mancini, P., and Pilo, A. (1970): A computer program for multiexperimental fitting by the peeling method. Comput. Biomed. Res., 3:1–14.

Petersen, O. H. (1974): Cell membrane permeability change: An important step in hormone action. *Experientia,* 30:1105–1108.

Prusiner, S., and Poe, M. (1970): Thermodynamic consideration of mammalian heat production. In: *Brown Adipose Tissue,* edited by O. Lindberg, pp. 263–282. Elsevier, New York, London, Amsterdam.

Rafael, J., Ludolph, H. J., and Hohorst, H. J. (1969): Mitochondria from brown adipose tissue: Uncoupling of oxydative phosphore relation by long chain fatty acids and recoupling by guanosin biphosphore. *Hoppe-Seylers Z. Physiol. Chem.,* 350:1121.

Rasmussen, H. (1970): Cell communication, calcium ion, and cyclic adenosine monophosphate. *Science,* 170:404–412.

Revel, J. P., and Sheridan, J. D. (1968): Electrophysiological and ultrastructural studies of intercellular junctions in brown fat. *J. Physiol. (Lond.),* 194:34P.

Sheridan, J. D. (1971): Electrical coupling between fat cells in newt fat body and mouse brown fat. *J. Cell Biol.,* 50:795–803.

Skala, J., Hahn, P., and Braun, T. (1970): Adenylcyclase activity in brown adipose tissue of young rats. *Life Sci.,* 9:1201.

Smith, R. E., and Roberts, J. C. (1964): Thermogenesis of brown adipose tissue in cold acclimatized rats. *Am. J. Physiol.,* 206:143–149.

Thoenen, H., and Tranzer, J. P. (1968): Chemical sympathectomy by selective destruction of adrenergic nerve endings with 6-hydroxydopamine. *Arch. Exp. Pathol. Pharmakol.,* 261:271–288.

Electrobiology of Nerve, Synapse, and Muscle,
edited by J. P. Reuben, D. P. Purpura, M. V. L. Bennett,
and E. R. Kandel. Raven Press, New York © 1976

Microelectrophoresis and Constant Current Sources

George M. Katz and Sidney Steinberg

Laboratory of Neurophysiology, Department of Neurology, College of Physicians and Surgeons, Columbia University, New York, New York 10032

With the advent of microelectrodes, the technique of electrophoresis has been extended so that materials may be selectively applied to biological preparations. In this manner, diffusional and enzymatic barriers can be bypassed and materials injected to the immediate environment of tissue sites or into the interior of cells. The injection of these microquantities can be controlled rapidly and with ease by an electric current. The technique has been used for micromarking the tip position of a microelectrode in the histological preparations (MacNichol and Svaetichin, 1958; Oikawa et al., 1959), for the injection of ions to change intracellular media (Araki et al., 1961; Coombs et al., 1955), and, most frequently, for the application of drugs to suitable areas (Diamond and Roper, 1973; Hill and Simmonds, 1973; Bloom, 1974; Engberg and Marshall, 1971; Nastuk, 1953). To illustrate the technique, Fig. 1 shows the effect on muscle tension of the extracellular and intracellular application of caffeine (Chiarandini et al., 1970).

The electrophoretic injection of substances from glass electrodes involves phenomena of both ionophoresis and electroosmosis. Ionophoresis is the movement of charged particles carrying the current. Electroosmosis, however, is the movement of solvent which carries along dissolved or particulate matter. This solvent movement is a consequence of the fixed charges on the inside surface of the glass. When a current is passed through a microelectrode, both phenomena are evoked. In a concentrated salt solution, particles will move primarily by ionophoresis whereas electroosmosis will be more significant if the micropipette contains a solution of low ionic strength.

The simplified equation for the efflux of a substance in an ideal case (Curtis, 1964) is:

$$M = M_i + M_0 = \frac{ni}{ZF} + \frac{C\mu i\rho}{10^3} \tag{1}$$

where M_i is iontophoretic flux in moles/sec; M_0 is electroosmotic flux in moles/sec, n is the transport number for the particular ion; i is the current in amps; Z is the valence; F is Faraday's constant; C is the concentration in moles/liter; μ is the electroosmotic mobility in cm/volt · sec; and ρ is the specific resistance of the solution in ohm · cm.

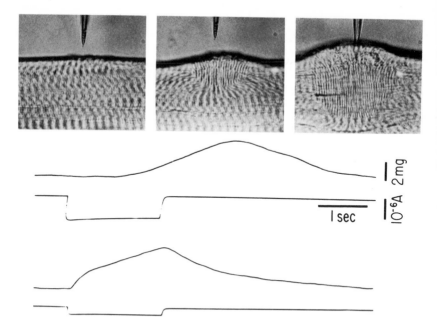

FIG. 1. Extra- and intracellular applications of caffeine to single muscle fibers. **Upper left:** the microelectrode filled with 10 mM caffeine and 50 mM KCl was positioned close to the fiber surface. **Center:** a localized tension was observed when a 2 sec pulse of outward current of 10^{-6} A was delivered. The first set of records in the bottom half of the figure shows the time course and amplitude of the evoked tension and the applied current recorded in another fiber. Note the delay in the onset of tension. **Right:** the fiber was impaled and the same pulse applied, resulting in a much larger contractile response. The lowest set of records show the tension induced when a current was applied. The intracellular application of caffeine that produced a tension comparable with that of the extracellular one required less current, and the delay in onset of tension was now negligible. (From Chiarandini et al., 1970, p. 643.)

Davies and Rideal (1961) have a more detailed analysis of the factors affecting electrophoretic flux. However, any equation concerning efflux from microelectrodes should be used with reservations. The concentration of the substance changes, particularly at the microelectrode tip due to diffusion and ionic movement. Hence, transport number n, electroosmotic mobility μ, and specific resistance ρ will also vary. Microelectrode resistances are usually voltage- and time-dependent.

For quantitative studies of the effects of electrophoretic injections, the amount of substance transferred should be experimentally evaluated. In a typical evaluation for a study of the effect of Ca^{2+} on muscle tension, Reuben et al. (*personal communication*) determined the transport number of electrophoretic injection of Ca^{2+}. A $^{45}Ca^{2+}$-labelled solution (0.1 M Tris-Ca EGTA) contained in a 1 μm tipped microelectrode was inserted into a beaker containing 0.1 M K-propionate at pH 7.0. The beaker solution approximated the intracellular concentration of a muscle fiber. On applying a pulse of constant current (0.5×10^{-6} A), but varying durations (2 to 5 min), the ejected $^{45}Ca^{2+}$ was measured and an average transport number of 0.20 ± 0.032 SD was determined. This transport number may be compared to the handbook value of 0.40 for Ca^{2+} in a $CaCl_2$ solution (MacInnes, 1961).

Even when a value is determined, it should be used with reservations. Several investigators (Chiarandini et al., 1970; Krnjevic et al., 1963) studied the rate of electrophoretic delivery *in vitro* and concluded that the ejecting capabilities with constant current varied considerably in different microelectrodes although prepared similarly and made from the same glass stock. Furthermore, there will presumably be additional variations due to the various degrees of blockage which might occur as the electrode passes through the tissue.

Although the transport number may be accurately determined, other problems exist. The concentration of the drug and its retention at the test site can only be estimated since diffusion occurs and geometrical factors affect the changing concentration. A retaining current may be required to eliminate the steady outward diffusion of the drug from the microelectrode. However, this continuous current will release a counter ion which may have physiological effects. In addition (but not finally), the ejection currents may cause an electrical response which may be interpreted instead as a response to the ejected substance. An excellent mini-review by Bloom (1974) and a check list by Salmoiraghi and Stefanis (1967) examine some of the technical problems intrinsic to microelectrophoresis that bear on the interpretation of data.

Because there are, in practice, large deviations from predicted values and there is no general way of assessing the concentration of drugs achieved, the qualitative effects of drugs are most often studied, i.e., describing the range of existing responses, inferring a transmitter, defining sites of drug interactions or determining antigonists and protogonists to pharmacological agents. Because the concentration can only be estimated, it is practical to express dosage in terms of the intensity and duration of the current used to eject the active ions (Salmoiraghi and Stefanis, 1967). However, not only is the ejecting current important. Bradshaw et al. (1973) studied the effect of the magnitude and duration of the retaining as well as the ejecting currents on neuronal responses. They found significant changes in the kinetics and time course of these responses with changes of the preejection currents. The authors concluded "that the time course of the responses to a particular drug is largely defined by the parameters of the electrophoretic currents (retaining and ejecting) and reproducible responses cannot be obtained unless these parameters are kept constant throughout the study." Therefore, a minimum requirement for reproducible results in microelectrophoresis is an accurately controlled, constant current of negative or positive polarity.

Our laboratory has used for several years three types of instruments designed to control and maintain constant currents through a microelectrode whereas resistance may vary by several orders of magnitude. Each will be discussed, emphasizing a different aspect of the circuit affecting the constancy or the response time of the circuit.

One of the instruments is shown in Fig. 2. In this circuit, A_1 is the current monitoring operational amplifier whose output voltage V_i is a measure of the current through the microelectrode and bathing solution. Since $i = V_i/R_c$, the current is the voltage V_i (in volts) times the scale factor on the current range switch.

The current monitoring voltage V_i is compared to the control voltage pulse V_c, and any error is amplified by A_2 to drive current through the microelectrode in such a direction and magnitude as to make the value of V_i approach that of V_c. The control voltage is shown as a pulse. However, a steady retaining potential of opposite polarity may be superimposed to minimize diffusion. A feedback system of this type is likely to be unstable unless some limiting time constant, τ_2, is incorporated. This is provided by the 0.0047 μF compensating capacitor on A_2.

The equations describing the system behavior is straightforward. Starting at the amplifier A_2 and using Laplace transforms

$$V_0 = \frac{(V_i - V_c)K_2}{\tau_2 s + 1} \tag{2}$$

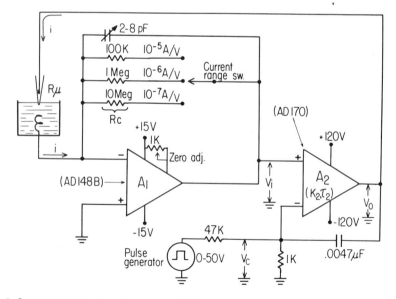

FIG. 2. Constant current feedback circuit. The current monitoring voltage V_i is compared to the control voltage V_c and the error is amplified by the amplifier A_2 to generate the controlled current through the microelectrode.

If the error voltage of the current monitoring amplifier is neglected (assuming the input is at virtual ground),

$$i = \frac{V_0}{R\mu} \tag{3}$$

where $R\mu$ is the microelectrode resistance, and finally

$$V_i = -R_c i \tag{4}$$

by combining the equations we get

$$i = -\frac{K_2 V_c}{\tau_2'(R\mu + K_2 R_c)\left(S + \dfrac{1}{\tau_2'}\right)} \tag{5}$$

where

$$\tau_2' = \frac{\tau_2}{1 + K_L}$$

and

$$K_L = K_2 \frac{R_c}{R\mu} \quad \text{(loop gain)} \tag{6}$$

If the control V_c is a step voltage, the current i will be

$$i_{(t)} = -\frac{K_2 V_c(1 - \epsilon^{-t/\tau_2'})}{R\mu + K_2 R_c} \tag{7}$$

An equivalent circuit of the feedback system (Fig. 3) clarifies the factors that affect the constancy and time course of the controlled current pulse. The voltage control pulse is replaced by an equivalent exponentially changing voltage with time constant τ_2' and a final value of $K_2 V_c$. This equivalent generator drives a current through the microelectrode in series with an equivalent resistance, $K_2 R_c$.

Two observations can be made. Firstly, if $K_2 R_c \gg R\mu$, the steady state current is V_c/R_c and is independent of the microelectrode resistance $R\mu$, or variations of $R\mu$. This is a reasonable condition since the gain K_2 of the

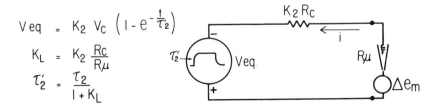

FIG. 3. An equivalent circuit of the feedback system.

AD 170 amplifier is 100,000. Secondly, the larger the value of $R\mu$, the smaller the value of loop gain, K_L. Therefore, it takes longer for the current to stabilize at its steady state value. Both aspects are shown in the oscilloscope recordings of Fig. 4. The upper trace is the voltage control pulse. The lower trace is the controlled current for microelectrode resistance $R\mu$ of 0.5, 100, and 1,000 MΩ. It can be seen that the current is essentially constant for a 2,000-fold increase in resistance and only the rise time is increased for larger values.

Another item should be noted. Occasionally, an injecting microelectrode may induce membrane potential changes. The effect of this potential change, Δe_m, on the controlled current is easily determined. In the equivalent circuit of Fig. 3, Δe_m is added in series with the microelectrode resistance $R\mu$ and $\Delta i = \Delta e_m / R\mu + K_2 R_c$. In practically all cases, this change of current from that caused by V_c is negligible since Δe_m is small compared to the equivalent driving voltage $K_2 V_c$.

There are several practical limitations of this feedback circuit:

(1) From Eq. (6) it is seen that as $R\mu$ approaches zero resistance, the loop gain K_L approaches infinity. (Actually, the maximum loop gain is the product of the individual gains, $K_1 K_2$.) This large loop gain may cause instability, and, as a precaution if low resistance microelectrodes are used, a limiting resistance of several megohms should be added in series with the electrode in the feedback loop.

(2) For a given microelectrode the largest current that can be generated is restricted by the maximum output voltage of A_2. The Analog Devices AD 170 operational amplifier has a maximum swing of only $\pm$ 100 V.

(3) The lowest current that can be controlled is limited by the input bias current of A_1. The FET Analog Devices AD 148B has a maximum input bias current of 25×10^{-12} A. For smaller controlled currents, another FET input operational amplifier with lower bias currents should be substituted.

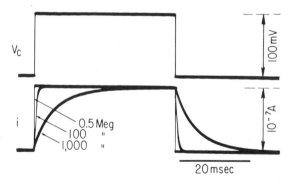

FIG. 4. Current response to a pulse of control voltage. *Upper trace:* control voltage. *Lower trace:* current with microelectrode resistances of 0.5, 100, and 1,000 mΩ. The longer time constant is associated with the larger microelectrode resistance.

(4) The functions and therefore the more important specifications of the two operational amplifiers have been separated. Amplifier A_1 requires a low bias current, whereas amplifier A_2 should have a large output swing.

(5) The microelectrode distributed capacitance in parallel with the microelectrode resistance introduces a leading time constant into this feedback system and may cause instability. A larger stabilizing capacitance in A_2 may be required to compensate for this leading time constant.

In this feedback configuration for generating constant current the bathing solution is not grounded. However, the bath will be at "virtual ground"; that is, a negligible potential will exist between the inputs of A_1. Therefore, normal single-ended membrane measurements with a voltage monitoring electrode can still be made. If the bath must be grounded, our laboratory has used a control circuit similar to that of Fig. 5.

In this circuit, the advantage of generating a current through a microelectrode into a grounded bathing solution is balanced by the disadvantage that the controlling voltage V_c must be isolated. However, isolation units are readily available. The operational amplifier should have a low bias current in order to control small constant current pulses. In addition, it must also be capable of withstanding large in-phase voltages at the input and have a large output swing. With 1 V pulses, this feedback circuit will generate current pulses whose value is indicated on the current range switch.

Again, an equivalent circuit of this feedback system (Fig. 6) shows the factors that affect the magnitude and time course of the controlled current pulses. The equivalent voltage consists of two components: a voltage pulse, $V_c(1 + K)$ and an opposing transient, $V_c\beta KE^{-t/\tau'}$, where

$$\beta = \frac{R\mu}{R\mu + R_c} \quad \text{and} \quad \tau' = \frac{\tau}{1 + (1 - \beta)K}.$$

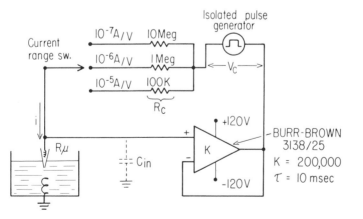

FIG. 5. Schematic representation of constant current generator for a grounded bath. The pulse generator V_c controlling the magnitude of the injected current must be isolated.

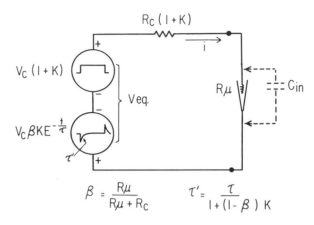

FIG. 6. An equivalent circuit for the current generator of Fig. 5. If $R_c(1 + K) \gg R\mu$, the steady-state value of current $i \cong V_c/R_c$.

The steady-state value of current from the equivalent circuit is

$$i = \frac{V_c(1 + K)}{R_c(1 + K) + R\mu} \tag{8}$$

and again as in the previous circuit, if $R_c(1 + K) \gg R\mu$, the final current value is

$$i = \frac{V_c}{R_c} \tag{9}$$

and is independent of the microelectrode resistance or its variations.

Theoretically, although the amplifier has a time constant of $\tau = 10$ msec, because of the amplifier gain, the transient voltage will decay and the current should reach steady-state value in microseconds. In practice, however, the input capacitance of the amplifier and the distributed capacitance of the microelectrode (lumped together as C_{in}) limit the response time of the current.

The combination of C_{in} and microelectrode resistance acts as a lagging time constant in this feedback configuration and has a stabilizing effect in preventing oscillations.

Another variation for injecting constant current into a grounded bathing solution is shown in Fig. 7. This circuit (sometimes called the Howland circuit) can be driven by two independent signals V_1 and V_2 which need not be isolated from ground. One voltage may be used for establishing the retaining, and the other the ejecting, pulse of current. Unlike the two previous circuits, the effect of an amplifier offset voltage, V_{os}, is included. Because the current range will vary with the application, symbols are used instead of resistance values.

For constant current, it is essential that the ratio $R_1/R_2 = R'_1/R'_2$ and al-

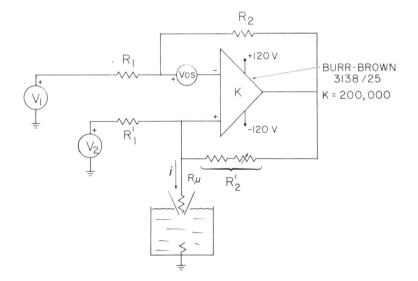

FIG. 7. The Howland circuit for driving a constant current into a grounded bath with single-ended driving sources V_1 and V_2. For constant current $R_1/R_2 = R_1'/R_2'$, and if the source resistance is large compared to the load resistance $R\mu$ (see text) $i = (V_1 - V_2)/R_1$.

though not necessary, the components are usually selected so that $R_1 = R_1'$. Under these conditions, the equivalent circuit of Fig. 8 for steady-state conditions can be derived. Neglecting the offset voltage V_{os}

$$i = \frac{V_2 \dfrac{R_0}{R_1} - KV_1 \overbrace{R_1\left(1 + \dfrac{R_2}{R_1} + K\right)}^{R_0}}{R_0 + R\mu} \tag{10}$$

where R_0 is the equivalent output resistance of the circuit. If $R_0 \gg R\mu$

$$i = \frac{V_2 - V_1}{R_i} \tag{11}$$

In this circuit, the ratio $R_1/R_2 \,(= R_1'/R_2')$ as well as the gain K, determine the effective source resistance, R_0, of the circuit. Figure 9 is a plot showing the variations of R_0/R_1 as a function of R_1/R_2 for operational amplifier gains, K, of 10^4 and 10^5. The maximum source resistance is obtained when $R_1/R_2 = 1$. However, for this condition the maximum voltage available for driving current through the microelectrode will be approximately half the available output voltage of the amplifier.

A deterioration in the equality of the ratio of $R_1/R_2 = R_1'/R_2'$ has a surprisingly significant effect on the magnitude of the source resistance, R_0. With

$$\frac{R_1}{R_2} = \beta \frac{R_1'}{R_2'} \tag{12}$$

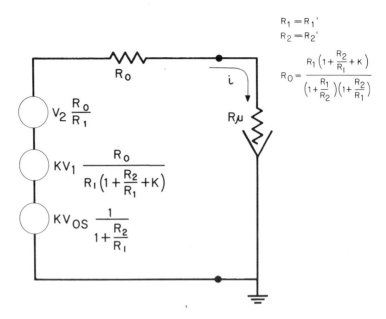

FIG. 8. An equivalent circuit for the Howland current generator.

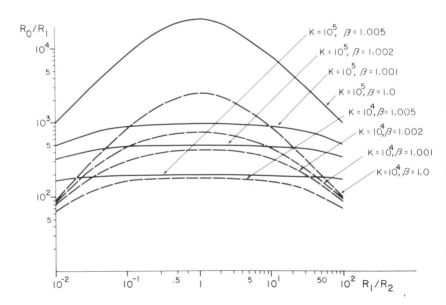

FIG. 9. Variation of R_0/R_1, with the ratio R_1/R_2 of Fig. 7. $R_1/R_2 = \beta R_1'/R_2'$.

the variations of R_0/R_1 are also plotted in Fig. 9 with variations in β. It is seen that a 0.1% change in the ratio can cause an approximately 25-fold reduction in the magnitude of the source resistance ($K = 10^5$). Therefore, care should be taken in the adjustment of the ratio (Fig. 7). It might be noted that $\beta \geq 1$. If β is less than 1, the positive feedback would be greater than the negative feedback and the circuit would be unstable.

ACKNOWLEDGMENTS

Work in the laboratory is supported in part by grants from the Muscular Dystrophy Associations of America, Inc.; by Public Health Service Research Grants (NS 03728 and HL 16082) from the NINDS and NHLI, respectively; and from a grant from the National Science Foundation (GB 31807X).

REFERENCES

Araki, T., Ito, M., and Oscarsson, O. (1961): The electrical properties of the motoneuron membrane. *J. Physiol.*, 130:291–325.

Bloom, F. E. (1974): To spritz or not to spritz: The doubtful value of aimless iontophoresis. *Life Sci.*, 14:1819.

Bradhsaw, C. M., Szabadi, E., and Roberts, M. H. J. (1973): The reflection of ejecting and retaining currents in the time-course of neuronal responses to microelectrophoretically applied drugs. *J. Pharmacol. Exp. Ther.* 25:513.

Chiarandini, D. J., Reuben, J. P., Brandt, P. W., and Grundfest, H. (1970): Effects of caffeine on crayfish muscle fibers. *J. Gen. Physiol.*, 55:640–687.

Coombs, J. S., Eccles, J. C., and Fatt, P. (1955): The electrical properties of the motoneurone membrane. *J. Physiol.*, 130:291–325.

Curtis, D. R. (1964): In: *Physical Techniques in Biological Research, Vol. 5, Part A*, edited by W. L. Nastuk, Academic Press, New York.

Davies, J. T., and Rideal, E. K. (1961): *Interfacial Phenomena*. Academic Press, New York and London.

Diamond, J., and Roper, S. (1973): Analysis of Mauthner cell responses to iontophoretically delivered pulses of GABA, glycine and L-glutamate. *J. Physiol.*, 232:113.

Engberg, I., and Marshall, K. C. (1971): Mechanism of noradrenaline hyperpolarization in spinal cord motor neurons of the cat. *Acta Physiol. Scand.*, 83:142.

Hill, R. G., and Simmonds, M. A. (1973): A method of comparing the potencies of GABA atagonists on single cortical neurones using micro-iontophoretic techniques. *Brit. J. Pharmacol.*, 48:1.

Krnjevic, K., Lavery, R., and Sharman, D. F. (1963): Iontophoretic release of adrenaline, noradrenaline, and 5-hydroxytryptamine from micropipettes. *Brit. J. Pharmacol.*, 20:491–496.

MacInnes, D. A. (1961): *The Principles of Electrochemistry*. Dover Publications, New York.

MacNichol, E. J. Jr., and Svaetichin, G. (1958): Electric responses from the isolated retinas of fishes. *Am. J. Ophtalmol.*, 46:26.

Nastuk, W. L. (1953): Membrane potential changes at a single muscle end-plate produced by transitory application of acetylcholine with an electrically controlled jet. *Fed. Proc.*, 12:102.

Oikawa, T., Ogawa, T., and Motokawa, K. (1959): Origin of so-called cone action potential. *J. Neurophysiol.*, 22:102–111.

Reuben, J. P., Brandt, P. W., and Grundfest, H. (1974): Regulation of myoplasmic calcium concentration in intact muscle fibers. *J. Mechanochem. Cell Motility*, 2:269–285.

Salmoiraghi, G. C., and Stefanis, C. N. (1967): A critique of iontophoretic studies of central nervous system neurons. *Int. Rev. Neurobiol.* 10:1.

Subject Index

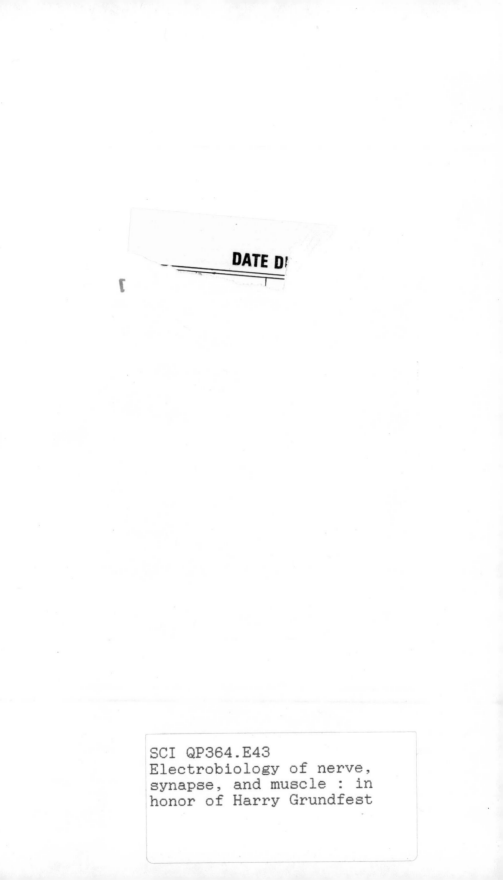